CELL BIOLOGY RESEARCH PROGRESS

OXIDATIVE STRESS AND THE CRITICALLY ILL PATIENT

CELL BIOLOGY RESEARCH PROGRESS

Additional books in this series can be found on Nova's website under the Series tab.

Additional E-books in this series can be found on Nova's website under the e-books tab.

PUBLIC HEALTH IN THE 21ST CENTURY

Additional books in this series can be found on Nova's website under the Series tab.

Additional E-books in this series can be found on Nova's website under the e-books tab.

CELL BIOLOGY RESEARCH PROGRESS

OXIDATIVE STRESS AND THE CRITICALLY ILL PATIENT

RAMÓN RODRIGO

AND

BETTINA VON DESSAUER

EDITORS

Nova Biomedical

New York

For permission to use material from this book please contact us:
Telephone 631-231-7269; Fax 631-231-8175
Web Site: http://www.novapublishers.com

LIBRARY OF CONGRESS CATALOGING-IN-PUBLICATION DATA

Oxidative stress and the critically ill patient / editors, Ramsn Rodrigo and Bettina von Dessauer.
p. cm.
Includes index.
ISBN 978-1-62081-576-2 (hardcover)
1. Oxidative stress. 2. Critically ill. I. Rodrigo, Ramon. II. Dessauer, Bettina von.
RB170.O9592 2012
362.17'5--dc23

2012011767

Published by Nova Science Publishers, Inc. † New York

CONTENTS

INTRODUCTION

The introduction and discussion of the concept of oxidative stress as causative of progressive physiologic derangement initiated by diverse factors, has caused a great impact in biological research. However, the inclusion of this metabolic systemic challenge in medical research and as part of the analysis of pathophysiologic mechanisms present in human diseases has been surprisingly delayed in time.

The complex processes occurring in vivo in clinical settings are meant to have absorbed the attention of the clinicians in relation to sepsis and shock in the intent to improve morbi-mortality. Together with the absence of easy available bedside biomarkers and precise therapeutic evidence-based measures, this could have made more difficult to include the analysis of biochemical effects of free radicals at the top of mind in daily practice.

Many beneficial effects have been reported for naturally occurring endogenous antioxidants, as well as for supplements of concentrated therapeutic compounds of one or more of them. The aim is to counterbalance the oxidative response. Although these effects should be expected to be related to the pathophysiological underlying mechanisms of structural and functional derangements associated with diseases, little effort has been made in the development of integrated perspectives leading to the understanding of the complete sequence of events ranging from the molecular triggers up to the clinical manifestations.

The use of pharmacological agents to act in some part of the process of the inflammatory and metabolic phenomena, together with the fact that physicians are not acquainted with the use of agents categorized as antioxidants, have decreased the possibility of using the latter with therapeutic purposes. This aspect is particularly relevant in the management of critically ill patients were the dynamic evolution and prognosis has proved to be strongly associated with the development of oxidative stress and further multiple organ dysfunction. In addition, oxidative stress may occur or increase associated to the use of some therapies, such us oxygen therapy, mechanical ventilation, vasoactive drugs, antibiotics, among others, causing metabolic impairments that may contribute to a worsening of the patients. Also it may occur in critically ill patients when treatment is delayed, including starving and fasting in stressed malnourished patients with an ongoing systemic inflammatory response. It is noteworthy that this focus has been historically neglected.

The novelty of the proposal included in "Oxidative stress and the critically ill patient" is the fact that it is forwarded to fulfill this default, providing the rationale scientific basis for an increase of the attention of clinicians in these topics including a rationale for an administration of safe specific substances in future guidelines, that could enable us to achieve an improvement in the outcome of these patients. Thus, this book is a practical guide in pathophysiology of oxidative stress linking them to the latest therapeutic advances meant to modulate the antioxidant defense in critically ill patients. In the near future, the pharmaceutical industry should give an appropriate response to this emergent need, through the development of oral and intravenous isolated or mixed products with antioxidant properties, as an adjunct therapy complementary to that available at the present.

The text is forwarded to a wide spectrum audience, including all members of the health team in contact with hospitalized patients, almost all of them at some extent in risk to develop an inflammatory response and shock, regardless of the primary basic diagnosis (trauma, infectious diseases, immunodeficiencies, metabolic diseases, surgical procedures, among others). In addition, medical students, basic science students and biomedical researchers are also part of the expectable audience.

In summary, this text will be not only an important reference for the teachers and students of biomedical sciences, but also it is thought to be used by medical doctors of any specialty, medical students, graduate and undergraduate students of biomedical and health science professions. Since the chosen language is clear enough to allow an adequate comprehension by a broad spectrum public from students up to experts, this book could be consulted even by non medical professionals interested in this field.

In: Oxidative Stress and the Critically Ill Patient
Editors: Ramón Rodrigo and Bettina von Dessauer
ISBN: 978-1-62081-576-2

Chapter I

FREE RADICALS: AN OVERVIEW

Osvaldo H. Berger
Faculty of Medicine, University of Chile

ABSTRACT

Reactive oxygen species and reactive nitrogen species, also known as free radicals, are products of normal cellular metabolism. They are species, capable of independent existence, which contains one or more unpaired electrons. That usually gives a degree of chemically reactivity to the free radical with the capacity of attacking biological structures.

Reactive oxygen species include superoxide, hydroxyl and hydrogen peroxide among others, and the most relevant reactive nitrogen species are nitric oxide and peroxynitrite. The sources of Reactive Species are mitochondria, enzymes like NADPH oxidase and xanthine oxidase, and the reactions with ion transition metals like iron and cupper. Free Radicals can act as physiological and pathophysiological agents, depending on their balance, and if the production is acute and reversible or chronic. The physiological functions include process like cellular signaling and immune response, and the pathological effects are as promoters and continuers of diverse diseases like cancer, cardiovascular diseases, inflammation and multi organ failure in the critical ill patient.

The antioxidant system consist of enzymes such as catalase, glutathione and superoxide dismutase, and scavengers like vitamins and flavonoids. This chapter provides a comprehensive review of the basis for the biochemical and physiological mechanisms involving reactive species.

ABBREVIATIONS

•OH	Hydroxyl radical
$^1O_2$	Oxygen singlet
-SH	Thiol group
8-OH-G	8-hydroxy Guanosine
Aβ	Beta amyloid

AD	Alzheimer´s disease
AGE	Advancedglycation end products
ALS	Amyotrophic lateral sclerosis
AOX	Antioxidants
AP-1	Activated Protein 1 transcription factor
apoE	Apolipoprotein E
ATP	Adenosine triphosphate
Bax	Bcl-2–associated X apoptotic protein
Bcl-2	B-cell lymphoma 2 apoptotic protein
BH_4	Tetrahydrobiopterin
C	Carbon molecule
Ca^{2+}	Calcium cation
CAT	Catalase
CCl_4	Carbon tetrachloride
Cl^-	Chloride anion
Co	Cobalt
C-P450	Cytochrome P450
Cu	Copper
cGMP	Cyclic guanosine monophosphate
DNA	Deoxyribonucleic acid
e^-	Electron
eNOS	Endothelial nitric oxide synthase
ESR	Electron spin resonance
ELAM-1	Endothelial cell leukocyte adhesion molecule-1
F_2IPs	F2-isoprostane
F_3IPs	F3-isoprostane
F_4IPs	F4-isoprostane
Fe^{2+}	Divalent Iron (ferrous)
Fe^{3+}	TrivalentIron (ferric)
FR	Free radical
FRAP	Ferric-reducing ability of plasma
GPx	Glutathione peroxidase
GSH	Glutathione
GSSG	Oxidized glutathione
H	Hydrogen
H_2O_2	Hydrogen peroxide
HDL	High density lipoprotein
Hg	Mercury
HIF-1	Hypoxia-inducible factor 1
HOCl	Hipochlorous acid
HNE	4-Hydroxynonenal
ICAM1	Inter-Cellular Adhesion Molecule 1 or CD45
ICAM2	Inter-Cellular Adhesion Molecule 2 or CD102
IGF-2	Insulin-like growth factor 2
IL-1	Interleukin 1
iNOS	Inducible Nitric oxide synthase

IPs	Isoprostanes
IRS-1	Insulin receptor substrate 1
JNK	c-Jun N-terminal kinases.
LDL	Low density lipoprotein
LDLox	Oxidized low density lipoprotein
MAPK	Mitogen-activated protein kinases
MDA	Malondialdehyde
Mg	Magnesium
MPO	Mieloperoxidase enzyme
NADPH	Reduced nicotinamide adenine dinucleotide phosphate
NF-kB	Nuclear factor kappa-light-chain-enhancer of activated B cells
Ni	Nickel
nNOS	Neuronal nitric oxide synthase
NO	Nitric oxide
NO^+	Nitrosonium cation
NO^-	Nitroxyl anion
NO_2	Nitrogen dioxide
NOS	Nitric oxide synthase
O	Oxygen element
O_2	Dyoxygen molecule
$O_2\bullet^-$	Superoxide radical
O_3	Ozone
$ONOO^-$	Peroxynitrite
p38	Protein 38 mitogen-activated protein kinases
p53	Protein 53 (tumor suppressor)
PDGF	Platelet-derived growth factor
PKC alpha	Protein kinase C alpha
PUFA	Polynsaturated fatty acid
RS	Reactive specie
ROS	Reactive oxygen species
RNS	Reactive nitrogen species
RH	Organic substrate
SOD	Superoxide dismutase
TNF-α	Tumor necrosis factor alpha
UV	Ultra violet
VCAM-1	Vascular cell adhesion protein 1
XO	Xantino oxidase
XOR	Xantinooxidoreductase
Zn	Zinc

2. INTRODUCTION

Free radicals (FR) or reactive species (RS), are receiving growing attention in view of the role that oxidative stress has been implicated in various pathological conditions involving cardiovascular disease, cancer, neurological disorders, diabetes, ischemia/reperfusion, inflammation and multi organ failure in the critical ill patient,..

The causes of the poisonous properties of oxygen were obscure prior to the publication of Gershman's free radical theory of oxygen toxicity in 1954, which states that the toxicity of oxygen is due to partially reduced forms of oxygen [1].

Numerous researchers are nowadays, inspired to investigate oxidative damage inflicted by radicals upon DNA, proteins, lipids, and other components of the cell. Important physiological functions that involve free radicals or their derivatives include the following: regulation of vascular tone, sensing of oxygen tension and regulation of functions that are controlled by oxygen concentration, enhancement of signal transduction from various membrane receptors, including the antigen receptor of lymphocytes, and oxidative stress responses that ensure the maintenance of redox homeostasis [2]. The most relevant free radicals in biological regulation are reactive oxygen (ROS), and nitrogen (RNS) species. They are products of normal cellular metabolism and they can be either harmful or beneficial to living systems.

In the structure of atoms and molecules, electrons occupy regions of space termed orbitals, each of which holds a maximum of two electrons. One electron in each pair has a spin quantum number of +1/2, and the other -1/2 (Figure 1). A free radical is any species capable of independent existence (hence the term "free") that contains one or more unpaired electrons, that is, one electron alone in an orbital (Figure 3). That usually gives a degree of chemically reactivity to the free radical, with the capability of attacking double bonds and other structures like sulfur clusters [3]. They may have positive, negative, or zero charge. Radicals may also be formed by single electron oxidation or reduction of an atom or molecule.

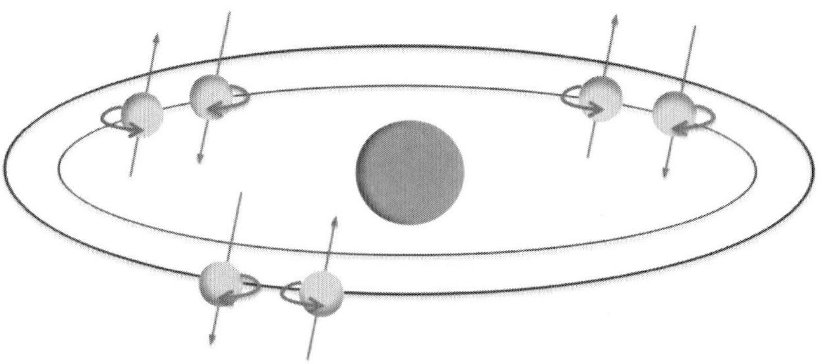

Figure 1. Normal distribution of electrons in orbitals. Only two electrons, because of their spin, can be associated with each orbital.

RS react with other molecules in a number of ways. If two radicals meet, they can combine their unpaired electrons and join to form a covalent bond (a shared pair of electrons). A free radical might donate its unpaired electron to another molecule, reducing it, or might take an electron from another molecule oxidizing it; a reactive radical may abstract a hydrogen atom from a C-H bond. If a radical reacts with a non-radical, then a new radical results and chain reactions may occur [4].

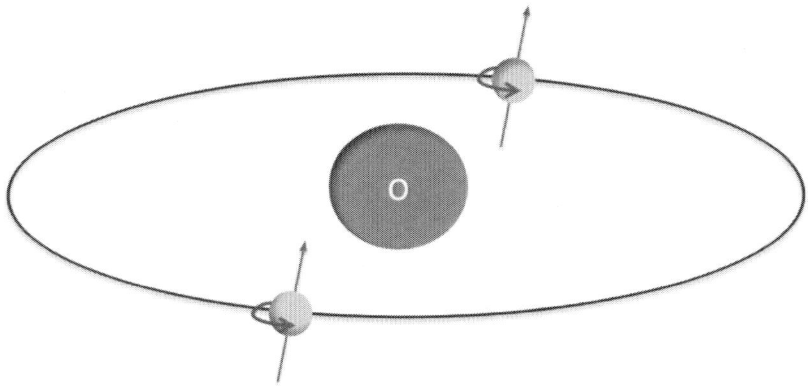

Figure 2. Oxygen atoms and unpaired electrons in the final orbital with the same spin orbital.

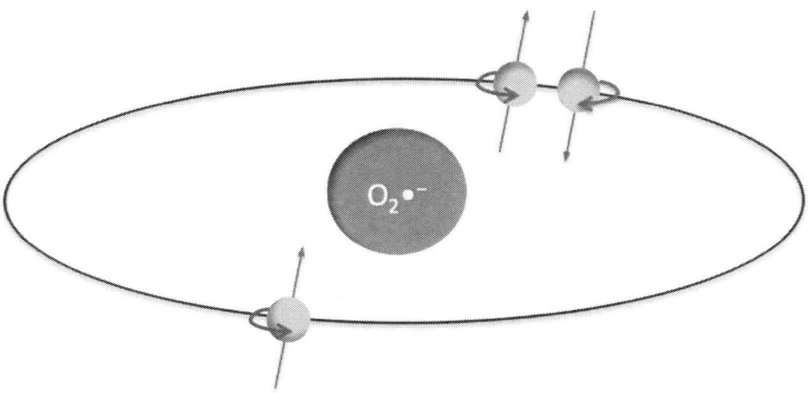

Figure 3. Superoxide representative molecule. Note the one unpaired electron.

Reactive species modifies phospholipids and proteins leading to peroxidation and oxidation of thiol groups [5]. The assaults by ROS lead to changes in membrane permeability, membrane lipid bilayer disruption and functional modification of various cellular proteins [1]. The simplest free radical is a hydrogen atom, because it only has one electron that must be unpaired [6]. A super script dot (•) is used to denote free radical species.

3. Types of Free Radicals

3.1. Reactive Oxygen Species

Not every oxidant reacts in the same way. Reactive oxygen species has widely different reactivity's. Some are strong and others are weak oxidants; some are non-radical species and cause two-electrons oxidation when others are free radicals and undergo one-electron reactions [7].

ROS is a term used to include not only oxygen radicals ($O_2•^-$) and hydroxyl radical, (•OH) but also some derivatives of O_2 that do not contain unpaired electrons, such as hydrogen peroxide (H_2O_2) and singlet $^1O_2$.

Molecular oxygen O_2 (dioxygen), has a unique electronic configuration and it is itself a free radical, containing two unpaired electrons (Figure 2). It should thus be written as $O_2\bullet$. Fortunately, the electronic arrangement in O_2 with the two electrons with the same spin quantum number, or parallel spin, makes this molecule unreactive despite its free radical nature [4].

Electronic excitation and rearranges of the electrons in the last orbitals of molecular oxygen, generates singlet oxygen. Singlet oxygen is not a radical specie, but unlike O_2 it is very reactive and has a half-life of 10^{-5} seconds. Nucleic acids, proteins, lipids, and sterols are the primary biological targets for singlet oxygen damage, and oxidation of these molecules has been implicated in skin cancer among other diseases.

a) Superoxide ($O_2\bullet^-$)

The addition of one electron (also called reduction in chemistry) to di-oxygen, forms the superoxide anion radical ($O_2\bullet-$) that has only one electron unpaired (Figure 3) [8]. This process is mediated by enzymes such as NADPH oxidases and xanthine oxidase or non-enzymically by redox reactive compounds such as the semi-ubiquinone compound of the mitochondrial electron transport chain [2].

$$O_2 + e^- \rightarrow O_2\bullet^-$$

Superoxide anion, arising either through metabolic processes or following oxygen "activation" by physical irradiation by ionizing radiation [9], is considered the "primary" ROS and can further interact with other molecules to generate "secondary" ROS, either directly or prevalently through enzyme or metal-catalyzed processes [10]. $O_2\bullet^-$has extremely limited permeability through lipid membranes and requireions channel to pass through the membrane [7]. Superoxide causes the inactivation of enzymes, including catalase (CAT) and glutathione peroxidase (GPx), and oxidation of intracellular components, such as DNA, lipids and proteins like glutathione, due to its long half-life (0,05 s in the absence of scavengers) [11].

b) Hydrogen peroxide (H_2O_2)

In biological tissues like in the organelle peroxisome, superoxide can also be converted by the enzyme superoxide dismutase (SOD) or non-enzymically into the non-radical species hydrogen peroxide (H_2O_2) and singlet oxygen ($^1O_2$).

$$2O_2\bullet^- + 2H^+ \rightarrow H_2O_2 + O_2$$

Hydrogen peroxide, which is a great diffusiblemolecule, is used to oxidize or reduce a variety of molecules but is poorly reactive. Can be converted into water by the enzymes catalase and glutathione peroxidase.

The danger of H_2O_2, comes from theconversion to the most reactive oxygen species, thehydroxyl radical (•OH), either by exposure to ultraviolet light or by interaction with a range of transition metal ions [3].

$$H_2O_2 + e^- \rightarrow \bullet OH$$

c) Hydroxyl Radical (•OH)

The hydroxyl radical is the neutral form of the hydroxide ion, consider the most reactive and harmful ROS with a very short *in vivo* half-life of approximate 10^{-9} seconds, therefore it reacts with molecules immediately after formation and release [12, 13].

Increases in free or non-protein-bound metal ion concentrations cause significant increases in •OH generation, because the primary source of cellular hydroxyl radical is from Fenton or Fenton-type reactions with copper and iron [12]. Hydroxyl radical formation causes oxidation of lipids, proteins, and nucleic acids; DNA strand breaks, base modifications, and DNA cross-linking have also been observed [14, 15].

3.2. Reactive Nitrogen Species

Nitric oxide (NO) is an abundant reactive radical that acts as an important oxidative biological signaling molecule in a large variety of diverse physiological processes. The NO radical (NO•) is produced by the oxidation of one of the terminal guanido-nitrogen atoms of L-arginine to citrulline. This process is catalyzed by a group of specific enzymes, called nitric oxide synthases (NOSs). NO has a half-life of only a few seconds in an aqueous environment. It is soluble in both aqueous and lipid media making it very diffusible through membranes.

Nitric oxide can be converted to various other reactive nitrogen species such as nitrosoniumcation (NO^+), nitroxyl anion (NO^-) or peroxynitrite ($ONOO^-$) [2].

Superoxide reacts fast with nitric oxide in a radical addition reaction:

$$O_2{\bullet}^- + NO{\bullet} \rightarrow ONOO^-$$

This reaction has one of the highest rate constant known, thus NO toxicity is predominantly linked to its ability to combine with superoxide anions [1].

Peroxynitrite are directly toxic to cells, causing DNA damage by fragmentation and lipid oxidation [16]. It might also decompose to form a range of toxic products, including some •OH

$$ONOO^- + H^+ \rightarrow {\bullet}OH,\ NO_2{\bullet},\ NO_2^+$$

4. Sources of Free Radicals

The consumption and utilization of oxygen in physiological processes result in the inevitable generation of ROS. In terms of human survival, probably the most important source of ROS is the immune system [17].

A reducing agent, or antioxidant, is a substance that donates electrons, whereas an oxidant, or pro-oxidant agent, is a substance that accepts electrons. Cells are constantly exposed to oxidants from both physiological processes, such as mitochondrial respiration and pathophysiological conditions such as inflammation, foreign compound metabolism, and radiation, among others [18].

ROS can be produced from both endogenous and exogenous sources. Endogenous sources include mitochondria, peroxisomes, and inflammatory cell activation [19].

A wide array of exogenous sources is also documented in literature, including environmental agents, ultraviolet radiation, thermal stress, radiation, therapeutic agents, tobacco smoke, inflammatory cytokines, ozone (O_3), nitrogen dioxide (NO_2), carbon tetrachloride (CCl_4), Paraquat, and chemotherapeutic drugs, among others.

Generation of radical species occurs by two types of processes:

a) "Accidental" Generation

This encompasses such mechanisms as "leakage" of electrons onto O_2 from mitochondrial electron transport chains, microsomal cytochromes P450 and their electron donating enzymes [20, 21]. It also includes autoxidation reactions, in which compounds such as catecholamines, ascorbic acid, and reduced flavins are alleged to react directly with O_2 to form $O_2•^-$ [20].

b) Deliberate Synthesis

The deliberate synthesis means that free radicals are needed for some kind of physiological function by the cells. Some example of this is the generation of ROS in the production of $O_2•^-$, HOCI, and H_2O_2 by activated phagocytes [22]. Hydrogen peroxideis additionally generated *in vivo* by several oxidase enzymes, such as glycolateoxidase, xanthineoxidase, and D-aminoacidoxidase.

Evidence is accumulating that $O_2•^-$ is also produced by several cell types other tan phagocytes, including lymphocytes, fibroblasts, and vascular endothelial cells. Such superoxide might be involved in intercellular signaling, and could serve important biologic functions [9].

4.1. Mitochondria

Energy production in mitochondria is dependent on oxygen metabolism, since O_2 is reduced to H_2O. Mitochondria take up O_2 and reduce 95% or more of it to water, a process achieved by cytochrome oxidase.

It removes one electron from each of four reduced (Fe^{2+}-haem) cytochrome c molecules, oxidizing them to ferric cytochrome c, and adds the four electrons onto O_2. Because the quantic characteristics of the oxygen, it is impossible to add to it four electrons at once and cytochrome oxidase must hold onto toxic partially reduced oxyden species until they can be fully reduced to water [23].

$$O_2 + e^- \rightarrow O_2•^-$$
$$O_2•^- + e^- \rightarrow H_2O_2$$
$$H_2O_2 + e^- \rightarrow •OH$$
$$OH + e^- \rightarrow H_2O$$

Some authors argue that this is part of an intracellular redox-signalling mechanism. More details of the relation between the mitochondria and free radicals will be presented in the chapter 4.

4.2. NADPH

The enzyme NADPH oxidaze, catalyzes the one electron reduction of O_2 to generate $O_2•^-$, using NADPH as the source of electrons. This enzyme has a complex function that is most easily understood in the context of the activated neutrophil, wherein it generates large amounts of toxic superoxide anion and other ROS important in the bactericidal function. In addition, it is also functional in membranes of vascular endothelial and vascular smooth muscle cells, and fibroblasts providing a constitutive source of $O_2•^-$. This enzyme consists of several membrane-bound subunits (gp91, Nox, and p22phox) and cytosolic subunits (p47phox, p67phox, p40phox, and Rac2). There appear to be at least three isoforms of NADPH oxidase expressed in the vascular wall [18].

$$NADPH + 2H_2 \leftrightarrow NADP^+ + O_2•^- + H^+$$

4.3. Xanthine Oxidase

The xanthine oxidase (XO) enzyme catalyzes the oxidation of hypoxanthine to xanthine and can further catalyze the oxidation of xanthine to uric acid, generating $O_2•^-$. This enzyme plays an important role in the catabolism of purines in some species, including humans. Under pathological conditions, such as tissue ischemia (like in septic shock), xanthine dehydrogenase can be converted to XO [18].

$$\text{Xanthine} + H_2O + O_2 \rightarrow \text{uric acid} + O_2•^-$$

4.4. Metal-Mediated Generation of ROS

Metal ions such as Cu^+, Fe^{2+}, Mg^{2+}, Zn^{2+}, Ni^{2+}, and Co^{2+} are required for biological processes such as oxygen transport, electron transfer, and catalysis [15]. Under normal conditions, the availability of metal ions to generate ROS is minimal due to sequestration and storage.

Iron reacts with endogenous H_2O_2 to generate •OH in the Fenton reaction:

$$Fe^{2+} + H_2O_2 \rightarrow Fe^{3+} + •OH + OH^-$$

Copper generates hydroxyl radical in a Fenton-type reaction 50 times faster than the reaction with iron:

$$Cu^+ + H_2O_2 \rightarrow Cu^{2+} + •OH + OH^-$$

H_2O_2 can contribute to Fenton chemistry not only by being one of the substrates but also by providing the other, e.g. by liberating iron from heme proteins [24].

$O_2\bullet^-$ also makes easier •OH production from H_2O_2 by making Fe^{2+} available from:

$$Fe^{3+} + O_2\bullet^- \rightarrow Fe^{2+} + O_2$$

In the Haber-Weiss reaction, the one-electron reduction of hydrogen peroxide by superoxide has also been invoked as a potential source of •OH:

$$O_2\bullet^- + H_2O_2 \rightarrow O_2 + \bullet OH + OH^-$$

4.5. Nitric Oxide Synthase

Three main iso-enzymes exist in mammals that are regulated by distinct genes: a constitutive neuronal NOS (nNOS) that performs an important role in intracellular communication, an endotoxin and cytokine inducible NOS (iNOS) that induce oxidative stress on pathogens, and a constitutive endothelial NOS (eNOS) which plays a major role in the regulation of vascular function.

Many tissues express one or more of these isoforms. However it has become clear, from studies with the purified enzyme, that eNOS may become uncoupled in the absence of the NOS substrate L-arginine or the cofactor tetrahydrobiopterin (BH_4).

Uncoupled state results in the production of $O_2\bullet^-$ rather than NO [25, 26].

4.6. Mieloperoxidase

The myeloperoxidase enzyme (MPO) produces hypochlorous acid (HOCl) from H_2O_2 and chloride anion (Cl^-) during the neutrophil's respiratory burst. It requires heme as a cofactor. In addition, it oxidizes tyrosine to tyrosyl radical usingH_2O_2 as oxidizing agent [27]. Both, HOCl and tyrosyl radical are cytotoxic, and used by the neutrophil to kill bacteria and other pathogens [18].

4.7. Cytochrome P450

The most common reaction catalyzed by the C-P450, is a monooxygenase reaction. This might be, for example, the insertion of one atom of oxygen into an organic substrate (RH) while the other oxygen atom is reduced to H_2O

$$RH + O_2 + 2H^+ + 2e \longrightarrow ROH + H_2O$$

One ROS-generating $O_2\bullet^-$ way is given by ferric P450.

5. *In Vivo* Effects of Free Radicals

The site or compartment where a reactive specie is generated is also an important determinant of how a cell responds to a free radical.

5.1. Physiological Functions

Numerous physiological functions are controlled by redox-responsive signaling pathways, nevertheless, in most cases are not yet well understood.

The surprisingly large number of NADPH oxidaseisoforms and NOS, is by itself a strong indication for the physiological relevance of redox signaling in biological regulation.

Free radicals play an essential role in the immune system. First, they help to kill some infecting organisms. Second they help to restrain the immune system (especially T-lymphocytes) from over-activation and prolonging inflammation once the threat has been eliminated [28].

Generationof $O_2•^-$, HOCI, and H_2O_2 by phagocytes in the called respiratory burst reactions, is known to play an important part in the killing of several bacterial and fungal strains [9].

NADPH oxidase is best characterized in neutrophils, where its production of $O_2•^-$generates the respiratory burst necessary for bacterial destruction.

Another killing mechanism used by neutrophils (but not macrophages) is the myeloperoxidase enzyme, which uses H_2O_2 to oxidize chloride ions into HOCI, a powerful oxidizing and chlorinating agent [4].

At sites of inflammation, H_2O_2 generated by activated phagocytes appears to modulate the inflammatory process, e.g. by up-regulating expression of adhesion molecules, controlling cell proliferation or apoptosis, and modulating platelet aggregation [29, 30].

In contrast to neutrophils, endothelial cells, fibroblasts and vascular smooth muscle cells produce superoxide radical, mainly intracellular.

Angiotensin II is known to enhance NADPH-mediated superoxide formation in vascular smooth cells and fibroblasts; thrombin, PDGF (platelet-derived growth factor) and TNF-α (tumor necrosis factor-α), stimulate NADPH-mediated superoxide formation in vascular smooth muscle cells; TNF- α, Interleukin- 1 (IL-1), and platelet-activating factor increase NADPH-mediated formation of superoxide in fibroblasts [1].

The production of thyroid hormones by the enzyme thyroid peroxidase requires hydrogen peroxide. H_2O_2 can induce expression of genes controlled by NF-κB [9].

Changes in oxygen concentration are sensed independently by several different ROS-producing proteins involving b-type cytochrome. Some other studies suggested that change in the rate of mitochondrial ROS may play a role in oxygen sensing by the carotid bodies [1].

Other responses to changes in oxygen tension include the control of ventilation by the carotid body and the regulated production of certain hormones such as erythropoietin, VEGF, and insulin-like growth factor II (IGF-II). All of these hormones are under transcriptional control of the transcription factor HIF-1 [31, 32].

NO• is known to be produced *in vivo* by vascular endothelial cells, by some cells in the brain, and by phagocytes. NO• performs useful physiologic functions, such as regulation of vascular smooth muscle tone (hence controlling blood pressure), insulin secretion, airway tone, peristalsis, and is involved in angiogenesis and in the development of nervous system [1].

cGMP which regulates the vascular tone, is known to be activated by both hydrogen peroxide and NO• radical. cGMP modulates the function of protein kinases, ion channels, and other physiologically important targets, the most important ones being the regulation of smooth muscle tone and the inhibition of platelet adhesion.

Peroxynitrite has been associated with the regulation of some physiological process like proteins functions, ischemic stress adaptation of the rat myocardium, mitochondrial translocation of PKC-alpha and activated cell survival pathways in U937 cells, and muscle relaxation, among others [33]. The role of NO in the vascular physiology will be discussed in the chapter 5.

Various types of non-phagocytic cells involving fibroblasts, vascular smooth muscle cells, cardiac myocytes, and endothelial cells are known to produce ROS by NADPH oxidase to regulate intracellular signaling cascades [34, 35]. Exposure of cells to sub-lethal oxidative stress results in the modulation of various signaling pathways (i.g Tyrosine Phosphatases, insulin receptor kinase, cytoplasmatic protein kinase, MAPK cascades, Ca^{2+}, transcription factor AP-1, NF-kB, etc).

Oxidants can activate and inactivate transcription factors as second messengers, membrane channels, and metabolic enzymes, and regulate calcium-dependent and phosphorylation signaling pathways. Oxidation and reduction of thiol proteins is thought to be the major mechanism by which reactive oxidants integrate into cellular signal transduction pathways [7].

Some intracellular signals of apoptosis are internal damage, mediated by ROS [2].

5.2. Pathophysiological Effects

Oxidative Damage

At high concentrations, RS can be important mediators of damage to cell structures, nucleic acids, lipids and proteins.

H_2O_2 at low micromolar levels also appears poorly reactiveas as we mentioned above. However, higher levels of H_2O_2 can attack several cellular energy-producing systems, e.g. by inactivating the glycolyticenzyme glycealdehyde-3-phosphate dehydrogenase [9].

It is usually thought that most or all of the toxicity of $O_2•^-$ and H_2O_2, involves their conversion into •OH.

If metal ions bound to a biological molecule that reacts with $O_2•^-$ and H_2O_2, •OH will be formed upon the molecule. This •OH-mediated damage is said to be "site specific". Binding metal ions to a target, means that any •OH generated will tend to react with that target rather than with any added scavenger.

It follows that a major determinant of the nature of the damage done by excessive generation of ROS *in vivo,* is the availability and location of metal ion catalysts of •OH radical formation (DNA, membrane lipids, proteins) [9].

The DNA damage, are considered as the most serious ROS-induced cellular modifications, as DNA is not synthesized *de novo* but copied, perpetuating by this way those modifications and hence inducing mutations and genetic instability [18].

The hydroxyl radical is known to react with all components of the DNA molecule, damaging both the purine and pyrimidine bases and also the deoxyribose backbone [36]. This is explained by the diffusion-limited •OH ability to add to double bonds of DNA bases, abstracting a hydrogen atom from the methyl group of thymine and each of the five carbon atoms of 2-deoxyribose [37].

The most extensively studied DNA lesion is the formation of 8-OH-G.

Permanent modification of genetic material resulting from these "oxidative damage" incidents represents the first step involved in mutagenesis, carcinogenesis, and ageing.

Reactive nitrogen species are able to cause DNA damage by basis deamination, endogenous formation of carcinogenic N-nitrosamine molecules and bases oxidation [18].

Another suggested hypothesis of DNA damage by RNS is based on the inhibition of the DNA repairing enzymatic systems, thereby making possible indirect damage. The RNS have a high affinity for the thiol group (-SH) of cysteine, and it is believed that those enzymes containing critic cysteine for their activity might be inhibited through RNS [38].

These mutations could result in the inactivation of suppressor tumor genes, and further activation of oncogenes, thus participating in various stages of carcinogenic process. The most evident example of this is given by the protein for p53 gene mutations, induced by NO and its methylation [38]. Further investigations also verified that there is a significant relation between the RNS activities and the mutations on p53 gene in early staged lung carcinoma [39].

Lipid peroxidation consists of three stages: initiation, propagation, and termination [40, 41]. OH• may abstract a hydrogen atom from a C–H bond, e.g. from a hydrocarbon side chain of a polyunsaturated fatty acid (PUFA) residue in a membrane. As H• has only one electron, an unpaired electron remains on the carbon.

Carbon-centered radicals react fast with O_2 (like many radicals do), to generate peroxyl-radicals, which are reactive enough to both oxidize membrane, proteins and attack adjacent PUFA side chains, propagating a chain reaction.

A new C• radical is formed to continue the chain, and a lipid hydroperoxide is generated. If the PUFA chain is long enough, the peroxyl-radicals can whip around and substract H• from the same PUFA, giving cyclic peroxides [42].

Some end products of lipid peroxidation have direct damaging effects. These include the isoprostanes (IPs), cyclic peroxides formed from PUFAs with at least three double bonds, including linolenic acid, arachidonic acid (F2 IPs), eicosapentaenoic acid (F3 IPs), and docosahexaenoic acid (F4 IPs, sometimes called neuroprostanes) [6].

Decomposition of lipid peroxides accelerated by iron and copper ions or by heating, generates a complex mixture of toxic products including epoxides, saturated aldehydes, unsaturated aldehydes, ketones, and hydrocarbons. Particularly toxic aldehyde include malondialdehyde (MDA) formed from peroxidation of linolenic, arachidonic, or docosahexaenoic acids, which can bind avidly to membrane proteins, inactivating enzymes and receptors, and attack DNA, forming mutagenic lesions [43]. Lipid peroxidation involves low-density lipoprotein (LDL), as well as high-density lipoprotein (HDL) oxidation. It is well known that the LDL oxidation is a key process in the pathogenesis of atherosclerosis. The oxidized cholesterol esters are directly incorporated into lipoproteins and transferred to endothelial cells via the LDL where they induce damage and start the sequence of events leading to atherosclerosis [18].

The side chains of all amino acid residues of proteins are susceptible to oxidation by theaction of ROS. The protein carbonyl group is generated by ROS through many different mechanisms and its concentration is a good measure of protein oxidation via oxidative stress. $ONOO^-$ is able to nitrosate the cysteine sulfhydryl groups of proteins, to nitrate tyrosine and tryptophan residues of proteins and to oxidize methionine residues to methionine sulfoxide [10]. Oxidation of proteins is associated with a number of age-related diseases and aging [44, 45].

Oxidative damage to the mitochondrial membrane can also occur, resulting in membrane depolarization and the uncoupling of oxidative phosphorylation, with altered cellular respiration [46] and activation of the Bcl-2 and Bax protein which makes "holes" in the outer mitochondrial membrane, causing cytochrome c to release from mitochondria, activation of caspases, and apoptosis [47]. The mitochondrial damage is an important hypothesis in the pathogenesis of the septic shock.

Sources, physiological functions and pathophysiological effects of RS are summarized in Table 1.

6. Antioxidant Defense Systems and Oxidative Stress

Defense mechanisms against free radical involve: preventative mechanisms, repair mechanisms, physical defenses, and antioxidant defenses. Some of these mechanisms are stimulated by an elevated concentration of reactive species. High levels of FR act as inhibitory feedback mechanisms of regulation.

Antioxidants are substances that are able, at relatively low concentrations, to compete with other oxidizable substrates and thus, to significantly delay or inhibit the oxidation of these substrates. [2]. Antioxidant substances can scavenge free radicals by accepting or donating an electron to eliminate the unpaired condition. Typically, this means that the antioxidant molecule becomes a free radical in the process of scavenging a FR to a more stable and less reactive molecule. In most cases the scavenger molecule provides hydrogen radical that combines with the free radical. Consequently, it is generated a new radical that has an enhanced lifetime compared with the starting one [18].

Antioxidants are produced during normal cellular metabolism, as well as in the pathophysiological states, or can be provided exogenously through diet or antioxidant supplements. They are divided in two types: enzymatic and non-enzymatic. Enzymatic antioxidant defenses include superoxide dismutase (SOD), glutathione peroxidase (GPx) and catalase (CAT). Non-enzymatic antioxidants are represented by ascorbic acid (Vitamin C), α - tocopherol (Vitamin E), glutathione (GSH), carotenoids, flavonoids, and others [1]. SOD converts superoxide anion to H_2O_2, which is a substrate for CAT and GPx. Catalase metabolizes H_2O_2 to water and oxygen and GPx reduces both H_2O_2 and organic hydroperoxides when reacting with GSH [48].

SOD GPx, CAT

$$O_2{\bullet}^- \rightarrow H_2O_2 \rightarrow H_2O$$

Table 1. Sources, physiological functions and pathophysiological effects of RS

Reactive specie	Source	Physiological functions	Pathophysiological effects
O_2	Atmosphere from photosynthesis	Oxygen is used in *mitochondria* to help generate adenosine triphosphate (ATP) during *oxidative phosphorylation*	Formation of FR
$^1O_2$	Leukocyte myeloperoxidase, UV reaction with some pigments	Respiratory burst by neutrophils Modification of important haemostatic factors (fibrinogen, factor V, factor VIII; factor X) and thus regulation of haemostasis. Inhibition of platelet agregation	Oxidation of LDL cholesterol, photohemolysis
$O_2•^-$	Reduction of dioxygen by NADPH oxidase and XO. Electron transport chain in mitochondria. Cytochrome P450. Uncoupled eNOS	Intracellular signaling cascades. Respiratory burst by neutrophils.	Oxidation of intracellular components, such as DNA, Lipids and proteins like glutathione, due to its long half-life. Formation of $ONOO^-$
H_2O_2	From $O_2•^-$ by SOD. *In* vivo by Glycolateoxidase, xanthineoxidase, and D-aminoacidoxidase.	Up-regulation of adhesion molecules, controlling cell proliferation or apoptosis and modulating platelet aggregation. Production of thyroid hormones. Induce expression of genes controlled by NF-κB. Intracellular signaling cascades.	Higher levels can attack several cellular energy-producing systems, e.g., by inactivating the glycolytic enzyme glycealdehyde-3-phosphate dehydrogenase.

Table 1. (Continued)

Reactive specie	Source	Physiological functions	Pathophysiological effects
•OH	Conversion from H_2O_2 by exposure to ultraviolet light or by interaction with a range of transition metal ions. (Fenton and Heber-Weiss reactions).	Apoptosis intracellular signaling.	Oxidation of lipids, proteins, and nucleic acids; DNA strand breaks, base modifications, and DNA cross-linking. Damaging both the purine and pyrimidine bases and also the deoxyribose backbone. Lipid peroxidation by abstract a hydrogen atom from a C–H bond.
NO	Oxidation of one of the terminal guanido-nitrogen atoms of L-arginine to citrulline by NOSs enzymes.	Signaling molecule. Regulation of vascular smooth muscle tone, insulin secretion, airway tone, and peristalsis, angiogenesis and in the development of nervous system and neurotransmission. Stimulates the soluble guanylatecyclase to generate the second messenger cyclic GMP. Regulation of cardiac contraction. Immune response in phagocytes.	p53 gen mutations. Deamination of DNA. Inhibition of the DNA repairing enzymatic systems.
$ONOO^-$	Reaction of NO with $O_2•^-$ Reaction of H_2O_2 with NO_2^-	Regulation of proteins functions.	DNA damage by fragmentation and lipid oxidation. Formation of •OH. Abstract H• from PUFA. Nitrosate the cysteine sulfhydryl groups of proteins, to nitrate tyrosine and tryptophan residues of proteins and to oxidize methionine residues to methionine sulfoxide.

The hydrophobic lipid interior of membranes requires a different spectrum of antioxidants. Fat-soluble vitamin E is the most important antioxidant in this environment, which protects it against the loss of membrane integrity.

Water-soluble antioxidants including vitamin C play a key role in scavenging ROS in the hydrophilic phase. Other small antioxidant molecules are also naturally present in the plasma, such as uricacid and bilirubin [18].

The oxidized form of glutathione is GSSG, glutathione disulphide. Glutathione is highly abundant in the cytosol (1–11mM), nuclei (3–15mM), and mitochondria (5–11mM) and is the major soluble antioxidant in these cell compartments [1].

GSH in the nucleus maintains the redox state of critical protein sulphydryls that are necessary for DNA repair and expression. Oxidized glutathione is accumulated inside the cells and the ratio of GSH/GSSG is a good measure of oxidative stress in organism [49, 50].

The main protective roles of glutathione against oxidative stress are [51]:

- Glutathione is a cofactor of several detoxifying enzymes against oxidative stress, e.g. glutathione peroxidase (GPx), glutathionetransferase and others.
- GSH participates in amino acid transport through the plasma membrane.
- GSH scavenges hydroxyl radical and singlet oxygen directly, detoxifying hydrogen peroxide and lipid peroxides by the catalytic action of glutathione peroxidase.
- Glutathione is able to regenerate the most important antioxidants, Vitamins C and E, back to their active forms; glutathione can reduce the tocopherol radical of Vitamin E directly, or indirectly, via reduction of semidehydroascorbate to ascorbate.

There are compounds that have a relatively low specific antioxidative activity, but, when present at high concentrations, can contribute significantly to the overall ROS scavenging activity. The most prominent examples of such high-level/low-efficiency antioxidants are free amino acids, peptides, and proteins [1].

Antioxidants should be managed carefully, because RS are involved as described above, in various normal cell functions, like tissue differentiation during development, so we must therefore be cautious in assuming that ROS are deleterious in pregnancy, newborns or during child development, and ensure that children and mothers are not overloaded with 'nutritional antioxidants [52].

Production of reactive species and antioxidant systems is balanced *in vivo*. The balance may be slightly tripped in favor of the RS, so that there is continuous low-level oxidative damage in the human body (Figure 4). This creates a need for repair or replace systems that can deal with oxidatively damaged molecules.

If the initial increase in RS is relatively small and occurs in a short period of time, the antioxidative response may be sufficient to compensate for the increase in RS and to reset the original balance between RS production and RS scavenging capacity (acute oxidative stress). These physiological manifestations of redox regulation, involve typically a temporary increase and/or a temporary shift of the intracellular thiol/disulfide redox state toward more oxidative conditions [2].

Pathological conditions may develop in more extreme cases of persistently high RS levels (Chronic oxidative stress). One important thing to know and measure is when an organism can reset to the original balance and when as entered in a no return point.

Oxidative stress is produced when the antioxidant defense systems are overwhelmed and there is a serious imbalance between the generation of reactive oxygen species and antioxidant protection in favor of the formation, causing excessive oxidative damage (Figure 5).

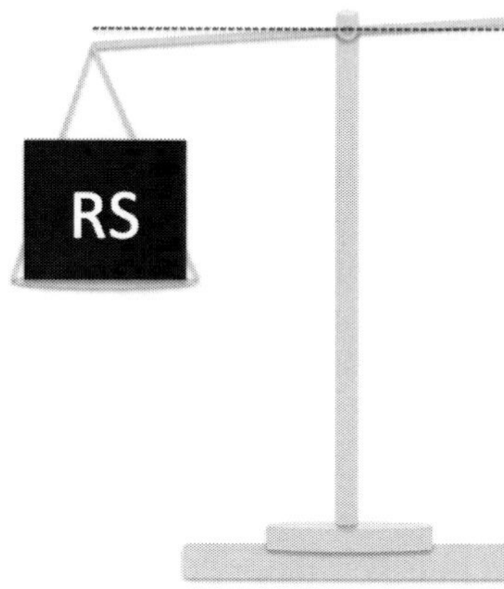

Figure 4. Normal physiological balance between RS and antioxidants. The balance may be slightly tripped in favor of the RS, so that there is continuous low-level oxidative damage in the human body.

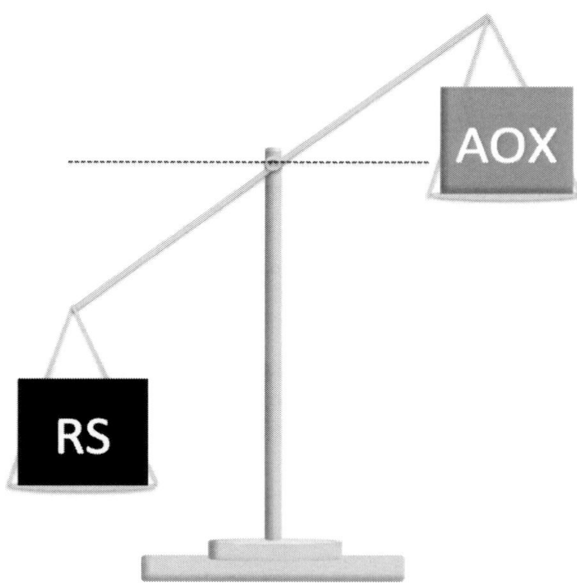

Figure 5. Oxidative stress duetoloss of physiological balancebetween RS and antioxidants. There is a serious imbalance between the generation of RS and antioxidant protection in favor of the former.

The antioxidants as a therapeutic approach for the critical ill patients will be presented in the chapter 12.

7. Biomarkers of Oxidative Stress

To establish the role of oxidative damage, it is therefore essential to be able to measure it accurately.

Essentially, there are two approaches to detecting transient RS [53]:

- Attempting to trap these species and measure the levels of the trapped molecules
- Measuring the levels of the damage done by RS, that is, the amount of oxidative damage.

Most RS persist for only a short time *in vivo* and cannot be measured directly.

The only technique that can 'see' free radicals directly and specifically is the electron spin resonance (ESR), because it detects the presence of unpaired electrons. However, ESR detects only fairly unreactive radicals, since the reactive ones, do not accumulate too high-enough levels to be measured [39]. Some reagentsused on ESR for trapping the RS are toxic in humans.

The easiest way to measure the concentration of RS *in vivo* is by measuring their effects or their chemical fingerprinting in some molecules. These biomarkers are very useful for measuring the oxidative damage and the effect of RS in some diseases. It is the damage caused by RS that is important rather than the total amount of each species generated.

Some frequently used Biomarkers are: ferric reducing ability of plasma (FRAP), MDA, HNE and Acrolein; Isoprostanes; Glutathione and S-Glutathionylated proteins; Tyrosine Oxidation, Nitration and Halogenation; Carbonylated proteins, and levels of antioxidant enzymes in erythrocytes (SOD, CAT, GPx, etc.)[54].

Some biomarkers are elevated in critically ill adult patients, showing a direct correlation between clinical severity and the level of elevation.

Whatever biomarkers is used, it is necessary know about how the method works, what is likely to confound it, and how quantitative it can be.

More information about the biomarkers of oxidative stress will be discussed in chapter 11.

8. Oxidative Stress and Diseases

Free radicals are widely believed to contribute to the development of several age-related diseases, and perhaps, even to the aging process itself.

These diseases fall into two groups: the first group involves diseases characterized by pro-oxidants shifting the thiol/disulphide redox state and impairing glucose tolerance the so-called "mitochondrial oxidative stress" conditions (cancer and diabetes mellitus); the second group involves disease characterized by "inflammatory oxidative conditions", and enhanced activity of either NADPH oxidase (leading to atherosclerosis and chronic inflammation) or xanthine oxidase-induced formation of ROS (implicated in ischemia and reperfusion injury) [1].

Convincing evidence for the association of oxidative/nitrosative stress and acute and chronic diseases lies on validated biomarkers of oxidative stress. [54]. Many studies have shown increased oxidative damage to all the major classes of biomolecules in the brains of Alzheimer's patients [55]. Other diseases in which oxidative damage has been implicated include cancer, atherosclerosis, other neurodegenerative diseases and diabetes [56 - 61].

The low level of antioxidants has been associated with certain pathologies. For example, the protective effects of SOD have been demonstrated in animal models where SOD significantly protects the heart and brain from ischemic injury [62, 63] and prevents alcohol-induced liver injury [64]. Mutations in SOD have been implicated in amyotrophic lateral sclerosis (ALS), increased susceptibility to Type 2 diabetes in humans, cancer, and Alzheimer's disease [12, 14, 64, 65, 66].

8.1. Cardiovascular Diseases

RS-induced oxidative stress plays a role in various cardiovascular diseases, such as atherosclerosis, ischemic heart disease, hypertension, cardiomyopathies, cardiac hypertrophy and congestive heart failure [67].

ROS are known to contribute to cardiac injury, both by oxidizing cellular constituents (mainly proteins, critical for excitation–contraction coupling), and by diminishing NO• bioactivity by direct inactivation [67].

Abnormalities in myocyte function due to increased oxidative stress are considered to be associated with the effects of ROS on subcellular organelles: inhibition of the ecto-ATPase activity and sarcolemmal ATP independient Ca^{2+} binding activity by Fe^{2+} and H_2O_2 [68].

Superoxide radical, hydroxyl radical, and nitric oxide have been reported to promote sarcoplasmic reticular Ca^{2+} release by the interaction with sulphydryl groups of the cardiac and skeletal ryanodine receptor [69]. Another source of Ca^{2+} is from membrane lipid peroxidation. The critical role of intracellular Ca^{2+} overload in the genesis of myocyte dysfunction has been well established [70].

Mitochondrial creatine kinase activity of rat heart was reported to decrease upon exposure to xanthine plus xanthine oxidase or hydrogen peroxide [71].

The major sources of oxidative stress in cardiovascular system involve: the enzymes xanthine oxidoreductase (XOR), NADPH oxidase and NOS, as well as the mitochondrial cytochromes and hemoglobin [72, 73].

Massive production of ROS during ischemia/reperfusion in turn lead to tissue injury causing thus serious complications in organ transplantation, stroke, and myocardial infarction [74]. During ischemia, oversized ATP consumption leads to the accumulation of the purine catabolites hypoxanthine and xanthine, which upon subsequent reperfusion and influx of oxygen are metabolized by xanthine oxidase to produce enormous amounts of superoxide radical and hydrogen peroxide [75]. Ischemia/reperfusion induced in a model of the rat heart was shown to activate the redox-sensitive transcription factors NF-κB and AP-1 and the MAPKs, JNK and p38 [76]. Activation of these transcription factors may be due to inflammatory responses and apoptotic cell death in the affected tissue [1].

8.2. Hypertension

Free radicals are thought to contribute to the pathogenesis of hypertension through an impairment of endothelial cells and through uncoupled eNOS.

Chronic oxidative stress causes senescence of endothelial cells. This is characterized by a detachment of endothelial cells or part of the endothelial cell membrane. With the persistence of oxidative stress, the capacity of neighboring endothelial cells to repair endothelial injury is limited. This is called endothelial dysfunction, which has been clearly associated with prognosis in patients with heart failure, essential hypertension, and peripheral artery disease [77]. This will be addressed in chapter 5.

Uncoupled eNOS is a significant superoxide source, and then $O_2 \bullet^-$ produced reduces NO bioavailability by inactivation, leading to $ONOO^-$ formation. The following $ONOO^-$ protonation will break off, liberating the highly peroxidant •OH. Endothelium is affected by this reaction in two ways: 1) NO scavenging impairs its vasodilating activity, leading to permanent high blood pressure and 2) Hydroxyl radical causes damage in endothelial cells, perpetuating by this way, resulting in a vicious cycle [78]. Superoxide promotes cell proliferation whereas hydrogen peroxide induces apoptosis. RS induced oxidative stress in hypertensive patients is accompanied by decreased levels of antioxidants such as Vitamin E, GSH, and SOD. It was also demonstrated that Angiotensin II-induced hypertension was associated with increased vascular superoxide production.

8.3. Atherosclerosis

In the thickening and hardening of the arterial walls, oxidative stress induces the expression of protein kinases such as focal adhesion kinase and intercellular adhesion molecules such as ICAM-1 leading to earlier invasion of monocytes and T-lynfocytes on the arterial wall [79].

Significant amounts of iron pool were found in atherosclerotic lesions, which may indicate that the iron-catalysed formation of free radicals (e.g. Fenton chemistry), may take place in the development process of atherosclerosis [80].

Oxidized low-density cholesterol (LDLox) mediated formation of RS also caused plaque formation [1].

8.4. Metabolic Syndrome and Diabetes

Chronic oxidative stress impairs insulin action, as was demonstrated in type 2 diabetics. This impairment might be due to several factors, such as membrane fluidity alterations, decreased availability of NO and increased intracellular calcium content [81].

The imbalance between the positive Insulin receptor substrates 1 (IRS-1), tyrosine phosphorylation, and the negative IRS-1 serine phosphorylation, is strongly stimulated by diabetogenic factors including free fatty acids, TNF αand oxidative stress, producing changes in the intracellular signaling of insulin [1]. All the metabolic pathways associated with the postprandial hyperglycemic spikes, increase free radical synthesis and worsen the oxidative state. Hyperglycemia in an organism stimulates ROS formation from a variety of sources. These sources include oxidative phosphorylation, glucose autooxidation, NADPH oxidase, lipooxygenase, cytochrome P450 monooxygenases, and nitric oxide synthase. Glucose itself, as well as its metabolites, is known to react with hydrogen peroxide in the presence of iron and copper ions to form hydroxyl radical.

Diabetic patients show, during the postprandial period, an increase in MDA plasma levels and a decrease in sulphydryl groups, α-tocopherol and total radical-trapping antioxidant parameter [82].

β-Cells are particularly sensitive to ROS, because they are low in free-radical quenching (antioxidant) enzymes such as catalase, glutathione peroxidase, and superoxide dismutase [1]. The intrinsically low levels of antioxidant activity of islets render them particularly at risk for ROS-induced damage. Several independent strategies that ameliorate mitochondrial ROS production were shown to prevent some of the typical secondary complications of the disease, including the activation of protein kinase C or NF-κB and the formation of advanced glycation end products (AGE)[83].

8.5. Neurodegenerative Diseases

The brain in Alzheimer´s disease (AD) is under increased oxidative stress and this may have a role in the pathogenesis of neuron degeneration and death in this disorder.

It has been found increased brain Fe, Al, Hg and Zn in AD, increased lipid peroxidation and increased protein and DNA oxidation. Also decreased cytochrome c oxidase levels, advanced glycation end products (AGE), malondialdehyde, carbonyls, peroxynitrite, heme oxygenase-1 and SOD-1 are found in neurofibrillary tangles and AGE, heme oxygenase-1, SOD-1 in senile plaques of AD brains. Also, a number of studies show that amyloid beta peptide is capable of generating free radicals [1, 18].

Cu^+ is a potent mediator of the highly reactive hydroxyl radical (•OH) and Aβ -associated Cu^+ may contribute to the elevated oxidative stress characteristic of AD brain. Cu^{2+} promotes the neuro-toxicity of Aβ, which correlates with metal reduction [$Cu^{2+} \rightarrow Cu^+$] and the generation of hydrogen peroxide [84]. In the presence of oxygen or H_2O_2, Cu^+ may catalyze free radical oxidation of the peptide via the Fenton reaction.

Apolipoprotein E (apoE), a lipid transport molecule that has been linked to the pathogenesis of AD, has been found to be subject to free radical attack and a direct correlation exists between Apo E peroxidation and Alzheimer's disease [55]. There is evidence that there are high levels of basal oxidative stress in the substantia nigra pars compacta in the normal brain, but this increases in Parkinson's disease patients [1].

Mitochondrial dysfunction associated with oxidative damage and abnormal protein accumulation (ubiquitin/proteosome pathway), is the key molecular mechanisms compromising dopaminergic neurons in familial Parkinson´s disease [18].

8.6. Cancer

It has been clearly demonstrated that ROS interfere with the expression of a number of genes and signal transduction pathways and are thus instrumental in the process of carcinogenesis [10, 85]. Cancer is characterized by a more reducing environment of the cell and can be considered as a disturbed balance between cell proliferation and cell death, shifted more greatly towards cell proliferation [86]. The redox imbalance is related to oncogenic stimulation. Modification of genetic material resulting from oxidative damage incidents represents the first step involved in mutagenesis, carcinogenesis and ageing. For example, iron–induced oxidative stress, is considered to be a principal determinant of human colorectal cancer [87]. Several studies documented that tumor cells from blood neoplasms, and also colon, breast, and pancreas cell lines have all been reported to express activated NF-κB [88]. Reactive oxygen species have been implicated as second messengers involved in the activation of NF-κB via tumor necrosis factor (TNF) and interleukin-1 [10, 85].

Many studies have been devoted to mutations in p53 caused by direct action of ROS or by carcinogenic metals [89]. In addition to the extensive studies devoted to the role of oxidative nuclear DNA damage in neoplasia, evidence about the involvement of mitochondrial oxidative DNA damage in the carcinogenesis process exists [10]. Besides from the DNA damage, lipid peroxidation has been suggested as carcinogenic too. MDA and HNE are mutagenic and carcinogenic in mammalian cells [1, 90].

8.7. Rheumatoid Arthritis

The pathogenesis of this disease is linked predominantly with the formation of free radicals at the site of inflammation. Oxidative injury and inflammatory status in various rheumatic diseases, was confirmed by increased levels of isoprostanes and prostaglandins in serum and synovial fluid compared to controls. T cells isolated from the synovial fluid of patients with rheumatoid arthritis show signs of decreased intracellular GSH level [91].

The migration of monocytes and lymphocytes into the rheumatoid arthritis synovium is mediated by the abnormal expression of several adhesion molecules (ELAM-1, VCAM-1, ICAM-1, ICAM-2) [92]; this can be explained by the abnormal induction of redox-sensitive signalling pathways.

8.8. Aging

Generally, there are two main theories describing the process of ageing: damage-accumulation theories and genetic theories [93]. In the damage accumulation theory, the RS play a key role in the fact that the formation of superoxide in the mitochondria generates DNA damage. The cells can repair much of the damage done to nuclear DNA but mitochondrial DNA cannot be fixed.

This damage accumulates over time and shuts down mitochondria, causing cells death and organism aging. It as been demonstrated in some species, that lowest calories intakes and work, is associated with lowest formation of RS and longest life [94]. Several more recent reports showed that telomere shortening could be induced in fibroblasts by mild oxidative stress [95 - 97]. Peroxynitrite has been implicated in aging due to damage of guanine repeats in telomeres and joint disease caused by decreased production of collagen [10, 98]. Evidence for RS implications in ageing and human disease is summarized in Table 2.

Table 2. Evidence for RS implications in ageing and human disease

Disease	Mechanisms	Reference
Cardiac Injury	Oxidizing proteins critical for excitation-contraction Diminishing NO bioactivity Inhibition of the ecto-ATPase and sarcolemmal ATP independent Ca^{2+} binding activity Sarcoplasmic release of Ca^{2+} by RS Decrease in the activity of mitochondrial creatine kinase in expose to XO	[99] [68] [69, 71]
Ischemia and reperfusion	Production of RS by XO Activation of transcription factors (NF-kB, AP-1, MAPK, JNK and p38)	[75] [76]
Hypertension	Endothelial dysfunction Inactivation of NO by superoxide leading to permanent vasoconstriction	[100] [78]
Atherosclerosis	RS induce expression of adhesion molecules leading the infiltration of macrophages and lynfocytes. Increased pool of Iron RS generated by LDLox leading to plaque formation	[79] [80]
Metabolic syndrome and Diabetes	Imbalance in phosphorylation of IRS Hyperglycemia stimulates RS formation Low concentration of antioxidant in β-cells	[101] [102] [103]
Alzheimer´s disease	Increased concentration of transition ions metals (Cu, Zn) RS Atack to ApoE	[84] [55]
Parkinson´s disease	Mitochondrial dysfunction Abnormal protein accumulation (ubiquitin/proteasome pathway)	[104] [105]
Glaucoma	Resistance to aqueous humor outflow increased by H_2O_2 RS related to neuronal death in optic nerve	[106]
Renal damage	Detection of Biomarkers in urine Protective effects of inhibition of ROS Alteration of the glomerulus structure by RS	[54] [107] [108]
Cancer	DNA damage by RS in nucleus and mitochondria Activation of transcription factor NF-kB, TNF and IL-1 Mutation in p53	[10] [85] [89]
Rheumatoid arthritis	High levels of isoprostanes and lows of GSH in synovial fluid of AR patients Abnormal expression of adhesion molecules	[91] [92]
Aging	Damage in mitochondrial DNA and low mitochondrial function Telomere shorting by RS	[109] [95 - 97]

CONCLUSION

From the exposed above, it is clear that reactive species act as signaling species in various normal physiological processes. It is also clear that excessive production of free radicals causes damage to biological material, and it is an essential event in the etiopathogenesis and progression of various diseases and ageing.

Overproduction of RS, most frequently either by excessive stimulation of NADPH by cytokines, or by the mitochondrial electron transport chain, and xanthine oxidase, results in oxidative stress.

Oxidative stress is a deleterious process, which can be an important mediator of damage to cell structures and consequently various disease states, including the multi organ failure and the septic shock in the critical ill patient.

In some diseases, such in the mechanism of carcinogenesis, the role of free radicals as primary species causing damage to DNA is clear, the primary role of ROS in the process of post-ischemic tissue injury and the criticall ill patient is controversial.

Learning how to stop the damage while preserving the useful functions of RS should be a major research priority. Treatments that enhance the antioxidant system are expected to effectively ameliorate cell damage.

REFERENCES

[1] Valko M, Leibfritz D, Moncol J, Cronin MT, Mazur M, Telser J. Free radicals and antioxidants in normal physiological functions and human disease. *Int. J. Biochem. Cell. Biol.* 2007; 39:44-84.

[2] Dröge W. Free radicals in the physiological control of cell function. *Physiol. rev.* 2002; 82:47-95.

[3] Halliwell B, Clement MV, Long LH. Hydrogen peroxide in the human body. *FEBS.* 2000a; 486:10-13.

[4] Halliwell B. Oxygen radicals, nitric oxide and human inflammatory joint disease. *Ann rheum. dis.* 1995; 54, 505-510.

[5] Molavi B, Mehta JL. Oxidative stress in cardiovascular disease: molecular basis of its deleterious effects, its detection, and therapeutic considerations. *Curr. Opin. Cardiol.* 2004;19:488-493.

[6] Halliwell B. Reactive species and antioxidants. Redox biology is a fundamental theme of aerobic life. *Plant physiol.* 2006; 141:312-322.

[7] Winterbourn CC, Hampton MB. Thiol chemistry and specificity in redox signaling. *Free. Rad. Biol. Med.* 2008; 45:549-61.

[8] Miller DM, Buettner GR, Aust SD. Transition metals as catalysts of "autoxidation" reactions. *Free Radic. Biol. Med.* 1990; 8:95–108.

[9] Halliwell B, Cross CE. Oxygen-derived species: their relation to human disease and environmental stress. *Environ health perspct.* 1994; 102: 5-12.

[10] Valko M, Rhodes CJ, Moncol J, Izakovic M, Mazur M. Free radicals, metals and antioxidants in oxidative stress-induced cancer. *Chem. Biol. Interact.* 2006; 160:1–40.

[11] Ambrosone CB, Freudenheim JL, Thompson PA, Bowman E, Vena JE, Marshall JR, Graham S, Laughlin R, Nemoto T, Shields PG. Manganese superoxide dismutase (MnSOD) genetic polymorphisms, dietary antioxidants, and risk of breast cancer. *Cancer Res.* 1999; 59:602-606.

[12] Battin EE, Brumaghim JL. Antioxidant activity of sulfur and selenium: a review of reactive oxygen species scavenging, glutathione peroxidase, and metal-binding antioxidant mechanisms. *Cell biochem. biophys.* 2009; 55:1-23.

[13] Pastor N, Weinstein H, Jamison E, Brenowitz M. A detailed interpretation of OH radical footprints in a TBP-DNA complex reveals the role of dynamics in the mechanism of sequence-specific binding. *J. Mol. Biol.* 2000, 304:55-68.

[14] Li F, Calingasan NY, Yu F, Mauck WM, Toidze M, Almeida CG, Takahashi RH, Carlson GA, Flint Beal M, Lin MT, Gouras GK. Increased plaque burden in brains of APP mutant Mn SOD heterozygous knockout mice. *J. Neurochem.* 2004; 89:1308–1312.

[15] Lippard SJ, Kopp DA, Berg EA, Costello CE. Structural features of covalently cross-linked hydroxylase and reductase proteins of soluble methane monooxygenase as revealed by mass spectrometric analysis. *J. Biol. Chem.* 2003; 278:20939-20945.

[16] Waris G, Ahsan H.Reactive oxygen species: role in the development of cancer and various chronic conditions.*J Carcinog.* 2006; 11:5-14.

[17] Lambeth JD. Nox enzymes, ROS, and chronic disease: an example of antagonistic pleiotropy. *Free Radic. Biol. Med.* 2007; 43:332–347.

[18] Rodrigo R, Toro J. *Oxidative Stress: Basic Overview*. IN: Oxidative stress and antioxidants: their role in human disease. Rodrigo R, Ed. Nova Bioscience. 1st ed. New York, US. 2009. pp. 1-24.

[19] Klaunig JE, Kamendulis LM. The role of oxidative stress in carcinogenesis. *Annu. Rev. Pharmacol. Toxicol.* 2004; 44:239-267.

[20] Fridovich I. Superoxide dismutases. An adaptation to a paramagnetic gas. *J. Biol. Chem.* 1989;264:7761-7764.

[21] Imlay JA, Fridovich I. Assays of metabolic superoxide production in Escherichia coli. *J. Biol. Chem.* 1991; 266:6957-6965.

[22] Babior BM, Woodman RC.Chronic granulomatous disease. *Semin. Hematol.* 1990; 27:247-259.

[23] Babcock GT. How oxygen is activated and reduced in respiration. *Proc. Natl. Acad. Sci. US.* 1999; 96:12971-12973.

[24] Puppo A, Halliwell B.Formation of hydroxyl radicals from hydrogen peroxide in the presence of iron. Is haemoglobin a biological Fenton reagent? *Biochem. J.* 1988; 249:185-190.

[25] Vásquez-Vivar J, Kalyanaraman B, Martásek P, Hogg N, Masters BS, Karoui H, Tordo P, Pritchard KA Jr.Superoxide generation by endothelial nitric oxide synthase: the influence of cofactors. *Proc. Natl. Acad. Sci. US.* 1998 4; 95:9220-9225.

[26] Xia Y, Zweier JL.Direct measurement of nitric oxide generation from nitric oxide synthase.*Proc Natl Acad Sci U S A*. 1997; 11:12705-12710.

[27] Heinecke JW, Li W, Francis GA, Goldstein JA.Tyrosyl radical generated by myeloperoxidase catalyzes the oxidative cross-linking of proteins. *J. Clin. Invest.* 1993; 91:2866-2872.

[28] Hultqvist M, Olsson LM, Gelderman KA, Holmdahl R.The protective role of ROS in autoimmune disease.*Trends Immunol.*2009; 30:201-208.

[29] Blouin E, Halbwachs-Mecarelli L, Rieu P. *Eur. J. Immunol.* 1999; 29:3419-3431.

[30] Naseem KM, Bruckdorfer KR. *Biochem. J.* 1995; 310:149-153.

[31] Semenza GL. HIF-1: Mediator of physiological and pathophysiological responses to hypoxia. *J. Appl. Physiol.* 2000; 88:1474–1480.
[32] Zhu H, Bunn HF.Oxygen sensing and signaling: impact on the regulation of physiologically important genes.*Respir Physiol.* 1999; 115:239-247.
[33] Ferdinandy P. Peroxynitrite: just an oxidative/nitrosative stressor or a physiological regulator as well? *Br. J. pharmacol.* 2006; 148:1-3.
[34] Jones SA, O'donnell, VB, Wood JD, Broughton JP, Hughes EJ, Jones OT. Expression of phagocyte NADPH oxidase components in human endothelial cells. *Am. J. Physiol. Heart Circ. Physiol.* 1996, 271:1626–1634.
[35] Thannickal VJ, Fanburg BL. Activation of an H_2O_2 generating NADH oxidase in human lung fibroblasts by transform-ing growth factor beta 1. *J. Biol. Chem.* 1995; 270:30334–30338.
[36] Halliwell B. Antioxidants and human disease: a general introduction. *Nutr. Rev.* 1997; *55*:44-52.
[37] Dizdaroglu M, Jaruga P, Birincioglu M, Rodriguez H. Free radicalinduced damage to DNA: mechanisms and measurement. *Free Radic. Biol. Med.* 2002; 32:1102–1115.
[38] Jourdhevil D, Idem FL, Feelisch M. Oxidation and nitrosation of thiols at low micromolar exposure to nitric oxide. Evidence for a free radical mechanism. *J. Biol. Chem.* 2000; 278:15720-15726.
[39] Fujimoto H, Sasaki J, Matsumoto M, Suga M, Ando Y, Iggo R, et al. Significant correlation of nitric oxide synthase activity and p53 gene mutation in stage I lung adenocarcinoma. Jpn. *J. Cancer Res.* 1998;89:696-702.
[40] Nyska A, Kohen R. Oxidation of biological systems: oxidative stress phenomena, antioxidants, redox reactions, and methods for their quantification. *Toxicol. Pathol.* 2002; 30:620–650.
[41] Pinchuk I, Schnitzer E, Lichtenberg D. Kinetic analysis of copper-induced peroxidation of LDL. *Biochim. Biophys. Acta.* 1998; 1389:155–172.
[42] Fam SS, Morrow JD.The isoprostanes: unique products of arachidonic acid oxidation a review.*Curr. Med. Chem.* 2003;10:1723-1740.
[43] Esterbauer H, Schaur RJ, Zollner H. Chemistry and biochemistry of 4- hydroxynonenal, malonaldehyde and related aldehydes. *Free Radic. Biol. Med.* 1991; 11:81–128.
[44] Levine RL, Stadtman ER. Oxidative modification of proteins during aging. *Exp. Gerontol.* 2001; 36:1495–1502.
[45] Stadtman ER. Protein oxidation in aging and age-related diseases. *Ann. NY Acad. Sci.* 2001; 928: 22–38.
[46] Nathan AT, Singer M. The oxygen trail: tissue oxygenation. *Br. Med. Bull.* 1999; 55: 96–108.
[47] Macdonald J, Galley HF, Webster NR. Oxidative stress and gene expression in sepsis. *Br. J. Anaesth.* 2003; 90: 221–232.
[48] Andreoli SP: Reactive oxygen molecules, oxidant injury and renal disease. *Pediatr. Nephrol.* 1991; 5:733-742.
[49] Jones DP, Carlson JL, Mody VC, Cai JY, Lynn MJ, Sternberg P. Redox state of glutathione in human plasma. *Free Radic. Biol. Med.* 2000, 28: 625–635.
[50] Nogueira CW, Zeni G, Rocha JBT. Organoselenium and organotellurium compounds: Toxicology and pharmacology. *Chem. Rev.* 2004; 104:6255–6285.

[51] Masella R, Di Benedetto R, Varì R, Filesi C, Giovannini C.Novel mechanisms of natural antioxidant compounds in biological systems: involvement of glutathione and glutathione-related enzymes. *J. Nutr. Biochem.* 2005; 16:577-586.

[52] Halliwell B. Free radicals and antioxidants - quo vadis? *Trends Pharmacol. Sci.* 2011; 32:125-30.

[53] Halliwell B, Whiteman M. Measuring reactive species and oxidative damage in vivo and in cell culture: how should you do it and what do the results mean? *Br. J. pharmacol.* 2004; 142: 231-55.

[54] Dalle-Donne I, Rossi R, Colombo R, Giustarini D, Milzani A. Biomarkers of oxidative damage in human disease. *Clin. chem.* 2006; 52:601-23.

[55] Butterfield DA, Castegna A, Lauderback CM, Drake J. Evidence that amyloid beta-peptide-induced lipid peroxidation and its sequelae in Alzheimer's disease brain contribute to neuronal death. *Neurobiol. Aging.* 2002; 23:655–664.

[56] Chowienczyk PJ, Brett SE, Gopaul NK, Meeking D, Marchetti M, Russell-Jones DL, Anggard EE, Ritter JM. Oral treatment with an antioxidant (raxofe- last) reduces oxidative stress and improves endothelial function in men with type II diabetes. *Diabetologia.* 2000; 43:974–977.

[57] Halliwell B. Lipid peroxidation, antioxidants and cardiovascular disease: how should we move forward? *Cardiovasc. Res.* 2000b; 47:410–418.

[58] Halliwell B. Role of free radicals in the neurodegenerative diseases: therapeutic implications for antioxidant treatment. *Drugs Aging.* 2001; 18: 685–716.

[59] Halliwell B. Vitamin E and the treatment and prevention of diabetes: a case for a controlled clinical trial. *Singapore Med.* 2002a; 43: 479–484.

[60] Halliwell B. Effect of diet on cancer development: is oxidative DNA damage a biomarker? *Free Radic. Biol. Med.* 2002b; 32:968–974.

[61] Parthasarathy S, Santanam N, Ramachandran S, Meilhac O. Potential role of oxidized lipids and lipoproteins in antioxidant defense. *Free Radic. Res.* 2000; 33:197–215.

[62] Keller JN, Kindy MS, Holtsberg FW, St Clair DK, Yen HC, Germeyer A, Steiner SM, Bruce-Keller AJ, Hutchins JB, Mattson MP. Mitochondrial manganese superoxide dismutase prevents neural apoptosis and reduces ischemic brain injury: Suppression of peroxynitrite production, lipid peroxidation, and mitochondrial dysfunction. *J. Neurosci.* 1998; 18:687–697.

[63] Wang P, Chen H, Qin H, Sankarapandi S, Becher MW, Wong PC, Zweier JL. Overexpression of human copper, zinc-superoxide dismutase (SOD1) prevents postischemic injury. *Proc. Natl. Acad. Sci. USA.* 1998; 95:4556–4560.

[64] Wheeler MD, Nakagami M, Bradford BU, Uesugi T, Mason RP, Connor HD, Dikalova A, Kadiiska M, Thurman RG. Overexpression of manganese superoxide dismutase prevents alcohol-induced liver injury in the rat. *J. Biol. Chem.* 2001; 276: 36664–36672.

[65] Tamai M, Furuta H, Kawashima H, Doi A, Hamanishi T, Shimomura H, Sakagashira S, Nishi M, Sasaki H, Sanke T, Nanjo K. Extracellular superoxide dismutase gene polymorphism is associated with insulin resistance and the susceptibility to type 2 diabetes. *Diab. Res. and Clin. Pract.* 2006; 71:140–145.

[66] Wheatley-Price P, Asomaning K, Reid A, Zhai R, Su L, Zhou W, Zhu A, Ryan DP, Christiani DC, Liu G. Myeloperoxidase and superoxide dismutase polymorphisms are

associated with an increased risk of developing pancreatic adenocarcinoma. *Cancer.* 2008, 112, 1037– 1042.

[67] Kim A, Joseph S, Khan A, Epstein CJ, Sobel R, Huang TT. Enhanced expression of mitochondrial superoxide dismutase leads to prolonged in vivo cell cycle progression and up-regulation of mitochondrial thioredoxin. *Free rad. biol. med.* 2010 48; 1501-1512.

[68] Kaneko M, Elimban V, Dhalla NS.Mechanism for depression of heart sarcolemmal Ca^{2+} pump by oxygen free radicals.*Am. J. Physiol.* 1989; 257:804-811.

[69] Stoyanovsky D, Murphy T, Anno PR, Kim YM, Salama G.Nitric oxide activates skeletal and cardiac ryanodine receptors.*Cell Calcium.* 1997; 21:19-29.

[70] Pérez NG, Gao WD, Marbán E.Novel myofilament Ca^{2+}-sensitizing property of xanthine oxidase inhibitors.*Circ. Res.* 1998; 83:423-430.

[71] Hayashi H, Iimuro M, Matsumoto Y, Kaneko M.Effects of gamma-glutamylcysteine ethyl ester on heart mitochondrial creatine kinase activity: involvement of sulfhydryl groups. *Eur. J. Pharmacol.* 1998; 349:133-136.

[72] Berry CE, Hare JM.Xanthine oxidoreductase and cardiovascular disease: molecular mechanisms and pathophysiological implications. *J. Physiol.* 2004; 555:589-606.

[73] Hare JM, Stamler JS.NO/redox disequilibrium in the failing heart and cardiovascular system. *J. Clin. Invest.* 2005;115:509-517.

[74] Kasparová S, Brezová V, Valko M, Horecký J, Mlynárik V, Liptaj T, Vancová O, Ulicná O, Dobrota D.Study of the oxidative stress in a rat model of chronic brain hypoperfusion.*Neurochem Int.* 2005; 46:601-11.

[75] Granger DN, Stokes KY, Shigematsu T, CerwinkaWH, Tailor A, Krieglstein CF. Splanchnic ischaemia-reperfusion injury: Mechanistic insights provided by mutant mice. *Acta. Physiol. Scand.* 2001; 173: 83–91.

[76] Lazou A, Bogoyevitch MA, Clerk A, Fuller SJ, Marshall CJ, Sugden PH. Regulation of mitogen-activated protein kinase cascade in adult rat heart preparations in vitro. *Circ. Res.* 1994; 75:932–941.

[77] Gokce N, Keaney JF, Hunter LM, Watkins MT, Nedeljkovic ZS, Menzoian JO, Vita JA. Predictive value of noninvasively determined endothelial dysfunction for long- term cardiovascular events in patients with peripheral vascular disease. *J. Am. Coll Cardiol.* 2003; 41:1769–1775.

[78] Mollnau H, Wendt M, Szocs K, Lassegue B, Schulz E, Oelze M, Li H, Bodenschatz M, August M, Kleschyov AL, Tsilimingas N, Walter U, Forstermann U, Meinertz T, Griendling K, and Munzel T. Effects of angiotensin II infusion on the expression and function of NAD(P)H oxidase and components of nitric oxide/cGMP signaling. *Circ. Res.* 2002; 90:58–65.

[79] Chien S, Li S, And Shyy Yj. Effects of mechanical forces on signal transduction and gene expression in endothelial cells. *Hypertension* . 1998;31:162–169.

[80] Yuan XM, Li W.The iron hypothesis of atherosclerosis and its clinical impact.*Ann. Med.* 2003; 35:578-591.

[81] Garg UC, Hassid A. Nitric oxide-generating vasodilators and 8-bromo-cyclic guanosine monophosphate inhibit mitogenesis and proliferation of cultured rat vascular smooth muscle cells. *J. Clin. Invest.* 1989; 83:1774–1777.

[82] Ceriello A, Lizzio S, Bortolotti N, Russo A, Motz E, Tonutti L, Crescentini A, Taboga C. Meal generated oxidative stress in type 2 diabetic patients. *Diabetes Care*. 1998; 21:1529-33.

[83] Nishikawa T, Edelstein D, Du Xl, Yamagishi S, Matsumura T, Kaneda Y, Yorek Ma, Beebe D, Oates Pj, Hammes Hp, Giardino I, And Brownlee M. Normalizing mitochondrial superoxide produc- tion blocks three pathways of hyperglycaemic damage. *Nature*. 2000; 404:787–790.

[84] Cuajungco MP, Goldstein LE, Nunomura A, Smith MA, Lim JT, Atwood CS, Huang X, Farrag YW, Perry G, Bush AI.Evidence that the beta-amyloid plaques of Alzheimer's disease represent the redox-silencing and entombment of abeta by zinc. *J. Biol. Chem*. 2000; 275:19439-19442.

[85] Poli G, Leonarduzzi G, Biasi F,Chiarpotto E. Oxidative stress and cell signalling. *Curr. Med. Chem*. 2004; 11:1163–1182.

[86] Schafer FQ, Buettner GR. Redox environment of the cell as viewed through the redox state of the glutathione disulfide/glutathione couple. *Free Radic. Biol. Med.* 2001; 30:1191–1212.

[87] Valko M, Morris H, Mazur M, Rapta P, Bilton RF. Oxygen free radical generating mechanisms in the colon: Do the semiquinones of Vitamin K play a role in the aetiology of colon cancer? *Biochim. Biophys. Acta*. 2001; 1527:161–166.

[88] Storz P. Reactive oxygen species in tumor progression. *Front Biosci.* 2005; 10:1881–1896.

[89] Hollstein M, Sidransky D, Vogelstein B, Harris CC. p53 mutations in human cancer. *Science*. 1991; 253:49–53.

[90] Marnett LJ. Lipid peroxidation DNA damage by malondialdehyde. *Mut. Res. Fund. Mol. Mech. Mutagen.* 1999; 424:83–95.

[91] Maurice MM, Nakamura H, van der Voort EA, van Vliet AI, Staal FJ, Tak PP, Breedveld FC, Verweij CL. Evidence for the role of an altered redox state in hyporesponsiveness of synovial T cells in rheumatoid arthritis. *J. Immunol.* 1997; 158:1458–1465.

[92] Cunnane G, FitzGerald O, Beeton C, Cawston TE, Bresnihan B. Early joint erosions and serum levels of matrix metalloproteinase 1, matrix metalloproteinase 3, and tissue inhibitor of metalloproteinases 1 in rheumatoid arthritis. *Arth. Rheumat.* 2001; 44: 2263–2274.

[93] Hayflick L. How and why we age. *Exp Gerontol.* 1998; 33: 639–653.

[94] Sohal RS, Mockett RJ, Orr WC.Mechanisms of aging: an appraisal of the oxidative stress hypothesis.*Free Radic. Biol. Med.* 2002;33:575-586.

[95] Sitte N, Saretzki G, Von Zglinicki T. Accelerated telomere shortening in fibroblasts after extended periods of confluency. *Free Radical Biol. Med.* 1997; 24:885–893.

[96] Von Zglinicki T, Nilsson E, Döcke W, Brunk Ut. Lipofuscin accumulation and aging of fibroblasts. *Gerontology*. 1995a; 41:95–109.

[97] Von Zglinicki T, Saretzki G, Döcke W, Lotze C. Mild hyperoxia shortens telomeres and inhibits proliferation of fibroblasts: a model for senescence? *Exp. Cell. Res.* 1995b; 220: 186–193.

[98] Afonso V, Champy R, Mitrovic D, Collin P, Lomr, A. Reactive oxygen species and superoxide dismutases: Role in joint diseases. *Joint Bone Spine*. 2007; 74:324–329.

[99] Khan SA, Lee K, Minhas KM, Gonzalez DR, Raju SV, Tejani AD, Li D, Berkowitz DE, Hare JM. Neuronal nitric oxide synthase negatively regulates xanthine oxidoreductase inhibition of cardiac excitation-contraction coupling. *Proc. Natl. Acad. Sci. USA*. 2004; 101:15944–15948.

[100] Deanfield JE, Halcox JP, Rabelink TJ. Endothelial function and dysfunction: testing and clinical relevance. *Circulation*. 2007; 115:1285–1295.

[101] Lawlor MA, Alessi DR. PKB/Akt: A key mediator of cell proliferation, survival and insulin responses? *J. Cell. Sci.* 2001; 114:2903–2910.

[102] Hink U, Li H, Mollnau H, Oelze M, Matheis E, Hartmann M, Skatchkov M, Thaiss F, Stahl RA, Warnholtz A, Meinertz T, Griendling K, Harrison DG, Forstermann U, Munzel T. Mechanisms underlying endothelial dysfunction in diabetes mellitus. *Circ. Res*. 2001; 88:14–22.

[103] Evans JL, Goldfine ID, Maddux BA, Grodsky GM. Are oxidative stress-activated signaling pathways mediators of insulin resistance and beta-cell dysfunction? *Diabetes*. 2003; 52:1–8.

[104] Andersen JK. Oxidative stress in neurodegeneration: Cause or consequence? *Nat. Rev. Neurosci*. 2004; 5:18–25.

[105] Mitsui T, Kuroda Y, Kaji R. Parkin and mitochondria. *Brain Nerve*. 2008; 60:923-929.

[106] Izzotti A, Bagnis A, Saccà SC. The role of oxidative stress in glaucoma. *Mutat. Res*. 2006; 612:105-114.

[107] Ishikawa I, Kiyama S, Yoshioka T. Renal antioxidant enzymes: their regulation and function. *Kidney Int*. 1994; 45:1–9.

[108] Klahr S. Oxygen radicals and renal diseases. *Miner Electrolyte Metab*. 1997; 23:140-143.

[109] Cadenas E, Davies KJ. Mitochondrial free radical generation, oxidative stress, and aging. *Free Radic. Biol. Med.* 2002; 29:222–230.

In: Oxidative Stress and the Critically Ill Patient
Editors: Ramón Rodrigo and Bettina von Dessauer
ISBN: 978-1-62081-576-2

Chapter II

Pathophysiology of Sepsis and Septic Shock

Jazmina Bongain
Staff member of the Pediatric Intensive Care Unit,
Doctor Roberto del Río Children´s Hospital, Santiago de Chile
Pediatrics and Intensive Care, University of Chile, Chile

Abstract

Sepsis has been recognized as an important public health problem and represents a major factor in morbidity and mortality in intensive care units worldwide in any age group. Recently, the American College of Chest Physicians and the Society of Critical Care Medicine (ACCP/SCCM) reaffirmed the criteria for diagnosing sepsis in order to improve patient care, allow the enrollment in clinical trials and improve communication between ICUs. In this consensus SIRS coined the term to refer to a process inflammatory independent of cause while the term sepsis represents the systemic inflammatory response to the presence of infection.

The host response to sepsis involves many concomitant, integrated, and often antagonistic processes that result both in exaggerated inflammation and immune suppression. The pathogenesis of this condition is now becoming better understood, allowing a greater understanding of the complex network of immune, inflammatory and hematological mediators, which may permit the development of rational and novel therapies. This chapter reviews the pathophysiology of the inflammatory process involved in sepsis and septic shock, laying the groundwork for better understanding of the origin in the generation of free radicals and oxidative stress.

Abbreviations

ATP	adenosine triphosphate
CARS	compensatory anti-inflammatory response syndrome

C5aR	C5a receptor
EF	ejection fraction
H_2O_2	oxygen peroxide
NFkB	nuclear factor kB
iNOS	inducible nitric oxide synthase isoform
LPS	lipopolysaccharide
MODS	multiple organ dysfunction syndrome
MHC	class II major histocompatibility complex
NO•	nitric oxide
NOS	nitric oxide synthase
O_2•−	superoxide
ONOO−	peroxynitrite
RNS	reactive nitrogen species
ROS	reactive oxygen species
SIRS	systemic inflammatory response syndrome
SOD	superoxide dismutase
TNF	tumor necrosis factor

2. Introduction

Sepsis has been recognized as an important public health problem and represents a major factor in morbidity and mortality in intensive care units worldwide at any age group. In the United Stated septic shock in adult patients causes more than 200,000 deaths and more than 750.000 sepses every year, with mortality rates as high as 40–60%. [1]. Despite prompt treatment with antibiotics, provision of adequate fluid resuscitation, and technological support of organ function, the mortality rate remains unacceptably high. In children it is also a major cause of mortality up to 80% in some developing countries [2]. In developed countries infant mortality due to sepsis has fallen significantly in recent years [3], but still remains one of the leading causes of morbidity and mortality being around 7% of all death [4].

Annually in the United States, there are 42,000 cases of pediatric severe sepsis, with a reported case fatality rate of 10.3% [4]. In the UK, infection accounts for more than 10% of deaths in children less than 4 years old [5] and approximately 1000 children with severe sepsis are admitted to pediatric intensive care units annually. In 1991, a consensus conference organized by the American College of Chest Physicians and Society of Critical Care Medicine (ACCP/SCCM) reaffirmed the criteria for diagnosing sepsis. It put forward a new syndrome, which was named the 'systemic inflammatory response syndrome' (SIRS) [6]. The concept of SIRS was coined to describe an inflammatory process, triggered by many factors including infections, trauma, surgery and others causing stress. Even though the definition has high sensitivity and low specificity, it has been helpful in improving patient care, allowing enrollment in clinical trials and improving communication between ICUs. Thus the term sepsis represents the systemic inflammatory response in relation to the presence of infection [7]. The clinical manifestations are the result of changes in pathophysiology at the capillary endothelial level and are characterized by the presence of fever, tachycardia, tachypnea and altered leukocyte counts with high suspicion of evidence of a presumed or known site of infection. Patients with sepsis and evidence of organ dysfunction such as respiratory or renal failure are considered to have severe sepsis.

Patients with severe sepsis, who additionally are on persistent hypotension refractory to fluid resuscitation, are in septic shock [7]. Progression of this continuum from sepsis to severe sepsis and septic shock is associated with increased morbidity and mortality. The pathogenesis of this condition, now better known, has allowed an improved understanding of the complex network of immune, inflammatory and hematological mediators that may allow the development of rational and novel therapies. Notwithstanding the foregoing, the mortality has remained high so that early recognition is still the best tool to decrease mortality and length of stay associated with multiple organ failure.

3. Pathophysiology of Sepsis

The normal host response to infection is to both identify and control pathogen invasion and to start immediate tissue repair when necessary. The host response to sepsis involves many concomitant, integrated, and often antagonistic processes that result both in exaggerated inflammation and immune suppression. These defense mechanisms include the release of cytokines, the activation of neutrophils, monocytes, and microvascular endothelial cells, as well as the activation of neuroendocrine reflexes and plasma protein cascade systems, such as the complement system, the intrinsic (contact system) and extrinsic pathways of coagulation, and the fibrinolytic system. The host response, rather than the nature of the pathogen, primarily determines the patient's outcome. Now it has been recognized that alterations to the patient's immune system, with an excessive systemic inflammatory response on one hand, and paralysis of cell mediated immunity on the other, appear to be the key elements in the pathogenesis of multiple organ failure, susceptibility to infection and associated mortality.

In sepsis, the inflammatory process becomes amplified leading in a continuum from a lowgrade systemic response associated with a self-limited infection to a marked systemic response, representing a spectrum of clinical and pathophysiologic severity. The intensity of the inflammatory response is determined by various host factors (e.g. comorbid diseases, nutritional status and genetics) as well as inciting infection related factors including virulence and bacterial load. [8] The intense and sustained inflammatory response can result in tissue damage and organ failure. Several factors are implicated in the pathogenesis of organ failure, such as the endocrine and immune systems, disseminated intravascular coagulation, genetic susceptibility and mitochondrial dysfunction and an acquired transient intrinsic defect in cellular respiration termed "cytopathic hypoxia" [9].

Following acute sepsis, a 'compensatory anti-inflammatory response syndrome' (CARS) develops, leading to immunosuppression [10]. This is an adaptive mechanism whose purpose is to regulate and protect against inflammatory injury, but with risk of newly acquired nosocomial infections and mortality in sepsis.

3.1. Basic Molecular Mechanisms of Inflammation in Sepsis

The innate immune system is the primordial and the first line of defense against invading pathogens [11]. Its function is thought to be the recognition of invading pathogens, the activation of inflammation to control the pathogen, and the subsequent activation of the acquired immune response. It includes cell types playing primary roles in phagocytosis and intracellular killing (polymorphonuclear cells), cytotoxic killing (natural killer cells), and antigen presentation (dendritic) cells [12]. The monocytes and their descendants play a key role in the activation and initiation of the innate immune response. Its function includes the recognition and phagocytosis of pathogens, secretion of mediators that modulate the overall immune response and presentation of digested peptides on its cell surface to activate the adaptive immune response. Once stimulated, monocytes engulf and destroy microbes, which then are processed into antigenic peptides. These are presented on the external surfaces of innate immune cells in conjunction with class II major histocompatibility complex molecules, such as HLA-DR. Antigens presented in this way, along with co-stimulatory input from the innate immune cells, activate the adaptive arm of the immune response [12].

3.1.1. Pathogen-Host Interaction

The recognition of microbial products by the innate arm of the immune system is an essential element for the setting of the host defense. After recognizing the pathogen, it occurs the production of cytokines and chemokines involved in the leukocyte promotion and recruitment to the infection focus, thus inducing their microbicidal activity.

The innate immune response begins with the recognition of the cellular constituents of the pathogen. This is accomplished through the presence of constitutively expressed receptors present on the plasma membranes of innate immune effectors cells. These receptors recognize broad classes of microbial constituents. These microbial components are known as pathogen-associated molecular patterns (PAMPs) and are key elements and constant in the structure of microorganisms [13].

These PAMPs are recognized by pattern recognition receptors (PRRs). These receptors also recognize eukaryotic cell key constituents released as a result of tissue damage and apoptosis. Such endogenous danger signals have been termed "alarmins" or danger-associated molecular patterns (DAMPs) [14]. Several families of PRRs, including Toll-like receptors and cytoplasm receptors, recognize distinct microbial components and directly activate immune cells [15]. This is accomplished through the presence of constitutively expressed receptors present on the plasma membranes of innate immune effector cells. These receptors mediated by phagocytes including macrophages and dendritic cells, initiate the innate immune response and regulate the adaptive immune response to infection. The TLR is the most important molecular mechanism by which the host recognizes the presence of a pathogenic organism and initiates the innate immune response. To date, almost 13 mammalian TLRs have been identified, and each is known to detect a specific intracellular signaling pathway. Toll-Like receptor 1,2,4,5 and 6 mainly recognize bacterial product, whereas TLR- 3, TLR-7 and TLR-8 are specific for viral detection. Toll like receptor 9 seems to be involved in both microbial and viral recognition, while TLR4 is the most important sensor of Gram-negative bacterial products [16], whereas TLR2 seems to be the key receptor in activating the immune system against Gram-positive bacteria [17]. TLR 4 may further contribute to the pathogenesis of sepsis by amplifying inflammatory responses through interaction with DAMPs released after tissue injury [18] besides acting as sensor of oxidative stress [19]. Binding of TLRs activates intracellular signal-transduction pathways that lead to the activation of cytosolic nuclear factor-kb (NF-κb). Activated NF-κb moves from the cytoplasm to the nucleus, binds to transcription sites and induces activation of hundreds of genes that are important in immune inflammatory responses [20]. These include genes for cytokines, adhesion molecules and chemokines, receptors required for neutrophil adhesion and transmigration across blood vessel walls, receptors involved in immune recognition, such as members of the major histocompatibility complex; and proteins involved in antigen presentation [21]. NF-κB also modulates antimicrobial and immunologic functions by controlling the survival of neutrophils and the proliferation and differentiation of B- and T-lymphocytes at the site of the infection [22].

3.1.2. Neutrophils

The neutrophil is an integral component of the innate immune system, the first and most abundant leukocyte to be delivered to a site of infection or inflammation [23].

These cells have a pivotal role in the defense against bacterial infections, as shown by neutropenia (eg, after chemotherapy), which increases the susceptibility to local infection and to sepsis. Bacterial elimination is dependent on the rapid recruitment of blood neutrophils into sites of infection. During inflammation, circulating bloodstream neutrophils contact and transiently interact with endothelial cell molecules resulting in a cell rolling on the blood vessel wall. This initial cell contact represents the first step in a cascade of molecular interactions leading to leukocyte extravasations, and is a critical prerequisite for a tighter interaction. Circulating neutrophils are attracted to the site of inflammation in response to chemoattractant mediators locally released such as the complement peptide C5a, leukotriene B4, platelet-activating factor, the bacterial peptide formyl-methionyl-leucyl-phenylalanine, and interleukin 8 [24]. The cells migrate from an area of low concentration (ie, blood vessel walls) to an area of high concentration (site of infection or inflammation), whereupon the chemotactic factors become potent neutrophil activators [25]. Once activated, neutrophils are able to phagocytose, release granular lytic enzymes and antimicrobial polypeptides into the phagolysosome, and to generate large amounts of reactive oxygen and nitrogen species, such as hydrogen peroxide (H2O2) and nitric oxide (NO), which are crucial products for the microbicidal activity of these cells.

Neutrophil priming causes an increase in the response of these cells to an activating agent and prolongs their lifespan by inhibiting apoptosis, as well as inducing an up-regulation in their expression of vascular adhesion molecules: the selectins and integrins [12]. Both families of adhesion molecules control the binding of neutrophils to the vascular endothelium. The selectins promote the initial rolling or tethering of the neutrophils to the endothelium under the shear force of blood flow, whereas the integrins induce firm adhesion [26].

Neutrophils are ideally suited to the elimination of pathogenic bacteria for their large stores of proteolytic enzymes and rapid production of reactive oxygen species to degrade internalyzed pathogens. If these lytic factor or pro-inflammatory cytokines are released in the tissue infiltrating neutrophils, local damage will ensue. By contrast, in severe sepsis local infection is accompanied by systemic neutrophil activation.

The overwhelming activation of neutrophils is known to elicit tissue damage. Clinical evidence related aberrant neutrophil activity with the organ failure of severe sepsis [27].

Removal of neutrophils by apoptosis is a homoeostatic mechanism preventing damage to healthy tissues that would otherwise occur after the lysis of necrotic cells. This process is central for the prevention and resolution of inflammation. Neutrophil apoptosis is inhibited in patients with systemic inflammation, systemic infections, severe sepsis, and those at risk of multiple organ failure [28].

3.1.3. Cytokines

Cytokines and chemokines are important components of the immune system that act as messages between cells, both in the innate and adaptive immune systems. So these molecules are the extracellular expression of the immune system.

The early phase of sepsis is dominated by a hyper-inflammatory state mediated by the systemic production of inflammatory cytokines. Interleukin 1 (IL-1), IL-6, tumor necrosis factor alpha (TNF-α), and gamma interferon (IFN-γ) have pro-inflammatory effects.

These cytokines and chemokines modulate the inflammatory response by recruiting and activating other immune effectors cells and activating non cellular aspects of the immune response, such as the complement and coagulation cascades [12, 29]. The most important pro-inflammatory cytokines are TNF and IL-1.

These cytokines have many local actions, including stimulation of synthesis of other cytokines, up-regulation of the expression of tissue factor and adhesion molecules on nearby cells, induction of certain enzymes (eg, phospholipase A2, cycloxygenase-2). TNF-α and other pro-inflammatory molecules can also activate downstream effectors of acute inflammation, for example, by up-regulating the expression of inducible nitric oxide synthase, which results in an increased release of NO and its attendant effects on the micro-vascular resistance and capillary flow, or by augmenting neutrophil cytotoxic mechanisms by inducing the release of oxygen radicals and proteolytic enzymes [29, 30].

TNF-α results in activation of nearby immune cells and pro-inflammatory changes in the vascular endothelium promoting cellular migration into the periphery. When this modulation becomes a systemic one, the clinical signs and symptoms of hyper-inflammation (fever, hemodynamic instability, capillary leak between others) become evident [12]. Concomitant with the initial hyper-inflammatory response, there is a nearly simultaneous production of anti-inflammatory cytokines, including IL-10, that serve to balance the inflammatory state.

Both, the inflammatory and anti-inflammatory phase, are coordinated to defend the host against invasion by pathogens. However, an excessive or sustained inflammatory response, an inadequate anti-inflammatory response, or perhaps an uncoupling of these 2 phases may contribute to tissue damage and cell death [29].

3.1.4. Coagulation Disorders in Sepsis

The coagulopathy in critical illness is biologically complex. Besides activating the inflammatory system, pathogens also trigger early activation of the contact system (factor XII, prekallikrein, and high-molecular-weight kininogen) and the complement cascade [31]. Blood coagulation is initiated by activation of the extrinsic pathway and is amplified through the intrinsic pathway.

Activation of the extrinsic pathway is initiated through tissue factor expressed on the surface of endothelial cells and monocytes, a process that can be induced by microbial products such as endotoxin, inflammatory cytokines or by integrin crosslinking [32].

The shift toward a procoagulant state results in excessive thrombin generation, fibrin formation, and consumption of clotting factors. Fibrin deposits isolate the source of infection in an attempt to prevent its spread. The disseminated intravascular coagulation in critically ill patients impedes an adequate oxygen delivery to tissues and can induce further inflammatory injury. Within the mechanisms involved in the amplification of the inflammatory response is hypoxia, as a factor indirectly related while the thrombin receptor activation and clustering of tissue factor directly stimulate the expression of multiple pro-inflammatory cytokine genes through the activation of nuclear transcription factor NFκB [33].

3.1.5. Endothelial Cells

Endothelial cells are the predominant lining cells in close and intimate contact with blood. Under normal conditions, the endothelium is highly active serving a variety of functions: among others it mediates vasomotor tone, regulates cellular and nutrient trafficking, maintains blood fluidity, contributes to the local balance of pro-inflammatory and anti-inflammatory mediators, participates in the generation of new blood vessels, and undergoes programmed cell death [34].

In recent years, it has been recognized that endothelial cells produce important regulators of both coagulation and inflammation, thus playing a key role in the pathophysiology of sepsis.

In fact, such a dysfunction could explain most of the clinical manifestations and complications of sepsis. In pro-inflammatory states the endothelial cells undergo functional changes. These changes occur after making contact with cytokines and other pro-inflammatory mediators and are known as endothelial activation. The activated endothelium produces an array of inflammatory mediators. Clearly, the endothelium should not be thought of as an inactive cell layer constituting the vessel wall but rather as a director orchestrating the inflammatory cascade. The physiologic goal of these changes, which are meant to occur locally and not systemically, is to wall off an infectious process.

There is evidence of significant microcirculatory disorders in the course of septic shock. A decrease of the density of perfused capillaries with sluggish or stop-flow perfusion patterns has been observed in septic patients [35]. The microvasculature responds to inflammatory stimuli mainly through activation of the endothelium. On the front line is the expression of adhesion molecules which will enhance endothelial–leukocyte interaction. P-selectin and E-selectin, intercellular adhesion molecule-1, or vascular cellular adhesion molecule-1 are up-regulated by gene-transcription under regulation of transcription factors such as NF-κβ [36]. Interaction of the endothelial adhesion molecules E-selectin with its ligand ESL-1 on leukocytes initiated a second phase of activation after it upregulated the alpha M beta2 integrin on neutrophils, allowing the interaction with RBCs and platelets. These interactions will in turn induce the production of ROS by neutrophils and lead to impairment of the capillary blood flow and vascular damage [37].

Other NF-κβ-regulated genes in endothelial cells include plasminogen activator inhibitor-1, cyclooxygenase-2, and inducible nitric oxide synthase, all involved in the microcirculatory blood flow regulation [36].

Among the factors involved in the alteration of the microcirculation are recognized red blood cells and platelets aggregation, endothelial cell swelling, arteriole vasoconstriction, injury of the endothelium, and increased microvascular permeability with interstitial edema [38]. Activation of the coagulation cascade is another hallmark of sepsis with the inflammatory response activating tissue factor on endothelial cells and monocytes, intravascular thrombin generation, depletion of anticoagulant factors, and alterations of the fibrinolytic system [39]. Alteration of the flow at the microcirculation causes initially a mismatch between cell oxygen demand and supply [40]. Tissue hypoxia stimulates the inflammatory pathways exacerbating the inflammatory state characteristic of this pathology.

Upon stimulation with cytokines such as TNF-α or IL-1, endothelial cells may produce another type of NO-synthase: the inducible NO-synthase. It´s expression likely explains the drop in blood pressure in sepsis [41]. Despite large amount of NO produced by inducible nitric oxide synthase during sepsis, generation of superoxide by adhesive leukocytes can decrease endothelium-derived NO bioavailability and compromise microcirculatory blood flow by inducing vasoconstriction or loose of vasodilatation [42].

Several mechanisms may contribute to endothelial damage during sepsis. *In vitro* experiments have shown that activated neutrophils that adhere to the endothelial cells via adhesion molecules are well able to injure the endothelial cells by producing oxygen radicals and proteinases such as elastase [43]. Another mechanism that may cause severe damage to the endothelium is apoptosis induced by TNF-α [44]. Cytokine-activated natural killer cells or cytotoxic T lymphocytes, together known as lymphokines, can adhere to and injure the endothelium, resulting, for example, in increased permeability [45].

3.1.6. Complement Activation

Complement is a complex series of self-assembling plasma proteins which play a major role in host defense against infection and in inflammation.

All three pathways of complement activation (classical, lectin and alternative) converge to generate the C3 convertase and C5 convertase, resulting in biologically active split products of C3 and C5. The major purpose of the complement pathway is to remove or destroy antigen by direct cell killing (complement-mediated lysis), opsonization and complement-dependent phagocytosis, elicitation of an inflammatory response (smooth muscle spasm, release of vasoactive amines, increase of vascular permeability, stimulation of neutrophils and macrophages, etc.), and stimulation of the immune response (such as antigen presentation, T-cell activation, B-cell activation, antibody responses and immunologic memory) [46].

C3b is known to be a vital opsonic product that coats bacteria and other microbes, resulting in uptake by phagocytic cells (neutrophils and macrophages), followed by oxygen-dependent intracellular killing of bacteria [47]. The C5a fragment of the complement is implicated as a particularly potent mediator of the inflammatory process, reacting with high affinity receptors on phagocytic cells, resulting in cell activation which causes generation of reactive oxygen species (O2•, H2O2, HO•) that are toxic to other cells, enzyme secretion from phagocytic cells, which results in tissue damage. C5a is highly chemotactic for phagocytic cells, especially neutrophils. Collectively, the outcome of C5a generation in vivo is induction of the acute inflammatory response characterized by increased vascular permeability and accumulation and activation of neutrophils and tissue macrophages [48].

3.2. Immunoparalysis

Almost concurrently with the initial hyper-inflammatory response, compensatory mechanisms play a role and shut down the immune system inflammatory response, often through the induction of anti-inflammatory cytokines. This phenomenon is referred to as the "compensatory anti-inflammatory response syndrome" (CARS) [12]. This period of transient immune suppression helps to counterbalance the inflammatory state avoiding a significant end-organ damage and death in a subset of patients [29].

The immunoparalysis represents a persistently severe form of CARS, which is associated with an increased frequency of nosocomial infections and mortality in sepsis. The immunoparalysis is characterized by a marked deterioration in the innate immune function, now recognized as a predictor of morbidity and mortality for children and adults [49, 50]. Clinical research in adults and children with septic shock and MODS have shown that survivors retain the ability to assemble and maintain an innate immune response, with expression of proinflammatory genes [51, 52].

The underlying mechanisms of immunoparalysis are poorly understood. Possible mechanisms responsible include inhibition of the proinflammatory transcription factor NFkB, through alteration of its subunit composition [53], up-regulation of its inhibitor IκBa [54], up-regulation of the NFκB pathway inhibitor IRAK-M, or impairment of TLR4 signaling [55].

This dysfunction is related to a reduction in the monocyte antigen presenting capacity, internalization of cell-surface HLA-DR molecules in normal human monocytes with co-incubation with serum from septic patients [50]. Fumeaux and colleagues [56] demonstrated internalization of cell-surface HLA-DR molecules in normal human monocytes with co-incubation with serum from septic patients. On the other hand, steroids may also play a role in the development or perpetuation of immunoparalysis. Le Tulzo et al [57] found an association between high levels of circulating cortisol and a reduction in monocyte HLA-DR expression in 48 septic patients on day 6 of illness. Others have shown that the administration of methylprednisolone in the setting of a cardiopulmonary bypass procedure resulted in an exacerbation of innate immunosuppression higher than that seen with a bypass alone [58].

In critically ill adults and children lymphocyte apoptosis and lymphopenia are common in ICU non-survivors. Programmed cell death (apoptosis) is a prominent feature in human and experimental sepsis, especially as it involves the lymphoid system with resulting immunoparalysis. In addition, sepsis is associated with strong activation of the complement system, resulting in the generation of the powerful anaphylatoxin, C5a, as well as the up-regulation of the C5a receptor (C5aR) in a variety of different organs.

The consequences of C5a interactions with C5aR can be directly linked to apoptosis of thymocytes and adrenal medullary cells in an experimental model after cecal ligation and puncture-induced sepsis in rodents, resulting in signaling paralysis of blood neutrophils and loss of their innate immune functions (phagocytosis, chemotaxis, respiratory burst), together with apoptosis of thymocytes [48, 59].

The temporal and causal relationship between the innate and adaptive immune dysfunction in critical illness remains incompletely understood.

During the past few decades several assays related to the measurement of immune responsiveness have been reported. Volk and colleagues have defined immunoparalysis in adults as prolonged monocyte HLA-DR expression below 30%, or reduction in whole blood ex vivo LPS-induced TNF-α response to 200 pg/mL for more than 5 days [60], while Hall and cols recently presented similar findings in children who present with a variety of secondary MODS [61].

4. Pathophysiology of Septic Shock

Septic shock is defined in adults as hypotension refractory to fluid resuscitation. In initial phases in children this may be absent. Its evolution is characterized by progressive hemodynamic and cardiovascular instability. At an early stage clinical signs include tachicardia, full bounding pulses, flushed skin, irritability or drowsiness, narrowed differential blood pressure and in a later stage hypotension, oliguria, clammy skin, low volume pulses, and the patients overall appear to be unstable in their basic condition.

During the initial stages of septic shock, reflex neurohumoral responses occur, that attempt to sustain perfusion by maintaining cardiac output and blood pressure. Activation of baroreceptor reflexes, release of catecholamines, activation of renin-angiotensin, release of antidiuretic hormone, and generalized sympathetic stimulation are included.

Two fundamental pathogenic processes contribute to the clinical manifestations of septic shock: cardiovascular dysfunction due to the combined effects of myocardial depression and systemic vasodilatation and inflammatory tissue damage. The concept of depressed myocardial function in sepsis emerged from studies performed with radionuclide ventriculograms in septic shock patients. Human septic myocardial depression is characterized by reversible biventricular dilatation, increased end diastolic volume, decreased ejection fraction, and decreased response to fluid resuscitation and catecholamine stimulation, despite a normal total cardiac output while compensated [62, 63].

Initial impaired left ventricular systolic and diastolic dysfunction may also be observed with similar alterations in right ventricular function. Different studies have shown that the decrease in EF is reversible with full functional recovery of cardiac function in survivors at 7–10 days after the episode. The presence of a cardiovascular dysfunction in adult sepsis is associated with a significantly increased mortality rate to 70% to 90% compared with 20% in septic patients without cardiovascular impairment. This has been corroborated with echocardiographies in other studies [64]. In this context, myocardial dysfunction was once considered as a preterminal event [63].

Cardiac depression during sepsis is probably multifactorial and involves multiple pathways. The first proposed mechanism is that of global ischemia, however studies in animals and humans showed a high coronary blood flow and diminished coronary artery–coronary sinus oxygen difference [65, 66]. Coronary sinus blood studies in patients with septic shock have also demonstrated increased lactate extraction, decreased free fatty acid extraction, and decreased glucose uptake. Furthermore, studies in animal models of sepsis have demonstrated the presence of normal high-energy phosphate levels in the myocardium. The absence of significant myocardial cell death and the reversible nature of myocardial dysfunction in sepsis support a prominent role for functional rather than anatomical abnormalities in the underlying pathophysiology mechanisms [67-69]. It has also been proposed that myocardial dysfunction in sepsis may reflect hibernating myocardium [70]. Furthermore, evidence of widespread myocardial necrosis has not been found in patients with septic shock. There is no evidence supporting global ischemia as an underlying cause of myocardial dysfunction in sepsis. Parrillo et al using rat cardiac myocytes exposed to serum from septic patients achieved correlating clinical severity quantitatively linked the clinical degree of septic myocardial dysfunction with the decrease in extent and velocity of myocyte shortening. These effects were not seen when serum from convalescent patients whose cardiac function had returned to normal was applied or when serum was obtained from other critically ill nonseptic patients [71]. From these studies the concept of circulating myocardial depressant factor was proposed for sepsis which could be responsible for this phenomenon. Subsequent studies identified cytokines such as TNF-α, IL-1b, and IL-6 as circulating causative factors of myocardial depression in sepsis. On the other hand Mink et al [72] demonstrated that lysozyme c, a bacteriolytic agent believed to originate mainly from disintegrating neutrophilic granulocytes and monocytes, mediates cardiodepressive effects during Escherichia coli sepsis. Early studies suggest a potential role for endothelin-1 (ET-1) in the development of sepsis-induced myocardial depression [73].

Among the factors involved in the myocardial depression of sepsis are nitric oxide, mitochondrial dysfunction, calcium, prostanoids such as thromboxane and prostacyclin and apoptosis. The most promising candidate is NO, which is produced in excessive amounts during sepsis as the consequence of induced expression of NOS in the myocardium. Effects of nitric oxide relevant to sepsis-induced myocardial dysfunction include vasodilation, the depression of mitochondrial respiration, and further release of pro-inflammatory cytokines. The NO also exerts its action indirectly through free radical peroxynitrite formed from NO and superoxide [74]. The description of the mechanisms involved in myocardial depression by the action of NO are beyond the scope of this chapter. In chapter 13 (myocardial dysfunction), these mechanisms are described, while in chapter 6 (multiorgan failure) the general mechanisms of mitochondrial dysfunction are described, along with cellular and organic dysfunction associated with inflammation and oxidative stress.

Calcium is thought to play an important role in the development of sepsis-induced myocardial depression. Current evidence suggests reductions in cytosolic calcium levels during sepsis leading to reduced contractility. Calcium signaling and metabolism is linked to mitochondrial function, which is also altered in sepsis.

Elevated levels of prostanoids such as thromboxane and prostacyclin, which have the potential to alter coronary autoregulation, coronary endothelial function, and intracoronary leukocyte activation, have been demonstrated in septic patients [75]. Unfortunately, studies in both septic patients and experimental animals have failed to demonstrate survival improvement.

Early septic shock is characterized by circulatory abnormalities that usually relate to intravascular volume depletion and vasodilation. As mentioned in the previous section of this chapter the normal function of the endothelium is to regulate the microcirculation by dictating the tonus of the arterioles, regulation of blood pressure (via their effects on arterioles), and regulation of vascular permeability. This function is performed through vasoactive compounds that regulate the tonus of the arterioles and hence have a great influence on blood pressure. These compounds include the vasodilating NO and prostacyclin and the vasoconstricting endothelins [76]. Inflammatory mediators strongly stimulate endothelial production of these molecules.

The production of NO can be regulated by two different mechanisms: constitutive NO-synthase, an enzyme that produces NO in a calcium-dependent manner, and inducible NO-synthase activated by the effect of proinflammatory cytokines, such as TNF-α or IL-1.This enzyme produces large quantities of NO in a calcium-independent manner. Expression of inducible NO synthase likely explains the drop in blood pressure in sepsis [77]. It is noticeable also that NO and prostacyclin also are potent inhibitors of platelet aggregation.

Early sepsis and septic shock are characterized by circulatory abnormalities that usually relate to intravascular volume depletion and vasodilation. This causes an oxygen supply-demand imbalance in various organ beds often reversed by fluid resuscitation when on-time. Insufficiently resuscitated animal models are therefore likely to evidence reduced cardiac performance [78]. Thus, in the early phase of shock, adequate volume replacement has proved to be far more effective for a successful resuscitation, than in later stages of shock, when the compensatory mechanisms have been overwhelmed. Aggressive volume administration as indicated by international guidelines without taking into account the myocardial compromise/depression may precipitate an additional cardiorespiratory dysfunction with pulmonary edema secondary to myocardial failure and a relative fluid overload for their underlying disease. Maitland et al in a study in critically ill children with impaired perfusion found that patients who received volume of 20 to 40 ml per kg according to guidelines presented significantly increased 48-hour mortality [79].

Conclusions and Future Goals

Sepsis and septic shock continue to be responsible for a considerable number of deaths in all age groups around the world. This is despite of advances in the comprehension of the underlying pathophysiologic mechanisms due to extensive research in the field. The aim of the research is to modify or stop the pathophysiologic mechanisms involved in the inflammatory and metabolic disorders to prevent the cellular damage responsible for MODS and deaths. Oxidative stress as part of the pathophysiological process, while extensively studied in biological research, has not just reached clinical settings with a successful therapeutic approach. Since the generation of ROS and RNS, and oxidative stress as a consequence of an imbalance of the oxidative –antioxidative response, play an important role in the pathophysiology of many diseases including sepsis and septic shock, enhancing the knowledge of clinicians about this topic and stimulating future research in the field must continue to be a goal.

References

[1] Angus DC, Wax RS. Epidemiology of sepsis: an update. *Crit. Care Med.* 2001; 29:S109-S116.

[2] Khilnani P, Sarma D, Zimmerman J. Epidemiology and peculiarities of pediatric multiple organ dysfunction syndrome in New Delhi, India. *Intensive Care Med.* 2006; 32:1856-1862.

[3] Brierley J, Carcillo JA, Choong K, Cornell T, Decaen A, Deymann A, Doctor A, Davis A, Duff J, Dugas MA, Duncan A, Evans B, Feldman J, Felmet K, Fisher G, Frankel L, Jeffries H, Greenwald B, Gutierrez J, Hall M, Han YY, Hanson J, Hazelzet J, Hernan L, Kiff J, Kissoon N, Kon A, Irazuzta J, Lin J, Lorts A, Mariscalco M, Mehta R, Nadel S, Nguyen T, Nicholson C, Peters M, Okhuysen-Cawley R, Poulton T, Relves M, Rodriguez A, Rozenfeld R, Schnitzler E, Shanley T, Kache S, Skippen P, Torres A, von Dessauer B, Weingarten J, Yeh T, Zaritsky A, Stojadinovic B, Zimmerman J, Zuckerberg A. Clinical practice parameters for hemodynamic support of pediatric and neonatal septic shock: 2007 update from American College of Critical Care Medicine. *Crit. Care Med.* 2009; 37:666-688.

[4] Watson RS, Carcillo JA, Linde-Zwirble WT, Clermont G, Lidicker J, Angus DC. The epidemiology of severe sepsis in children in the United States. *Am. J. Respir. Crit. Care Med.* 2003; 167:695-170.

[5] Bryce J, Boschi-Pinto C, Shibuya K, Black RE, WHO Child Health Epidemiology Reference Group. WHO estimates of the causes of death in children. *Lancet.* 2005; 365:1147-1152.

[6] American college of chest physicians/society of critical care medicine consensus conference: definitions for sepsis and organ failure and guidelines for the use of innovative therapies in sepsis. *Crit. Care Med.* 1992; 20:864-874.

[7] Bone RC, Balk RA, Cerra FB, Dellinger RP, Fein AM, Knaus WA, Schein RM, Sibbald WJ. Definitions for sepsis and organ failure and guidelines for the use of innovative therapies in sepsis. The ACCP/SCCM Consensus Conference Committee. American College of Chest Physicians/Society of Critical Care Medicine. *Chest.* 1992; 101:1644-1655.

[8] van der Poll T, Opal SM. Host-pathogen interactions in sepsis. *Lancet Infect. Dis.* 2008; 8:32-43.

[9] Brown KA, Brain SD, Pearson JD, Edgeworth JD, Lewis SM, Treacher DF. Neutrophils in development of multiple organ failure in sepsis. *Lancet.* 2006; 368:157-169.

[10] Bone RC. Sir Isaac Newton, sepsis, SIRS, and CARS. *Crit. Care Med.* 1996; 24:1125-1128.

[11] Janeway CA Jr, Medzhitov R. *Annu. Rev. Immunol.* 2002; 20:197-216.

[12] Frazier WJ, Hall MW. Immunoparalysis and adverse outcomes from critical illness. *Pediatr. Clin. North Am.* 2008; 55:647-668.

[13] Janeway CA, Medzhitov R. Introduction: The role of innate immunity in the adaptive immune response. *Semin. Immunol.* 1998; 10:349-350.

[14] Bianchi ME. DAMPs, PAMPs and alarmins: all we need to know about danger. *J. Leukoc. Biol.* 2007; 81:1-5.

[15] Akira S, Uematsu S, Takeuchi O. Pathogen recognition and innate immunity. *Cell.* 2006; 124:783-801.

[16] Poltorak A, Ricciardi-Castagnoli P, Citterio S, Beutler B. Physical contact between lipopoly-saccharide and Toll-like receptor 4 revealed by genetic complementation. *Proc. Nat. Acad. Sci. US.* 2000; 97:2163-2167.

[17] Schwandner R, Dziarski R, Wesche H, Rothe M, Kirschning CJ. Peptidoglycan- and lipoteichoic acid-induced cell activation is mediated by Toll-like receptor 2. *J. Biol. Chem.* 1999; 274:17406-17409.

[18] Mollen KP, Anand RJ, Tsung A, Prince JM, Levy RM, Billiar TR. Emerging paradigm: Toll-like receptor 4-sentinel for the detection of tissue damage. *Shock.* 2006; 26:430-437.

[19] Imai Y, Kuba K, Neely GG, Yaghubian-Malhami R, Perkmann T, van Loo G, Ermolaeva M, Veldhuizen R, Leung YH, Wang H, Liu H, Sun Y, Pasparakis M, Kopf M, Mech C, Bavari S, Peiris JS, Slutsky AS, Akira S, Hultqvist M, Holmdahl R, Nicholls J, Jiang C, Binder CJ, Penninger JM. Identification of oxidative stress and Toll-like receptor 4 signaling as a key pathway of acute lung injury. *Cell.* 2008; 133:235-249.

[20] Zingarelli B, Sheehan M, Wong HR. Nuclear factor-□B as a therapeutic target in critical care medicine. *Crit Care Med. 2003*; 31:S105-S111.

[21] Zingarelli B. Nuclear factor-kappaB. *Crit. Care Med.* 2005; 33:414-416.

[22] Caamaño J, Hunter CA. NF-kappaB family of transcription factors: central regulators of innate and adaptive immune functions. *Clin. Microbiol. Rev.* 2002; 15:414-429.

[23] Seely AJ, Pascual JL, Christou NV. Science review: Cell membrane expression (connectivity) regulates neutrophil delivery, function and clearance. *Crit. Care.* 2003; 7:291-307.

[24] Brown KA, Brain SD, Pearson JD, Edgeworth JD, Lewis SM, Treacher DF. Neutrophils in development of multiple organ failure in sepsis. *Lancet.* 2006; 368:157-169.

[25] Bokoch GM. Chemoattractant signaling and leukocyte activation. *Blood.* 1995; 86:1649-1660.

[26] Barreiro O, Sanchez – Madrid F. Signals emanating from leukocyte-endothelium interactions during inflammation. *An. R.Acad. Farm.* 2008; 74:1-16.

[27] Brown KA, Brain SD, Pearson JD, Edgeworth JD, Lewis SM, Treacher DF. Neutrophils in development of multiple organ failure in sepsis. *Lancet.* 2006; 368: 157-169.

[28] Martins PS, Kalla EG, Neto MC, Dalboni MA, Blecher S, Salamao R. Upregulation of reactive oxygen species generation and phagocytosis and an increased apoptosis in human neutrophils during severe sepsis and septic shock. *Shock.* 2003; 20:208-212.

[29] Muenzer JT, Davis CG, Chang K, Schmidt RE, Dunne WM, Coopersmith CM, Hotchkiss RS. Characterization and Modulation of the Immunosuppressive Phase of Sepsis. *Infect. Immun.* 2010; 78:1582-1592.

[30] Mallick AA, Ishizaka A, Stephens KE, Hatherill JR, Tazelaar HD, Raffin TA. Multiple organ damage caused by tumor necrosis factor and prevented by prior neutrophil depletion. *Chest.* 1989; 95:1114-1120.

[31] Aird WC. Vascular bed-specific hemostasis: role of endothelium in sepsis pathogenesis. *Crit. Care Med.* 2001; 29:S28-S35.

[32] Esmon CT. Possible involvement of cytokines in diffuse intravascular coagulation and thrombosis. *Baillieres Best Pract Res Clin Haematol.* 2000; 12:343-359.

[33] McGilvray ID, Rotstein OD. Signaling pathways of tissue factor expression in monocytes and macrophages. *Sepsis.* 1999; 3:93-101.

[34] Cines DB, Pollak ES, Buck CA, Loscalzo J, Zimmerman GA, McEver RP, Pober JS, Wick TM, Konkle BA, Schwartz BS, Barnathan ES, McCrae KR, Hug BA, Schmidt AM, Stern DM. Endothelial cells in physiology and in the pathophysiology of vascular disorders. *Blood.* 1998; 91:3527-3561.

[35] Boerma EC, van der Voort PH, Spronk PE, Ince C. Relationship between sublingual and intestinal microcirculatory perfusion in patients with abdominal sepsis. *Crit. Care Med.* 2007; 35:1055-1060.

[36] De Martin R, Hoeth M, Hofer-Warbinek R, Schmid JA. The transcription factor NF-kappa B and the regulation of vascular cell function. *Arterioscler. Thromb. Vasc. Biol.* 2000; 20:E83-E88.

[37] Tyml K, Li F, Wilson JX. Septic impairment of capillary blood flow requires nicotinamide adenine dinucleotide phosphate oxidase but not nitric oxide synthase and is rapidly reversed by ascorbate through an endothelial nitric oxide synthase-dependent mechanism. *Crit. Care Med.* 2008; 36:2355-2362.

[38] Balestra GM, Legrand M, Ince C. Microcirculation and mitochondria in sepsis: getting out of breath. *Curr. Opin. Anaesthesiol.* 2009; 22:184-190.

[39] Opal SM, Garber GE, LaRosa SP, Maki DG, Freebairn RC, Kinasewitz GT, Dhainaut JF, Yan SB, Williams MD, Graham DE, Nelson DR, Levy H, Bernard GR. Systemic host responses in severe sepsis analyzed by causative microorganism and treatment effects of drotrecogin alfa (activated). *Clin. Infect. Dis.* 2003; 37:50-58.

[40] Ince C, Sinaasappel M. Microcirculatory oxygenation and shunting in sepsis and shock. *Crit Care Med.* 1999; 27:1369-1377.

[41] Petros A, Bennett D, Vallance P. Effect of nitric oxide synthase inhibitors on hypotension in patients with septic shock. *Lancet.* 1991; 338:1557-1558.

[42] Marshall J. Inflammation, coagulopathy, and the pathogenesis of multiple organ dysfunction syndrome. *Crit. Care Med.* 2001; 29:S99-S106.

[43] Harlan JM. Leukocyte-endothelial interactions. *Blood.* 1985; 65:513-525.

[44] Deshpande SS, Angkeow P, Huang J, Ozaki M, Irani K. Rac1 inhibits TNF-alpha-induced endothelial cell apoptosis: dual regulation by reactive oxygen species. *FASEB J.* 2000; 14:1705-1714.

[45] Damle NK, Doyle LV, Bender JR, Bradley EC. Interleukin 2-activated human lymphocytes exhibit enhanced adhesion to normal vascular endothelial cells and cause their lysis. *J. Immunol.* 1987; 138:1779-1785.

[46] Haeney MR. The role of the complement cascade in sepsis. *J Antimicrob Chemother.* 1998; 41 (Suppl A):41-46.

[47] Walport MJ. Complement. First of two parts. *N. Engl. J. Med.* 2001; 344:1058-1066.

[48] Ward PA. Sepsis, apoptosis and complement. *Biochem. Pharmacol.* 2008; 76:1383-1388.

[49] Ho YP, Sheen IS, Chiu CT, Wu CS, Lin CY. A strong association between down-regulation of HLA-DR expression and the late mortality in patients with severe acute pancreatitis. *Am. J. Gastroenterol.* 2006; 101:1117-1124.

[50] Monneret G, Lepape A, Voirin N, Bohe J, Venet F, Debard AL, Thizy H, Bienvenu J, Gueyffier F, Vanhems P. Persisting low monocyte human leukocyte antigen-DR expression predicts mortality in septic shock. *Intensive Care Med.* 2006; 32:1175-1183.

[51] Pachot A, Lepape A, Vey S, Bienvenu J, Mougin B, Monneret G. Systemic transcriptional analysis in survivor and nonsurvivor septic shock patients: a preliminary study. *Immunol. Lett.* 2006; 106:63-71.

[52] Hall MW, Gavrilin MA, Knatz NL, Duncan MD, Fernandez SA, Wewers MD. Monocyte mRNA phenotype and adverse outcomes from pediatric multiple organ dysfunction syndrome. *Pediatr. Res.* 2007; 62:597-603.

[53] Bohuslav J, Kravchenko VV, Parry GC, Erlich JH, Gerondakis S, Mackman N, Ulevitch RJ. Regulation of an essential innate immune response by the p50 subunit of NF-kappaB. *J. Clin. Invest.* 1998; 102:1645-1652.

[54] Wahlstrom K, Bellingham J, Rodriguez JL, West MA. Inhibitory kappaB alpha control of nuclear factor-kappaB is dysregulated in endotoxin tolerant macrophages. *Shock.* 1999; 11:242-247.

[55] Medvedev AE, Lentschat A, Wahl LM, Golenbock DT, Vogel SN. Dysregulation of LPS-induced Toll-like receptor 4-MyD88 complex formation and IL-1 receptor-associated kinase 1 activation in endotoxin-tolerant cells. *J. Immunol.* 2002; 169:5209-5216.

[56] Fumeaux T, Pugin J. Role of interleukin-10 in the intracellular sequestration of human leukocyte antigen-DR in monocytes during septic shock. *Am. J. Respir. Crit. Care Med.* 2002; 166:1475-1482.

[57] Le Tulzo Y, Pangault C, Amiot L, Guilloux V, Tribut O, Arvieux C, Camus C, Fauchet R, Thomas R, Drénou B. Monocyte human leukocyte antigen-DR transcriptional downregulation by cortisol during septic shock. *Am. J. Respir. Crit. Care Med.* 2004; 169:1144-1151.

[58] Volk T, Schmutzler M, Engelhardt L, Döcke WD, Volk HD, Konertz W, Kox WJ. Influence of aminosteroid and glucocorticoid treatment on inflammation and immune function during cardiopulmonary bypass. *Crit. Care Med.* 2001; 29:2137-2142.

[59] Hotchkiss RS, Tinsley KW, Swanson PE, Chang KC, Cobb JP, Buchman TG, Korsmeyer SJ, Karl IE. Prevention of lymphocyte cell death in sepsis improves survival in mice. *Proc. Natl. Acad. Sci. U S A.* 1999; 96:14541-14546.

[60] Volk HD, Reinke P, Docke WD. Clinical aspects: from systemic inflammation to 'immunoparalysis'. *Chem. Immunol.* 2000; 74:162-177.

[61] Hall MW, Knatz NL, Vetterly C, Tomarello S, Wewers MD, Volk HD, Carcillo JA. Immunoparalysis and nosocomial infection in children with multiple organ dysfunction syndrome. *Intensive Care Med.* 2011; 37:525-532.

[62] Calvin JE, Driedger AA, Sibbald WJ. An assessment of myocardial function in human sepsis utilizing ECG gated cardiac scintigraphy. *Chest.* 1981; 80:579-586.

[63] Parker MM, Shelhamer JH, Bacharach SL, Green MV, Natanson C, Frederick TM, Damske BA, Parrillo JE. Profound but reversible myocardial depression in patients with septic shock. *Ann. Intern. Med.* 1984; 100:483-490.

[64] Charpentier J, Luyt CE, Fulla Y, Vinsonneau C, Cariou A, Grabar S, Dhainaut JF, Mira JP, Chiche JD. Brain natriuretic peptide: A marker of myocardial dysfunction and prognosis during severe sepsis. *Crit. Care Med.* 2004; 32:660-665.

[65] Cunnion RE, Schaer GL, Parker MM, Natanson C, Parrillo JE. The coronary circulation in human septic shock. *Circulation.* 1986; 73:637-644.

[66] Herbertson MJ, Werner HA, Russell JA, Iversen K, Walley KR. Myocardial oxygen extraction ratio is decreased during endotoxemia in pigs. *J. Appl. Physiol.* 1995; 79:479-486.

[67] Dhainaut JF, Huyghebaert MF, Monsallier JF, Lefevre G, Dall'Ava- Santucci J, Brunet F, Villemant D, Carli A, Raichvarg D. Coronary hemodynamics and myocardial metabolism of lactate, free fatty acids, glucose, and ketones in patients with septic shock. *Circulation.* 1987; 75:533-541.

[68] Solomon MA, Correa R, Alexander HR, Koev LA, Cobb JP, Kim DK, Roberts WC, Quezado ZM, Scholz TD, Cunnion RE, Hoffman WD, Bacher J, Yatsiv I, Natanson C. Myocardial energy metabolism and morphology in a canine model of sepsis. *Am. J. Physiol.* 1994; 266:H757-H768.

[69] Van Lambalgen AA, van Kraats AA, Mulder MF, Teerlink T, van den Bos GC. High-energy phosphates in heart, liver, kidney, and skeletal muscle of endotoxemic rats. *Am J Physiol.* 1994; 266:H1581-H1587.

[70] Levy RJ, Piel DA, Acton PD, Zhou R, Ferrari VA, Karp JS, Deutschman CS. Evidence of myocardial hibernation in the septic heart. *Crit. Care Med.* 2005; 33:2752-2756.

[71] Parrillo JE, Burch C, Shelhamer JH, Parker MM, Natanson C, Schuette W. A circulating myocardial depressant substance in humans with septic shock: septic shock patients with a reduced ejection fraction have a circulating factor that depresses in vitro myocardial cell performance. *J. Clin. Invest.* 1985; 76:1539-1553.

[72] Mink SN, Jacobs H, Duke K, Bose D, Cheng ZQ, Light RB. N, N', N'' - triacetylglucosamine, an inhibitor of lysozyme, prevents myocardial depression in Escherichia coli sepsis in dogs. *Crit. Care Med.* 2004; 32:184-193.

[73] Konrad D, Oldner A, Rossi P, Wanecek M, Rudehill A, Weitzberg E. Differentiated and dose-related cardiovascular effects of a dual endothelin receptor antagonist in endotoxin shock. *Crit. Care Med.* 2004; 32:1192-1199.

[74] Massion PB, Feron O, Dessy C, Balligand JL. Nitric oxide and cardiac function: ten years after, and continuing. *Circ Res.* 2003; 93:388-398.

[75] Reines HD, Halushka PV, Cook JA, Wise WC, Rambo W. Plasma thromboxane concentrations are raised in patients dying with septic shock. *Lancet.* 1982; 2:174-175.

[76] Cines DB, Pollak ES, Buck CA, Loscalzo J, Zimmerman GA, McEver RP, Pober JS, Wick TM, Konkle BA, Schwartz BS, Barnathan ES, McCrae KR, Hug BA, Schmidt AM, Stern DM. Endothelial cells in physiology and in the pathophysiology of vascular disorders. *Blood.* 1998; 91:3527-3561.

[77] Gross SS, Kilbourn RG, Griffith OW. NO in septic shock: Good, bad or ugly? Learning from iNOS knockouts. *Trends Microbiol.* 1996; 4:47-49.

[78] Chagnon F, Bentourkia Mh, Lecomte R, Lessard M, Lesur O. Endotoxin-induced heart dysfunction in rats: Assessment of myocardial perfusion and permeability and the role of fluid resuscitation. *Crit. Care Med.* 2006; 34:127-133.

[79] Maitland K, Kiguli S, Opoka RO, Engoru C, Olupot-Olupot P, Akech SO, Nyeko R, Mtove G, Reyburn H, Lang T, Brent B, Evans JA, Tibenderana JK, Crawley J, Russell EC, Levin M, Babiker AG, Gibb DM; FEAST Trial Group. Mortality after Fluid Bolus in African Children with Severe Infection. *N. Engl. J. Med.* 2011; 364:2483-2495.

In: Oxidative Stress and the Critically Ill Patient
Editors: Ramón Rodrigo and Bettina von Dessauer
ISBN: 978-1-62081-576-2

Chapter III

INFLAMMATION

Rodrigo Castillo
Pathophysiology Program, Institute of Biomedical Sciences
Faculty of Medicine, University of Chile, Chile

ABSTRACT

Sepsis occurs with an exacerbated inflammatory response that damages tissues and impairs bioenergetic processes. Nitric oxide and cytokines constitute the molecular markers and the intracellular messengers of inflammatory conditions that are derived from the activation of the NF-kappaB pathway and the transcription of proinflammatory genes. The current hypothesis for the molecular mechanism that links systemic and cellular inflammation is based on the enhanced nitric oxide (NO) production by mitochondrial NOS that lead to excessive peroxynitrite production and protein nitration in the mitochondrial matrix, which causes mitochondrial dysfunction and organ failure. The mechanism of the development and progression of sepsis and multi-organ failure involves inflammation and ROS production.

This chapter presents the mediators and mechanisms that are associated with the condition or the pro-inflammatory "status" that can be found in a critically ill patient.

ABBREVIATIONS

TLR:	Toll-like receptors
PRR:	Pattern-recognition receptors
HMGB1:	High-mobility-group-box-1
LT:	Leukotriene
LX:	Lipoxin
NO:	Nitric oxide
TNF-α:	Tumor necrosis factor –alpha

COX:	Cyclooxygenase
NF-κB:	Nuclear factor-kappaB
iNOS:	Inducible nitric oxide
AA:	Arachidonic acids
EPA:	Eicosapentaenoic acids
DHA:	Docosaexaenoic acids
NOS:	Nitric oxide synthase
ALI:	acute lung injury
PAMPs:	Pathogen-associated molecular patterns
GSH:	Glutathione
Trx:	Thioredoxin
APACHE:	Acute Physiology and Chronic Health Evaluation
STAT:	Signal transducers and activators of transcription
CLP:	Cecal ligation and puncture procedure
PCT:	Procalcitonin
CRP:	C-reactive protein
LBP:	Lipopolysaccharide binding protein
MMPs:	Matrix metalloproteinases
TIMPs:	inhibitors of matrix-metalloproteinases

2. Introduction

Although the systemic inflammatory response syndrome predominates in early sepsis, the compensatory anti-inflammatory response syndrome causes immunosuppression associated with late mortality. Toll-like receptors (TLR), the inflammasomes and other pattern-recognition receptors (PRR) initiate the host response after the recognition of invading pathogens and endogenous signals of danger. The TLR-regulated pro-inflammatory cytokines macrophage migration inhibitory factor and high-mobility-group-box-1 (HMGB1) protein are promising treatment targets. Controversy on intensive insulin therapy, steroids, and activated protein C in sepsis has led to a re-evaluation of these immunomodulatory strategies. Interestingly, the anticoagulant protein C also exerts cytoprotective effects by neutralizing extracellular DNA. Endotoxin removal devices, TLR4-inhibitors, and restoration of sepsis-induced immunosuppression are other strategies being evaluated in septic patients.

3. Current Concepts of the Inflammatory Response

3.1. Cellular Mediators

Mononuclear cells play a central role in the inflammatory response due to the releasing of proinflammatory cytokines and other products, such as lipid mediators (i.e., tissue factors, prostaglandins, and platelet activating factors) and nitric oxide. The primary aim of this mediator release is the enhancement of leukocyte migration to the infective site to combat the infecting organism and to limit the area of infection. This release also involves endothelial activation, increased neutrophil migration, and neutrophil-mediated killing [1]. The release of tissue factors determines the activation of the coagulation cascade and, in severe sepsis, can lead to the development of a consumptive coagulopathy. The activation of the complement system is associated with the production of complement C5a, which enhances the production of cytokines and chemokines in sepsis. The release of nitric oxide produces local vasodilatation, which may lead to hypotension. This mediator is secreted during the transition of the inflammatory response to infection and reflects the overactive status of the immune response. The effector phagocytic cells of the immune system (i.e., neutrophils and macrophages) respond to these mediators by releasing granular enzymes and producing reactive oxygen species, such as H_2O_2, which facilitate the elimination of the infecting bacteria. Products such as H_2O_2 are capable of causing tissue damage, which ultimately leads to increased vascular permeability and organ injury. This phase of the proinflammatory response can lead to refractory hypotension, endothelial leakage with severe edema, and, ultimately, organ failure and death. In later stages of sepsis, antiinflammatory mediators, such as interleukin (IL)-10, transforming growth factor-b, and IL-13, are produced, which lead to the suppression of the production of many proinflammatory mediators. This suppression, in turn, often leads to the suppression of various functions of the immune system, especially those of neutrophils, which results in a depressed host defense system [2].

3.1.1. Neutrophils

Neutrophils have been viewed as the final effector cells of the acute inflammatory response and have a primary role in the clearance of extracellular pathogens. However, recent evidence has extended the functions of these cells. The newly discovered repertoire of effector molecules in the neutrophil armamentarium includes a broad array of cytokines, extracellular traps and effector molecules of the humoral arm of the innate immune system. In addition, neutrophils are involved in the activation, regulation and effector functions of innate and adaptive immune cells [3].

Neutrophils are generally considered passive components of the resolution process of inflammation, and the fate of these cells is death followed by rapid and silent elimination. However, recent evidence suggests that neutrophils are also involved in the active induction of the resolution through the production of pro-resolving lipid mediators.

During the late, final phases of the acute inflammatory response, neutrophils switch their eicosanoid biosynthesis from leukotriene B4 (LTB4) to lipoxin A4 (LXA4), which can inhibit neutrophil recruitment through its interaction with some superficial receptors (e.g., G protein-coupled receptor) [4]. Neutrophils can also contribute to the biosynthesis of resolvins (such as resolvins E1, E2, D1 and D2) and protectin D1, which are derived from omega-3 essential polyunsaturated fatty acids. These pro-resolving lipid mediators and the recently described macrophage-derived compound, maresin 1, inhibit neutrophil transendothelial migration and tissue infiltration [5].

3.1.2. Macrophages

The macrophage is a prominent inflammatory cell that is found in wounds, but the role of these cells in the healing process remains incompletely understood. Macrophages have many functions in wounds, which include host defense, the promotion and resolution of inflammation, the removal of apoptotic cells, and the support of cell proliferation and tissue restoration following injury.

Recent studies suggest that macrophages exist in several different phenotypic states within the healing wound and that the influence of these cells on each stage of repair varies with the specific phenotype. Although the macrophage is beneficial in contributing to the repair of normally healing wounds, this pleotropic cell type may promote excessive inflammation or fibrosis under certain circumstances.

Within three to five days after injury, macrophages are the most prominent cells in the healing tissue, and Lucas et al. [6] demonstrated that depletion of macrophages during the inflammatory phase resulted in a significant delay in wound repair in a mouse model. Macrophages are important for the clearance of senescent cells and debris within a wound, and, in the case of a pathogen that is spreading within the wound bed, macrophages can phagocytose these pathogens and present their antigens to T-cells. Macrophages that are involved in the clearance of cells in dead tissues apoptose. However, some macrophages survive and do not apoptose; these cells remain in the wound-bed area and exert other functions, including the stimulation of collagen production, angiogenesis and reepithelization. This change in functional activity appears to be initiated predominantly by the phagocytosis of apoptotic cells [7].

Moreover, it has recently been reported that macrophages can phenotypically convert from an M1 to an M2 phenotype [8], and a phenotype switch of bone-marrow-derived macrophages in an atherosclerosis model in apolipoprotein E KO mice due to environmental changes in cytokine expression has been clearly demonstrated. Macrophages play a pivotal role in the transition from the inflammatory to the proliferative phase of wound healing, where they coordinate and sustain wound-healing events.

3.1.3. Other Cells

It has been documented that trauma impairs the immune response and consequently predisposes the host to sepsis. The immunologic alterations that occur after trauma and the subsequent septic challenge require further investigation. Kupffer cells are specialized macrophages that line the hepatic sinusoids and represent 80% of the body's fixed macrophage population. Previously, Kupffer cells were shown to mediate the responses to endotoxins, burns, and sepsis [9], but these cells also produce important inflammatory mediators that include tumor necrosis factor (TNF-α), interleukin-1, prostaglandin E2, O_2 and nitric oxide (NO).

In addition, enhanced Kupffer cell numbers have been associated with major mortality after trauma because these cells exert a pro-inflammatory imbalance in the development of sepsis. Interestingly, Kupffer-cell depletion improved hepatic microcirculation after sepsis and sequential stress by reducing the hypercontractile response to vasoconstrictors such as endothelin-1.

Recent evidence has demonstrated that trauma causes little overt, imbalanced gene expression of the hepatic vasoactive mediators, and this change increases the susceptibility of the liver to subsequent septic injury.

In particular, when trauma is combined with a septic insult, Kupffer cells develop exaggerated TNF-α and COX-2 expression levels and up-regulated expression of vasodilators but not of vasoconstrictors. These findings suggest that the activation of Kupffer cells might contribute to hepatic microvascular dysfunction after a sequential stress [10].

3.2. Cytokines, Chemokines and Lipid Mediators

Cytokines play a central role in the development of the systemic inflammatory response that occurs after an infection and/or trauma. The activation of some receptors by bacteria leads to the activation of nuclear factor-kappaB (NF-κB), which subsequently triggers the intracellular transcription of various proinflammatory cytokines such as tumor necrosis factor-alpha (TNF-α); IL-1; IL-6; IL-8; and other cytokines, which include IL-12, IL-15, and IL-18.

The cytokines TNF-α and IL-1 play a synergistic role in the development of the inflammatory response. These factors activate neutrophils, lymphocytes, and vascular endothelial cells, up-regulate the expression of adhesion molecules, enhance the pro-coagulant activity of vascular endothelial cells and trigger the production of inducible nitric oxide synthetase (iNOS), which causes the local production of nitric oxide (NO) in immune and vascular cells. NO-induced local vasodilatation slows blood flow and, with the increased expression of adhesion molecules, leads to enhanced adhesion of neutrophils to the tissue wall. These factors also induce the synthesis of lipid mediators of sepsis (i.e., prostaglandins), the production of acute phase proteins and fever [11].

Interleukin-8 is a prototypical chemokine that is locally produced at the site of infection. This factor is important as an activator and chemoattractant for neutrophils to migrate on the vessel wall and enter the area of infection. The cytokine IL-6 is often elevated in patients with severe sepsis; however, IL-6 levels, but not TNF-α levels, have been shown to predict a fatal outcome in patients with septic shock [12]. However, studies in humans and animals have not shown a causal role for this cytokine in septic shock. IL-6 is also considered an antiinflammatory cytokine because it can induce the release of IL-10, which is thought to be a classic anti-inflammatory cytokine [13]. The cytokines IL-12 and IL-18 are important in the production of interferon (IFN)-γ, which enhances phagocytosis and free radical production and increases the bactericidal activity of macrophages and neutrophils. In animal models of sepsis, interferon-γ blockage is associated with decreased systemic inflammation and a better prognosis [14]. Interleukin-12 also plays a major role in the defense against polymicrobial sepsis, whereas IL-18 is important in infections that are caused by gram-negative organisms. Moreover, IL-18 neutralization in an animal model of sepsis resulted in protection against endotoxemia [15].

3.2.1. Lipid Mediators

Local-acting lipid mediators that are involved in the regulation of inflammation are derived from the semi-essential polyunsaturated fatty acids, such as the arachidonic acids (AA), eicosapentaenoic acids (EPA) and docosaexaenoic acids (DHA). Oxidation of these substrates by cyclooxygenase, lipoxygenase, and cytochrome P-450, respectively, produces prostaglandins, leukotrienes, lipoxins, resolvins and protectins. These mediators act as intercellular signaling molecules that cause either pro- or anti-inflammatory effects.

While most AA-derived mediators aggravate inflammation, n-3-derived compounds display reduced inflammatory effects. EPA or DHA influence the magnitude and course of inflammation using the same metabolic pathways and enzymes that metabolize AA. Omega 3-derived mediators are capable of binding the same receptors as the AA-derived metabolites but possess considerably less-potent inflammatory effects [16].

Additionally, it is known that an effective immune response is based on the availability of n-6 and n-3 fatty acids and their metabolites. This information may be interesting when considering different ratios of fatty acids, especially those of n-6 and n-3 fatty acids, in lipid emulsions because a balanced and effective immune response may be achieved by providing the optimal ratio of n-6 and n-3 fatty acids.

Lately, anti-inflammatory and pro-resolving acting lipid mediators have been a focus of research. These mediators were termed resolvins because they were first discovered during the resolution phase of acute inflammation.

Their synthesis is based on the interaction of two different cell types [17]: the compounds that are derived from EPA are designated as E-series resolvins, and the mediators that are derived from DHA are called D-series resolvins and (neuro) protectins. The biosynthesis of E-series resolvins involves the di-oxygenation of EPA by endothelial COX-2 or cytochrome (Cyt) P450 and then by 5-lipoxygenase, which is found in neutrophils [18].

3.2.1.1. Resolvins Improve the Course of Inflammation

Resolvins dampen the course and enhance the resolution of inflammation via several different mechanisms. These factors reduce neutrophil extravasation and invasion to inflammatory sites by attenuating the expression of adhesion molecules and stimulating endothelial nitric oxide synthase (eNOS) [19]. Resolvins are also associated with the reduced activation of NF-κB and the anti-inflammatory effect that is reflected by the number of minor neutrophils. Furthermore, resolvins are capable of reducing the activity of proteases and ROS, which leads to reduced tissue injury and edema formation. A special role of resolvins occurs during the resolution phase of inflammation. At the end of the inflammatory process, resolvins facilitate the removal of macrophages via lymphatic vessels. The results of experiments in animals show that these factors may present new options to treat diseases that are associated with an uncontrolled immune response [21], which includes acute lung injury (ALI) and pneumonia [22], chronic airway inflammation [23], asthma [24], peritonitis and sepsis [19].

3.2.2. Novel Cytokines

High-mobility group box 1 (HMGB1) is a highly conserved protein that was previously thought to be a DNA-binding protein involved in the maintenance of nucleosome structure and the regulation of gene transcription [25]. Recently, this protein was found to act as a potent proinflammatory cytokine during infection, and levels of HMGB1 increased in serum and tissues during infection, especially during sepsis [26].

Various studies have revealed that HMGB1 is also a proinflammatory cytokine because it can be released from activated monocytes/macrophages, is related to delayed endotoxin lethality, activates macrophages and stimulates proinflammatory cytokine release. HMGB1 that is obtained from the serum of septic patients can up-regulate TNF-α mRNA and protein expression in a dose-dependent manner in human primary blood mononuclear cells [27]. Recently, clinical evidence indicated higher HMGB1 levels at the site of local tissue infection and trauma, and Ueno found that high HMGB1 levels were present in the pulmonary epithelial lining fluid of patients with sepsis [28,29]. Indeed, HMGB1 serum levels increased during sepsis, independent of the primary source of infection, except in urinary tract infections, where the secretion of HMGB1 into the circulation was delayed when compared with that of patients with pneumonia and peritonitis [30]. Currently, it is not known to what extent local HMGB1 release contributes to serum HMGB1 levels or how much this release contributes to damage at the site of infection and to distant organs in patients with sepsis. The following several important areas require more research: the mechanisms that regulate HMGB1 release from cells, the surface receptors that interact with HMGB1 and the intracellular signal transduction pathways through which HMGB1 functions as a proinflammatory cytokine.

3.3. The Role of Toll-Like Receptors

The complement system is also important in the initial immune response to bacteria. The deposition of complement C3b (opsonin) on gram-positive or gram-negative bacteria facilitates neutrophil-mediated bacterial killing, whereas the terminal complex that is formed by complements C5 to C9 can also destroy gram-negative bacteria. If a pathogen is able to evade these mechanisms, it is exposed to the immune cells that recognize certain preserved bacterial motifs. These pathogen-associated molecular patterns (PAMPs) are recognized by pattern-recognition receptors on the immune cells, which then trigger the sepsis cascade [31].

One family of pattern-recognition receptors, the TLRs, plays a central role in the initiation of the immune response. A variety of TLRs have been identified in humans, and these extracellular receptors recognize various microbial ligands. Another important pattern-recognition receptor recognizes peptidoglycan, which is present in both gram-positive and gram-negative organisms. The recognition of a subunit of peptidoglycan (i.e., muramyl dipeptide) by receptors that contain ligand-sensing, leucine-rich repeat regions leads to the activation of the immune system through connected signaling components that are termed nucleotide-binding oligomerization domains [32].

The best-studied microbial ligand that initiates sepsis in humans is LPS, which is also known as endotoxin and is found in the outer cytoplasmic membranes of gram-negative bacteria. The recognition of LPS by the pattern-recognition receptors of the immune system triggers sepsis during various gram-negative infections, and the initiation of this process occurs when LPS is bound by the host-derived lipopolysaccharide-binding protein after a bacterium enters into the host. This protein transfers bound LPS to the opsonin receptor CD14 on the cell surface, and the binding of LPS to CD14 leads to the association of CD14 with the Toll-like receptor TLR4 and initiates TLR stimulation [33]. This stimulation leads to the initiation of the intracellular signaling cascade and recruitment of a signaling protein termed myeloid differentiation primary response protein (MyD88). MyD88 subsequently facilitates the release of transcription factors, such as nuclear factor-κB release, the transcription of various inflammatory genes and the release of various cytokines and other molecules [34].

In contrast, gram-positive infections involve the recognition by TLRs of gram-positive cell wall components, lipoteichoic acid (LTA), and peptidoglycans. The lipoprotein components of LTA are recognized by Toll-like receptor 2 (TLR2), and the activation of TLR2 results in signal transduction and the subsequent release of cytokines. Another important feature of sepsis that results from infection by gram-positive organisms is the production of potent exotoxins. Exotoxins have properties of superantigens and are able to bind to the major histocompatibility complex class II and T-lymphocyte receptors. This activity causes a massive T-cell activation and release of various cytokines independent of the

TLR pathways [11]. An example of this type of toxin is the toxic shock syndrome toxin 1, which is produced by certain strains of *Staphylococcus aureus*.

3.3.1. Clinical Aspects

The TLRs can detect the structural components of microorganisms that occur inside and outside of cells (i.e., intra- and extracellular TLRs). Some studies show that trauma reduces, but a severe infection increases, the expression of TLRs that recognize bacterial antigens (e.g., LPS, peptidoglycan). Furthermore, the expression of TLR4 in the monocytes of trauma patients was reduced when compared to those of healthy people [35]. Therefore, it is tempting to postulate that the increased expression of TLRs could have a beneficial effect in trauma patients. Polymorphisms of TLRs were factors that increased the susceptibility of patients to infections that were caused by particular bacteria, but these changes did not significantly affect the course or outcome of infection in patients with mixed-severe infections. In some experimental studies, a lack of TLRs increased the susceptibility of mice to infections [36] and caused disorders in inflammatory mediator secretion and in phagocytosis and antigen presentation [37]. Intraperitoneal administration of living *Escherichia coli* bacteria or TLR4 had a significant impact on the phagocytic activity of peritoneal macrophages. When no TLR2 was present, the TLR4 on macrophages caused disorders in bacterial phagocytosis (i.e., for *E. coli and S. aureus*). The experimental findings suggest that TLR4 plays a key role in regulating the expression of inflammatory cytokines in the lung during endotoxic shock [38]. Six hours of LPS administration induced a significant increase in pulmonary TNF-a, IL-1b and IL-6 mRNA in control ($TLR4^+$) mice, when compared to TLR4-deficient mice, and recent studies showed that apoptotic macrophages could have a protective function in septic shock that is caused by LPS administration in mice [39]. This study, for the first time, demonstrated that the administration of apoptotic cells could protect mice against LPS-induced death, even when the apoptotic cells were administered 24 h after the LPS challenge.

After partially successful attempts to block LPS-binding receptors in septic patients and to block the signaling pathway proteins that are associated with the antibacterial immune response (e.g., suppression of HMGB1), modulating the response by immunonutrition seems to be a new and promising re-direction of studies. To date, several randomized clinical trials have evaluated the efficacy of arginine, glutamine, omega-3 fatty acids, nucleotides and trace elements with antioxidant properties in critically ill patients with trauma and/or infections, but the basic molecular mechanisms that are responsible for attenuating the overwhelming inflammatory response in sepsis are still unclear [40]. In malnourished surgical patients, the “first-line’’anti-bacterial defense may be disorders of PAMPs (e.g., LPS, peptidoglycan, teichoic acids, or bacterial DNA), which change the recognition patterns of innate immunity cells. The increased activation of receptors that take part in PAMP recognition can facilitate the occurrence of severe infections, and the hypothesis that one of the main reasons for false recognition of bacterial antigens by immune system cells, mainly by phagocytic cells, is malnutrition is highly probable. The deficiency of immunoactive nourishing substances (e.g., glutamine, fatty acids or trace elements such as selenium and zinc) can intensify disorders involving the expression of bacterial antigens that bind extracellular receptors and intracellular proteins/receptors. Furthermore, the excessive accumulation of bacterial wall fragments and proliferating microorganisms in tissues intensify the inflammatory response and increase the release of cytokines into the blood.

3.4.1. Nuclear Factor kappaB

The transcriptional regulatory factor NF-κB is a central participant in modulating the expression of many of the immunoregulatory mediators that are involved in sepsis. Signaling pathways that are initiated by the engagement of TLRs, such as TLR2 and TLR4, by bacterial products or cytokine receptors, which include those for TNF-α and IL-1, induced the nuclear accumulation of NF-κB and enhanced the transcription of genes that are responsible for the expression of cytokines, chemokines, adhesion molecules, apoptotic factors and other mediators of the inflammatory response that are associated with sepsis [41].

NF-κB is a dimer that is composed of members of the Rel family. In vertebrates, this family includes RelA (p65), RelB, c-Rel, NF-κB1 (p50) and NF-κB2 (p52) [42]. Any homo- or heterodimer is considered NF-κB, although the most common complex that is found in activated cells, RelA/NF-κB1 (p65/p50), is a heterodimer and is often referred to as a 'classic' NF-κB. All of these proteins share a highly conserved Rel homology domain that is composed of two immunoglobulin-like domains. The 'classical' NF-κB factor can vary and can have different effects on gene regulation, depending upon the specific combination of proteins.

A schematic representation of the NF-κB pathway is illustrated in Figure 1. The interaction of NF-κB with specific binding sequences in gene promoters can be induced by multiple stimuli, such as endotoxins, cytokines (such as TNF-α and IL-1h), ROS (especially hydrogen peroxide) [43], protein kinase C activators, viruses, UV light and ionizing radiation.

However, it should be noted that the presence of an NF-κB binding site in a gene does not necessarily imply regulation by that factor. Feedback loops have been identified that might amplify the response to the initial stimulus (positive feedback) or regulate NF-κB activation (negative feedback) [44]. In addition, LPS could induce the synthesis of anti-inflammatory cytokines, such as IL-10, IL-4 and IL-13, thereby blocking NF-κB activation and inhibiting cytokine production, which would provide an extracellular mechanism for negative feedback.

3.4.1.1 Nuclear Factor kappaB and Oxidative Stress

Regulation of NF-κB involves cascades of phosphorylation and dephosphorylation, but it may also be controlled by the redox status of the cell. The major intracellular regulator of redox homeostasis is GSH, which acts via reversible oxidation of an active thiol group. NF-κB has been implicated in the up-regulation of the rate-limiting enzyme for GSH synthesis, γGCS, in response to various stimuli that include inflammatory cytokines (i.e., IL-1h and possibly TNF-α) [45].

Another important thiol-containing compound that is involved in redox homeostasis is thioredoxin (Trx). Thioredoxin possesses a large number of functions other than its originally identified role as a hydrogen donor for ribonucleotide reductase. After the dissociation of IκB, the reduction of NF-κB by Trx is necessary for the binding of NF-κB to DNA in the nucleus. However, Trx appears to play dual and opposing roles in the regulation of NF-κB. In the cytoplasm, Trx interferes with the signal to IκB kinases and blocks the degradation of IκB [46]. Thioredoxin also contributes indirectly to AP-1 activation via the nuclear redox factor

Ref-1 (redox factor 1). Therefore, cells respond to adverse conditions by modulating their antioxidant levels, stimulating new gene expression and modifying proteins.

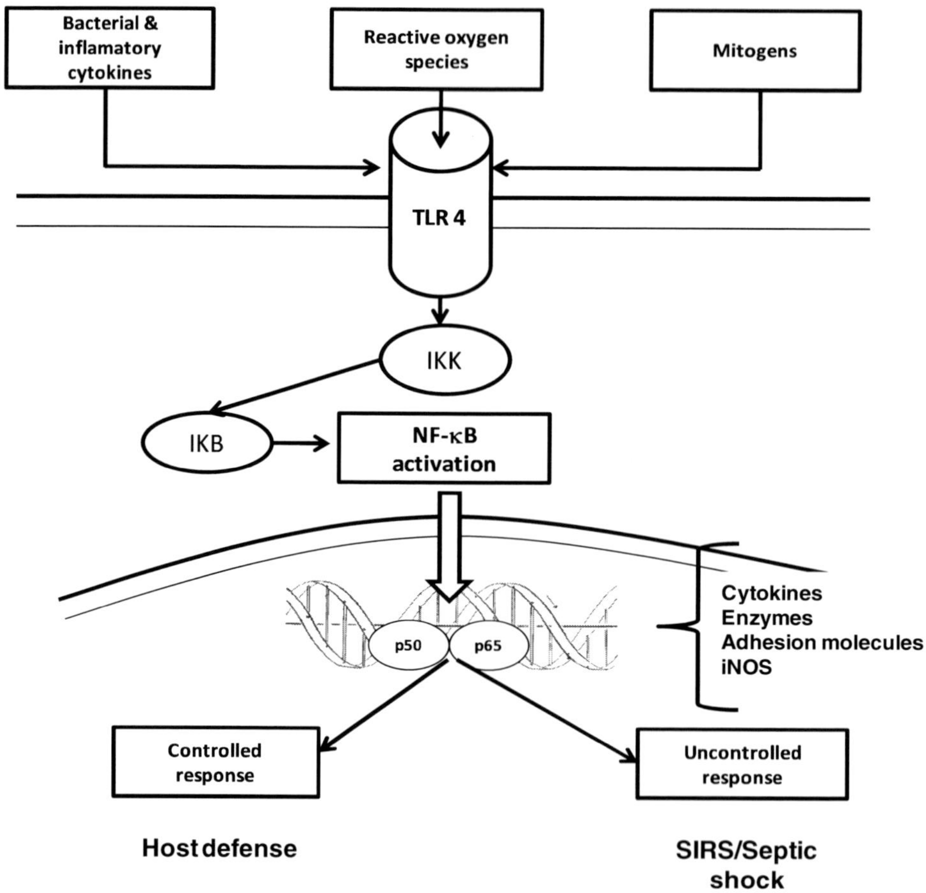

Figure 1. A schematic representation of the NF-κB pathway in SIRS/Septic shock. TLR4, toll like receptor-4; IKK, I kappa B kinase; IKB, inhibitory factor kappa B; p50/p65 rel, catalytic subunits of NF-kappaB factor; iNOS, inducible nitric oxide synthase; SIRS, Systemic inflammatory response syndrome.

At least two transcription factors, NF-κB and AP-1, have been identified as being regulated by the intracellular redox state and may have important roles in the inflammatory response [47]. The redox regulation of transcription factors appears to occur via highly conserved cysteine residues in their DNA-binding domains.

In general, in intact cells, antioxidant and oxidant species appear to have opposite roles: antioxidants decrease NF-κB activation while dramatically increasing AP-1 activation (AP-1 acts as a secondary antioxidant response factor), and oxidant species strongly activate NF-κB while moderately activating AP-1 [48].

The relative importance of steps within the NF-κB activation pathway that are amenable to redox influence remains to be determined. It has been postulated that NF-κB regulation via redox activities might occur at various sites, which include specific kinase (i.e., NIK/IKK/MAPKs) and phosphorylation steps, protease activity, nuclear translocation and gene transcription. Therefore, NF-κB is a transcription factor that is required for the gene expression of many inflammatory mediators and is a therapeutic target in critical care medicine.

3.4.1.2. Nuclear Factor kappaB and SIRS/Sepsis

Several in vitro and animal studies have demonstrated a link between sepsis and NF-κB activation and oxidative stress. In a recent animal study, LPS administration resulted in NF-κB activation in several organs and was associated with an increase in lung tissue mRNA and protein expression of a variety of NF-κB-regulated cytokines, which included TNF-α and IL-6 [49]. Because oxidative stress regulates NF-κB activation and evidence of such stress has been demonstrated in patients with sepsis, it is expected that increased NF-κB and, hence, up-regulation of cytokines, will occur in these patients, in animal models of sepsis, or in in vitro cell cultures [50]. Several studies have demonstrated increased NF-κB activity in isolated leukocytes from patients with sepsis, which was associated with non-survival [51]. Bohrer et al. [52] reported that increased NF-κB activity was comparable to the Acute Physiology and Chronic Health Evaluation (APACHE II) score as a predictor of outcome and mortality from sepsis. These findings were confirmed by Arnalich et al. [53], who found that NF-κB activity was significantly higher in non-survivors and correlated strongly with the APACHE II score. These authors also found that the IL-1 receptor antagonist had a predictive value for mortality, although this receptor is an anti-inflammatory mediator with no known effects that are exerted via NF-κB. Furthermore, Paterson et al. reported increased NF-κB activation in critically ill patients who later died. In addition, the activation of this factor was inhibited by the antioxidant N-acetyl-cysteine [54]. Recently, it has been demonstrated that plasma that had been isolated from patients with septic shock after being admitted to an ICU for 24 h had higher NF-κB activity than that of patients who had not been admitted to an ICU [55]. Finally, a number of agents have been used in experimental and clinical settings with the aim of reducing oxidative stress, presumably by inhibiting the activation of transcriptional factors (mainly NF-κB) that attenuate the inflammatory response. Because NF-κB occupies a central role in signaling pathways that are important in sepsis, the modulation of NF-κB may be an appropriate therapeutic target in patients with sepsis.

3.4.2. STAT-3

STAT3 is a member of the signal transducers and activators of transcription (STAT) transcription factor family, which functions with the janus kinases (JAK) in the JAK-STAT signaling networks that are commonly activated by cytokines. Activation of STAT3 appears to be essential for the anti-inflammatory actions of IL-10 [56]. The serum concentrations of TNFα and the cytokines IL-10, IL-6, IFNγ, and IL-1β were all substantially elevated after LPS administration to STAT3−/− mice, whose STAT3 expression was specifically knocked out in macrophages and neutrophils with the cre-lox P system. The mutant mice were highly susceptible to LPS-induced sepsis, presumably because the anti-inflammatory actions of IL-10 on macrophages and neutrophils were greatly suppressed. Additional STAT family members showed importance in sepsis. In mice, the cecal ligation and puncture procedure (CLP), which is different with respect to the injection of LPS, induces severe septic peritonitis. STAT4−/− and STAT6−/− mice that had been subjected to CLP exhibited fewer complications that developed into severe sepsis (i.e., 50% dead on day four versus 50% dead on day 2 in wild type mice) [57]. STAT4 and STAT6 are activated by the cytokines IL-12 and IL-13, respectively.

In STAT6−/− mice, bacterial levels were much lower than in wild type mice after CLP was performed. STAT6−/− mice also had higher peritoneal IL-12, TNFα, macrophage-derived chemokines, and C10, which are mediators that are known to enhance bacterial clearance, after the CLP was performed. The main cytokines and transcriptional factors that are associated with and involved in the inflammatory response are shown in Table 1.

Table 1. Summary of protein function

Toll like receptors	Receptor family, at least 10 members, TLR4 present on most cell types binds LPS, resulting in activation of NFkB and pro-inflammatory gene transcription.
IL-1	Interleukin-1 is a major pro-inflammatory cytokine, produced by macrophages, activates NF-kB.
IL-8	This is a chemokine that is produced locally at the site of infection. It is important as an activator and chemoattractant for neutrophils to marginate on the vessel wall and enter the area of infection.
IL-6	IL-6 is an interleukin that acts as both a pro-inflammatory and anti-inflammatory cytokine. It is secreted by T cells and macrophages to stimulate immune response, e.g. during infection and after trauma, especially burns or other tissue damage leading to inflammation.
TNF-α	Tumor necrosis factor - α is a major pro-inflammatory cytokine, released from macrophages, controlling cellular survival/apopotosis.
HMGB1	High-mobility group box 1, a proinflammatory cytokine. Recently, it has been found to act as a potent proinflammatory cytokine during infection responses. Levels of HMGB1 increase in serum and tissues during infection, especially in sepsis.
Chemokines	Generally small peptide hormones, which bind to G-protein coupled receptors present on many cell types, have profound effects of leukocyte biology, stimulating chemotaxis, proteolytic enzyme release and superoxide production.
Lipid mediators	Local-acting lipid mediators involved in the regulation of inflammation are derived from the semi-essential polyunsaturated fatty acids AA, EPA and DHA. It has been showing that depending of concentration and saturation grade these compounds would be involved in pro-inflammatory and anti-inflammatory pathways.
MAPK	The mitogen activated protein kinase family composed of 12 members grouped into five subfamilies. These kinases are activated by many signaling pathways, regulating gene transcription, and many other functions.
NF-κB	Transcription factor particularly important in inflammation, transcription of many pro- inflammatory gene products requires NF-κB, believed to play important role in sepsis.
JAK-STAT	Janus kinase-signal transducers and activators of transcription are tyrosine phosphorylated transcription factors activated by JAKs activated by various cytokine receptors. Four JAKs, and seven STATs are known.
PI3K	Catalyze conversion of phosphatidyl inositol 4,5 bisphosphate to membrane delimited second messenger phosphatidyl inositol-3,4,5-trisphosphate. Several forms are known regulated by distinct mechanisms, intimately involved in neutrophil activation.
G proteins	Family of some 20 members, transduce the activity of seven transmembrane G protein coupled receptors.

AA, arachidonic acids; EPA, eicosapentaenoic acids; DHA, docosaexaenoic acids.

4. The Relationship between ROS Production and the Inflammatory Response in Critical Patients

Reactive oxygen species affect many signaling events, protein kinase networks, and downstream transcription factors. Activated neutrophils, such as those that infiltrate the lungs and other organs of septic animals, produce large amounts of ROS. Under these conditions, neutrophil-derived ROS may initiate signaling events in other cell populations in addition to their direct, destructive effects on host tissues. Recent evidence demonstrates that activated PKB/Akt protects lung tissue from oxidant-induced lung injury and reduces death in mice [58]. It is believed that hyperoxic pulmonary damage is caused by the production of ROS.

4.1. Gene Expression

Oxidants have been shown to regulate gene expression by their effects on transcription factors such as NF-κB, c-fos, and c-jun. The evidence that ROS can activate the transcription factor NF-κB may be directly relevant to leukocyte responses during acute inflammation. NF-κB is ubiquitously expressed and mediates the fast induction of the expression of genes that are involved in the acute inflammatory response, which include cytokines, cytokine receptors, adhesion molecules, MHC antigens, acute-phase proteins, and several viral enhancers [59].

There are several important implications of NF-κB activation in neutrophils. First, NF-κB is involved in the transcriptional regulation of several key cytokines and chemokines, including IL-1, IL-6, IL-8, and MIP-2, which are produced by neutrophils in an inflammatory milieu. Second, macrophages generate ROS in response to LPS, and, in this case, it is possible that ROS may participate in LPS-induced NF-κB activation in these cells, which is an effect that would have important consequences for the inflammatory and immune responses. Third, cytokines such as TNF-α and IL-1 can result in NF-κB activation, which is mediated by a pro-oxidant imbalance that is induced by TNF-α [60]. Evidence for a role of mitochondrial-derived ROS in TNF-mediated signaling has been provided by studies on the cytotoxic effects of TNF in fibrosarcoma cells [61]. Taken together, these observations provide a basis for a mitochondrion–nucleus regulatory pathway in which ROS participate as physiological signaling molecules.

4.2. Paracrine Effects of ROS

ROS that are produced by leukocytes may act in a paracrine manner to influence other cells. The majority of oxidizing equivalents (e.g., ROS) that are produced by the respiratory burst oxidase are released into the extracellular space. Because ROS are membrane permeates, these substances may influence intracellular signaling pathways in cells such as other leukocytes and other cell types that are present in the inflammatory milieu.

The vascular endothelium, by virtue of its location, is a prime target for such oxidant effects. During their migration through the endothelium, neutrophils may release ROS, which may trigger responses in endothelial cells. Indeed, the exposure of endothelial cells to exogenous hydrogen peroxide has been shown to activate phospholipase D, an enzyme that catalyzes the hydrolysis of phospholipids [62]. Additionally, studies have demonstrated that ROS induce human endothelial cells to express P-selectin and bind neutrophils [63].

Thus, ROS that are produced by neutrophils can influence signaling pathways in adjacent cells, other neutrophils, macrophages, or resident tissue cells such as fibroblasts, endothelial, or epithelial cells. The accumulation of activated neutrophils has been implicated in the pathogenesis of acute lung injury, which is characterized by inflammatory injury to the endothelium and epithelium.

Based on the evidence that is outlined above, ROS that are produced by the leukocyte NAD(P)H oxidase may contribute to the amplification of inflammatory injury in this disorder. ROS may also influence the reparative phase of inflammation and, in particular, the deleterious repair, from the physiologic point of view, which leads to fibrosis.

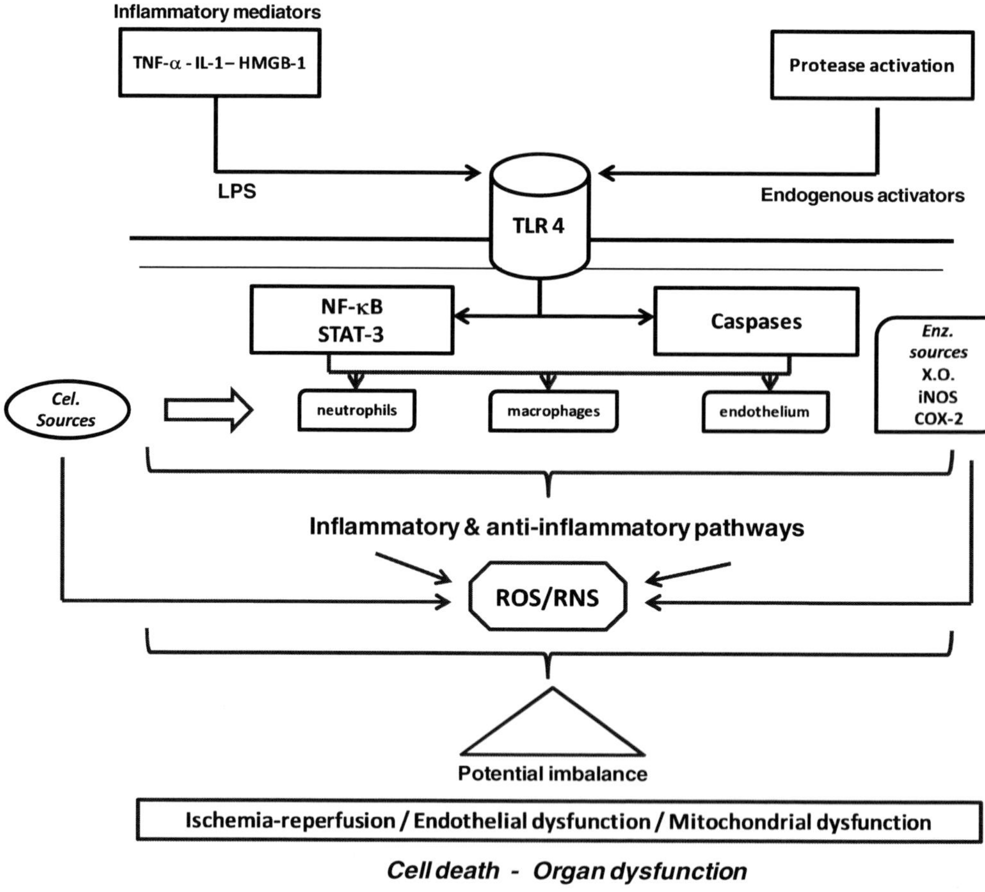

Figure 2. Schematic representation of the relationship between ROS production and inflammatory response in critical patients. TNF-α, Tumoral necrosis factor-α; IL-1, Interleukin-1; HMGB1, High-mobility group box 1; LPS, Lypopolysaccharide; STAT-3, Signal transducer and activator of transcription 3; X.O., xanthine oxide-reductase; iNOS, inducible nitric oxide synthase; COX, cyclo-oxygenase.

5. Biomarkers of the Inflammatory Response in Critically Ill Patients

Differentiating between sepsis and SIRS is of utmost importance, and doing so is a common dilemma for the intensivist. Many biomarkers have been proposed and tested in a clinical setting, but this search has not provided, until recently, a test that is widely accepted and enables the bedside clinician to confidently confirm or reject the diagnosis of sepsis. The most commonly used biomarkers in clinical laboratories and applied research are the following: i) procalcitonin (PCT), ii) C-reactive protein (CRP)/IL-6, and iii) lipopolysaccharide binding protein (LBP).

i) Procalcitonin (PCT) serum levels are elevated in patients with sepsis, and the usefulness of PCT in diagnosing sepsis has been studied extensively but has conflicting results because the biological function of PCT is not known. Normal serum levels are below 0.5 ng/mL, patients with levels above 2 ng/mL are thought to be at risk for sepsis [64], and the serum half-time is 24–36 h.

In a recent meta-analysis of 33 studies that included nearly 4,000 patients, Uzzan et al., [65] concluded that PCT is superior to CRP in differentiating between sepsis and SIRS, and these authors favored the routine use of PCT in differentiating between SIRS and sepsis. On the contrary, Tang et al. [66] reviewed 18 studies, which included 2,097 patients, and concluded that PCT could not reliably differentiate sepsis from other causes of SIRS. This group also argued against the routine of using of PCT in differentiating sepsis from SIRS.

ii) *C-reactive protein/IL-6*. Interleukin-6 is an important mediator of the acute phase reaction in response to inflammation in sepsis and is produced in response to TNF-α stimulation. In the liver, IL-6 induces the synthesis of acute phase proteins like C-reactive protein (CRP). The normal range of the serum concentration of this protein is <5.9 pg/mL. Following inflammation, serum levels of IL-6 have been shown to rise within one hour before CRP levels and even before the onset of fever. Interleukin-6 values above 500 pg/mL were found in patients with sepsis [64].

iii) Another acute phase protein is the lipopolysaccharide binding protein (LBP), which is produced by the liver in response to circulating bacterial endotoxins or LPS. Lipopolysaccharide is a constituent of the outer coat of Gram-negative bacteria. LBP facilitates the binding of LPS to the LPS receptor on monocytes, which results in monocyte activation and cytokine production (e.g., TNF-α and IL-6).

Elevated levels of serum LBP have been reported in Gram-negative, Gram-positive, and fungal infections, but not in viral infections.

The normal range of LBP serum concentration is 5 to 10 μg/mL, but in patients with sepsis, LBP levels rise to over 50 μg/mL in approximately 36 hours.

The C-reactive protein is produced by the liver in response to stimulation by several cytokines (e.g., IL-6), and it is measured routinely in hospitalized patients, although it is generally recognized to not be specific for sepsis or infection because it is elevated in infectious and noninfectious states [67].

5.1. Clinical Trials that Support the Prognostic Values of Procalcitonin

Serum PCT levels have also been noted to increase with increasing severity of sepsis and organ dysfunction. This increase has led to interest in using PCT as a prognostic indicator in critical care patients, and a number of studies have been performed to test the utilization of PCT in this manner. One of the largest studies was performed by Jensen et al. [68, 69]. This study prospectively looked at daily PCT measurements in 1,200 critical care patients and correlated the results with all-cause mortality in a 28-day study period (i.e., the primary end-point was death from any cause at day 28). The authors concluded that procalcitonin-guided antimicrobial escalation in the intensive care unit did not improve survival and led to organ-related harm and prolonged admission to the intensive care unit.

The PRORATA trial is the largest randomized PCT trial to establish the effectiveness of an algorithm, which is based on the biomarker procalcitonin, to reduce antibiotic exposure in this setting [70]. Primary endpoints were mortality at days 28 and 60 (i.e., non-inferiority analysis) and the number of days without antibiotics by day 28 (i.e., superiority analysis). The mortality of patients in the procalcitonin group was not less than that of patients in the control group at days 28 and 60.

The authors concluded that a procalcitonin-guided strategy to treat suspected bacterial infections in non-surgical patients who were in intensive care units could reduce antibiotic exposure and selective pressure with no apparent adverse outcomes.

5.2. Others Proposed Biomarkers in Critical Ill Patients

Eosinopenia is an attractive potential biomarker in sepsis, as the eosinophil count is serially measured in routine clinical practice and the additional costs would therefore be minimal negligible. In a recent trial, Abidi and colleagues [71] showed that eosinopenia could be useful to differentiate between no infection and infection in patients recently admitted to an ICU. However, the association of eosinopenia with infections is not new and has been described previously.

Changes of the biomarkers of coagulation have also been demonstrated in severe sepsis, with activated partial thromboplastin time waveform analysis appearing to have notable clinical potential. Differences in the magnitude of the abnormality and in the rate of normalization of the markers were clearly observed when parsed by 28-day survival of patients with severe sepsis. Non-survivors had greater derangement and less normalization of hemostasis, endothelial injury, and inflammation.

These observations, drawn from a large number of patients selected with consistent entry criteria, supported the hypothesis that an out-of-control host response of coagulopathy and inflammation in severe sepsis may lead to multiorgan failure syndrome and death.

The enzyme group of matrix metalloproteinases (MMPs) and their inhibitors, so-called tissue inhibitors of matrix-metalloproteinases (TIMPs), are crucial mediators responsible for wound repair after parenchymal damage. Little is known about the role of MMPs and TIMPs in severe sepsis. Hoffmann et al. [72] investigated the role of these enzymes in a study of 37 patients with severe sepsis and 37 healthy controls. MMP-9, TIMP-1, TIMP-2 and IL-6 were significantly higher in ill patients; TIMP-1 was also found to be significantly higher in those who died compared with survivors and IL-6 were significantly higher in ill patients; TIMP-1 was also found to be significantly higher in those who died compared with survivors.

The above studies, whilst not representing an exhaustive review of non-PCT biomarkers in sepsis, demonstrate the wide range of potentially clinically useful biomarkers currently being investigated.

As has already been demonstrated to some extent in a few studies, to be highly predictive of sepsis and/or clinical outcome, it is likely that a combined panel of novel biomarkers, with or without traditional markers of sepsis, will be required.

Conclusions and Perspectives

An optimal therapeutic plan for severe sepsis and septic shock remains a major unmet medical need. Novel treatments to regulate the disordered inflammatory response in sepsis are needed if improved outcomes for sepsis in the future. Current therapy is primarily supportive and includes timely administration of antibiotics, source control of infection, aggressive fluid resuscitation, organ support and use of activated protein C in adults when indicated. Bacterial mediators including endotoxin, superantigens and endogenous proinflammatory cytokines are critical to the pathogenesis of sepsis-induced organ failure and are being targeted with numerous molecules; some with pluripotent activity such as inter-alpha inhibitor proteins, lipid mediators and estrogen-receptor ligands are also being investigated. Efforts are underway to re-establish microbial clearance mechanisms and allow immune reconstitution following sepsis-induced immune suppression. In this purpose, novel biomarkers have been included in the clinical evaluation such as procalcitonin and eosinopenia, who are a reliable marker of sepsis on admission to medical intensive care units. These help to increase the accuracy of diagnostic tools and thus reduce the use of invasive treatments.

References

[1] Wiersinga W J. Current insights in sepsis: from pathogenesis to new treatment targets. *Curr. Opin. Crit. Care* 2011;17:480–486.

[2] Orman M A, Ierapetritou M G, Berthiaume F, Androulakis I P. The dynamics of the early inflammatory response in double-hit burn and sepsis animal models. *Cytokine* 2011; 56:494–502.

[3] Mantovani A, Cassatella M A, Costantini C, Jaillon S. Neutrophils in the activation and regulation of innate and adaptive immunity. *Nat. Rev. Immunol.* 2011;25:519–531.

[4] Serhan C N, Chiang N, Van Dyke T E. Resolving inflammation: dual anti-inflammatory and pro-resolution lipid mediators. *Nature Rev. Immunol.* 2008;8:349–361.

[5] Serhan C N, Yang R, Martinod K, Kasuga K, Pillai P S, Porter T F, Oh S F, Spite M. Maresins: novel macrophage mediators with potent antiinflammatory and proresolving actions. *J. Exp. Med.* 2009;206:15–23.

[6] Lucas T, Waisman A, Ranjan R, Roes J, Krieg T, Muller W, Roers A, Eming S A. Differential roles of macrophages in diverse phases of skin repair. *J. Immunol.* 2010;184:3964–3977.

[7] Stout R D. Editorial: macrophage functional phenotypes: no alternatives in dermal wound healing?. *J. Leukoc. Biol.* 2010;87:19–21.

[8] Khallou-Laschet J, Varthaman A, Fornasa G, Compain C, Gaston A T, Clement M, Dussiot M, Levillain O, Graff-Dubois S, Nicoletti A, Caligiuri G. Macrophage plasticity in experimental atherosclerosis. *PLoS One* 2010;25:e8852.

[9] Antoniades C G, Berry P A, Wendon J A, Vergani D. The importance of immune dysfunction in determining outcome in acute liver failure. *J. Hepatol.* 2008;49:845–861.

[10] Lee S H, Clemens M G, Lee S M. Role of Kupffer cells in vascular stress genes during trauma and sepsis. *J Surg Res* 2010;158:104–111.

[11] Sriskandan S, Altmann D M. *The immunology of sepsis. J. Pathol.* 2008;214:211–223.

[12] Ley K, Laudanna C, Cybulsky M I, Nourshargh S. Getting to the site of inflammation: the leucocyte adhesion cascade updated. *Nat. Rev. Immunol.* 2007;7:678–689.

[13] Dinarello C A. Proinflammatory and anti-inflammatory cytokines as mediators in the pathogenesis of septic shock. *Chest* 1997;112:321S–329S.

[14] Qiu G, Gribbin E, Harrison K, Sinha N, Yin K. Inhibition of gamma interferon decreases bacterial load in peritonitis by accelerated peritoneal fibrin deposition and tissue repair. *Infect. Immun.* 2003;71:2766–2774.

[15] Hochholzer P, Lipford G B, Wagner H, Pfeffer K, Heeg K. Role of interleukin-18 (IL-18) during lethal shock: decreased lipopolysaccharide sensitivity but normal superantigen reaction in IL-18-deficient mice. *Infect. Immun.* 2000;68:3502–3508.

[16] Mayer K, Seeger W. Fish oil in critical illness. *Curr. Opin. Clin. Nutr. Metab. Care* 2008;11 121–127.

[17] Serhan C N. Systems approach to inflammation resolution: identification of novel anti-inflammatory and pro-resolving mediators. *J. Thromb. Haemost* 2009;7:44–48.

[18] Prescott S M, Stenson W F. Fish oil fix. *Nat. Med.* 2005;11:596–598.

[19] Spite M, Norling L V, Summers L, Yang R, Cooper D, Petasis N A, Flower R J, Perretti M, Serhan C N. Resolvin D2 is a potent regulator of leukocytes and controls microbial sepsis, *Nature* 2009;461:1287–1291.

[20] Flower R J, Perrett M. Controlling inflammation: a fat chance?, *J. Exp. Med.* 2005;201:671–674.

[21] Bannenberg G L, Chiang N, Ariel A, Arita M, Tjonahen E, Gotlinger KH, Hong S, Serhan CN. Molecular circuits of resolution: formation and actions of resolvins and protectins. *J. Immunol.* 2005;174:4345–4355.

[22] Seki H, Fukunaga K, Arita M, Arai H, Nakanishi H, Taguchi R, Miyasho T, Takamiya R, Asano K, Ishizaka A, Takeda J, Levy B D. The anti-inflammatory and proresolving mediator resolvin E1 protects mice from bacterial pneumonia and acute lung injury, *J. Immunol.* 184; 2009:836–843.

[23] Haworth O, Levy B D. Endogenous lipid mediators in the resolution of airway inflammation. *Eur. Respir. J. 2007*:30:980–992.

[24] Levy BD, Kohli P, Gotlinger K, Haworth O, Hong S, Kazani S, Israel E, Haley KJ, Serhan CN. Protectin D1 is generated in asthma and dampens airway inflammation and hyperresponsiveness, *J. Immunol.* 2007;178:496–502.

[25] Yang H, Tracey K J. High mobility group box 1 (HMGB1). *Crit. Care Med.* 2005;33:S472-S474.

[26] Huang W, Tang Y, Li L. HMGB1, a potent proinflammatory cytokine in sepsis. *Cytokine* 2010;51:119–126.
[27] Andersson U, Wang H, Palmblad K, Aveberger AC, Bloom O, Erlandsson-Harris H, Janson A, Kokkola R, Zhang M, Yang H, Tracey KJ. High mobility group 1 protein (HMG-1) stimulates proinflammatory cytokine synthesis in human monocytes. *J. Exp. Med.* 2000;192:565–570.
[28] Ueno H, Matsuda T, Hashimoto S. Amaya F, Kitamura Y, Tanaka M, Kobayashi A, Maruyama I, Yamada S, Hasegawa N, Soejima J, Koh H, Ishizaka A. Contributions of high mobility group box protein in experimental and clinical acute lung injury. *Am. J. Respir. Crit. Care Med.* 2004;170:1310–1316.
[29] Takahata R, Ono S, Tsujimoto H, Hiraki S, Kimura A, Kinoshita M, Miyazaki H, Saitoh D, Hase K. Postoperative serum concentrations of high mobility group box chromosomal protein-1 correlates to the duration of SIRS and pulmonary dysfunction following gastrointestinal surgery. *J. Surg. Res.* 2011;170:135-140.
[30] van Zoelen M A, Laterre P F, van Veen S Q, van Till JW, Wittebole X, Bresser P, Tanck MW, Dugernier T, Ishizaka A, Boermeester MA, van der Poll T. Systemic and local high mobility group box 1 concentrations during severe infection. *Crit. Care Med.* 2007;35:2799–2804.
[31] Rittirsch D, Flierl M A, Ward P A. Harmful molecular mechanisms in sepsis. *Nat. Rev. Immunol.* 2008;8:776–787.
[32] Inohara C, McDonald C, Nunez G. NOD-LRR proteins: role in host–microbial interactions and inflammatory disease. *Annu. Rev. Biochem.* 2005;74:355–383.
[33] Lu Y C, Yeh W C, Ohashi P S. LPS/TLR4 signal transduction pathway. *Cytokine* 2008;42:145–151.
[34] Chaurasia B, Mauer J, Koch L, Goldau J, Kock A S, Brüning J C. Phosphoinositide-dependent kinase 1 provides negative feedback inhibition to Toll-like receptor-mediated NF-kappaB activation in macrophages. *Mol. Cell Biol.* 2010:4354–4366.
[35] Adib-Conquy M, Moine P, Asehnoune K, Edouard A, Espevik T, Miyake K, Werts C, Cavaillon JM. Toll-like receptor-mediated tumor necrosis factor and interleukin-10 production differ during systemic inflammation. *Am. J. Respir. Crit. Care Med.* 2003;168:158–164.
[36] Qureshi S T, Medzhitov R. Toll-like receptors and their role in experimental models of microbial infection. *Genes. Immun.* 2003;4:87–94.
[37] Blander J M, Medzhitov. Regulation of phagosome maturation by signals from Toll-like receptors. *Science* 2004;304:1014–1018.
[38] Baumgarten G, Knuefermann P, Wrigge H, Putensen C, Stapel H, Fink K, Meyer R, Hoeft A, Grohé C. Role of Toll-like receptor 4 for the pathogenesis of acute lung injury in Gram-negative sepsis. *Eur. J. Anaesthesiol* 2006;23:1041–1048.
[39] Ren Y, Xie Y, Jiang G Fan J, Yeung J, Li W, Tam P K, Savill J. Apoptotic cells protect mice against lipopolisaccharide-induced shock. *J. Immunol.* 2008;180:4978–4985.
[40] Słotwiński R, Słotwińska S, Kędziora S, Bałan B J. Innate immunity signaling pathways: links between immunonutrition and responses to sepsis. *Arch. Immunol. Ther. Exp. (Warsz)* 2011;59:139-50.
[41] Victor V M, Rocha M, De la Fuente M. Immune cells: free radicals and antioxidants in sepsis. *Int. Immunopharmacol.* 2004;4:327–347.

[42] Oeckinghaus A, Hayden M S, Ghosh S. Crosstalk in NF-κB signaling pathways. *Nat. Immunol.* 2011;19:695–708.

[43] Ma X, Becker Buscaglia L E, Barker J R, Li Y. MicroRNAs in NF-kappaB signaling. *J. Mol. Cell Biol.* 2011;3:159–166.

[44] Poligone B, Baldwin A S. Positive and negative regulation of NF-kappaB by COX-2: roles of different prostaglandins. *J. Biol. Chem.* 2001;276:38658–38664.

[45] Oakley A. Glutathione transferases: a structural perspective. *Drug Metab. Rev.* 2011;43:138–51.

[46] Heilman J M, Burke T J, McClain C J, Watson W H. Transactivation of gene expression by NF-κB is dependent on thioredoxin reductase activity. *Free Radic. Biol. Med.* 2011;51:1533–1542.

[47] Callister M E, Pinhu L, Catley M C, Westwell A D, Newton R, Leaver S K, Quinlan G J, Evans T W, Griffiths M J, Burke-Gaffney A. PMX464, a thiol-reactive quinol and putative thioredoxin inhibitor, inhibits NF-kappaB-dependent proinflammatory activation of alveolar epithelial cells. *Br. J. Pharmacol.* 2008;155:661–672.

[48] Meyer D M, Crottet P, Maco B, Degtyar E, Cassel D, Spiess M. Oligomerization and dissociation of AP-1 adaptors are regulated by cargo signals and by ArfGAP1-induced GTP hydrolysis. *Mol. Biol. Cell* 2005;16:4745–4754.

[49] Ansaldi D, Hod E A, Stellari F, Kim J B, Lim E, Roskey M, Francis K P, Singh R, Zhang N. Imaging pulmonary NF-kappaB activation and therapeutic effects of MLN120B and TDZD-8. *PLoS One* 2011;6:e25093.

[50] Victor V M, Rocha M, De la Fuente M. N-acetylcysteine protects mice from lethal endotoxemia by regulating the redox state of immune cells. *Free Radic. Res.* 2003;37:919– 29.

[51] Hotta N, Ichiyama T, Shiraishi M, Takekawa T, Matsubara T, Furukawa S. Nuclear factor-kappaB activation in peripheral blood mononuclear cells in children with sepsis. *Crit Care Med* 2007;35:2395–2401.

[52] Bohrer H, Qiu F, Zimmermann T, Zhang Y, Jllner T, Männel D, Böttiger B W, Stern D M, Waldherr R, Saeger H D, Ziegler R, Bierhaus A, Martin E, Nawroth P P. Role of NFκB in the mortality of sepsis. *J. Clin. Invest.* 1997; 100:972– 985.

[53] Arnalich F, Garcia-Palomero E, Lopez J, Jimenez M, Madero R, Renart J, Vázquez J J, Montiel C. Predictive value of nuclear factor nB activity and plasma cytokine levels in patients with sepsis. *Infect. Immun.* 2000;68:1942–1945.

[54] Paterson R L, Galley H F, Dhillon J K, Webster N R. Increased nuclear factor nB activation in critically ill patients who die. *Crit. Care Med.* 2000;28:1047–1051.

[55] van Hees H W, Schellekens W J, Linkels M, Leenders F, Zoll J, Donders R, Dekhuijzen P R, van der Hoeven J G, Heunks L M. Plasma from septic shock patients induces loss of muscle protein. *Crit. Care* 2011;15:R233.

[56] Schaefer A, Unterberger C, Frankenberger M, Lohrum M, Staples K J, Werner T, Stunnenberg H, Ziegler-Heitbrock L. Mechanism of interferon-gamma mediated down-regulation of interleukin-10 gene expression. *Mol. Immunol.* 2009;46:1351–1359.

[57] Matsukawa A, Kaplan M H, Hogaboam C M, Lukacs N W, Kunel S L. Pivotol role of signal transducer and activator of transcription (STAT4) and STAT6 in the innate immune response during sepsis. *J. Exp. Med.* 2001;193:679–688.

[58] Horowitz J C, Rogers D S, Sharma V, Vittal R, White E S, Cui Z, Thannickal V J. Combinatorial activation of FAK and AKT by transforming growth factor-beta1 confers an anoikis-resistant phenotype to myofibroblasts. *Cell Signal* 2007;19:761–771.

[59] Celec P. Nuclear factor kappa B--molecular biomedicine: the next generation. Biomed Pharmacother 2004;58:365–371.

[60] Gauss K A, Nelson-Overton L K, Siemsen D W, Gao Y, DeLeo F R, Quinn M T. Role of NF-kappaB in transcriptional regulation of the phagocyte NADPH oxidase by tumor necrosis factor-alpha. *J. Leukoc. Biol.* 2007;82:729–741.

[61] Tanaka H, Hoshikawa Y, Oh-hara T, Koike S, Naito M, Noda T, Arai H, Tsuruo T, Fujita N. PRMT5, a novel TRAIL receptor-binding protein, inhibits TRAIL-induced apoptosis via nuclear factor-kappaB activation. *Mol. Cancer Res.* 2009;7:557-569.

[62] Disse J, Vitale N, Bader M F, Gerke V. Phospholipase D1 is specifically required for regulated secretion of von Willebrand factor from endothelial cells. *Blood* 2009;113:973–980.

[63] Millar T M, Phan V, Tibbles L A. ROS generation in endothelial hypoxia and reoxygenation stimulates MAP kinase signaling and kinase-dependent neutrophil recruitment. *Free Radic. Biol. Med.* 2007;42:1165–1177.

[64] Reinhart K, Meisner M, Brunkhorst FM."Markers for sepsis diagnosis: what is useful?" *Critical Care Clinics* 2006;22:503–519.

[65] Uzzan B, Cohen R, Nicolas P, Cucherat M, Perret GY. Procalcitonin as a diagnostic test for sepsis in critically ill adults and after surgery or trauma: a systematic review and meta-analysis. *Crit. Care Med.* 2006;34:1996– 2003.

[66] Tang B M, Eslick G D, Craig J C, McLean A S. Accuracy of procalcitonin for sepsis diagnosis in critically ill patients: systematic review and meta-analysis. *Lancet Infect. Dis.* 2007;7:210–217.

[67] Meynaar I A, Droog W, Batstra M, Vreede R, Herbrink P. In Critically Ill Patients, Serum Procalcitonin Is More Useful in Differentiating between Sepsis and SIRS than CRP, Il-6, or LBP. *Crit. Care Res. Pract.* 2011;2011:594645.

[68] Preas H L, Nylen E S, Snider R H, Becker K L, White J C, Agosti J M, Suffredini A F. Effects of anti-inflammatory agents on serum levels of calcitonin precursors during human experimental endotoxaemia. *J. Infect. Dis.* 2001;184: 373–376.

[69] Jensen J U, Hein L, Lundgren B, Bestle M H, Mohr T T, Andersen M H, Thornberg K J, Løken J, Steensen M, Fox Z, Tousi H, Søe-Jensen P, Lauritsen AØ, Strange D, Petersen PL, Reiter N, Hestad S, Thormar K, Fjeldborg P, Larsen K M, Drenck N E, Ostergaard C, Kjær J, Grarup J, Lundgren J D. Procalcitonin And Survival Study (PASS) Group. Procalcitonin-guided interventions against infections to increase early appropriate antibiotics and improve survival in the intensive care unit: a randomized trial. *Crit. Care Med.* 2011;39:2048–2058.

[70] Bouadma L, Luyt C E, Tubach F Cracco C, Alvarez A, Schwebel C, Schortgen F, Lasocki S, Veber B, Dehoux M, Bernard M, Pasquet B, Régnier B, Brun-Buisson C, Chastre J, Wolff M; PRORATA trial group. Use of procalcitonin to reduce patients' exposure to antibiotics in intensive care units (PRORATA trial): a multicentre randomised controlled trial. *Lancet* 2010;375:463–474.

[71] Abidi K, Khoudri I, Belayachi J, Madani N, Zekraoui A, Zeggwagh A A, Abouqal R. Eosinopenia is a reliable marker of sepsis on admission to medical intensive care units. *Crit. Care* 2008,12:R59.

[72] Hoffmann U, Bertsch T, Dvortsak E Liebetrau C, Lang S, Liebe V, Huhle G, Borggrefe M, Brueckmann M. Matrix-metalloproteinases and their inhibitors are elevated in severe sepsis: prognostic value of TIMP-1 in severe sepsis. *Scand. J. Infect. Dis.* 2006;38:867–872.

In: Oxidative Stress and the Critically Ill Patient
Editors: Ramón Rodrigo and Bettina von Dessauer
ISBN: 978-1-62081-576-2

Chapter IV

MITOCHONDRIAL DYSFUNCTION

Víctor Molina
Faculty of Medicine, University of Chile, Chile

ABSTRACT

Adequate mitochondrial function is essential for proper cell and organ performance. Critically ill patients are exposed to a variety of conditions likely to result in mitochondrial malfunctioning. In the past years most of the therapeutic measures applied to these patients were focused on increasing the oxygen delivery to tissues by treating hypoxemia, shock, anemia and other related conditions. However, it became progressively clear that in some cases impairment in oxygen utilization, rather that inadequate oxygen delivery was a more relevant issue. This phenomenon was called 'cytopathic hypoxia'. From this finding, numerous studies, particularly related with sepsis, have provided evidence pointing to a major role of mitochondrial dysfunction as a common feature of the deleterious conditions contributing to disease progression and organ damage. In turn, mitochondrial dysfunction and its maintenance could arise from the effects of increased reactive oxygen and nitrogen species. Oxidative stress, a consequence consistent with mitochondrial dysfunction, could give rise to further mitochondrial damage, thus constituting a self-sustaining cycle. Consequently, bioenergetic derangement, apoptosis and oxidative stress may result. Accordingly, in the last years a lot of attention has been paid to the potential therapeutic utility of mitochondria-directed antioxidant therapy. Available promising data have been obtained from animal models, but large-scale studies in humans are still lacking.

ABBREVIATIONS

ADP	adenosine diphosphate
AIF	apoptosis-inducing factor
APAF-1	apoptosis protease-activating factor 1
ATP	adenosine triphosphate

CLP	cecal ligation and puncture
CoQ	coenzyme Q or ubiquinone
Cyt-c	cytochrome c
DD	death domain
DIABLO	direct inhibitors of apoptosis proteins binding protein with low isoionic point
DISC	death-inducing signaling complex
DR	death receptor
FAD	flavin adenine dinucleotide
$FADH_2$	reduced flavin adenine dinucleotide
FMN	flavin mononucleotide
GSH	glutathione
H^-	hydride anion
H^+	hydrogen proton
H_2O_2	oxygen peroxide
HIF-1	hypoxia inducible factor-1
IAP	inhibitors of apoptosis proteins
iNOS	inducible nitric oxide synthase isoform
LPS	lipopolysaccharide
MODS	multiple organ dysfunction syndrome
MOMP	mitochondrial outer membrane permeabilization
mtNOS	mitochondrial nitric oxide synthase isoform
NADH	reduced nicotinamide adenine dinucleotide
$NO^\bullet$	nitric oxide
NOS	nitric oxide synthase
O_2	molecular oxygen
$O_2^{\bullet-}$	superoxide
$ONOO^-$	peroxynitrite
PARP	poly ADP-ribose polymerase
RET	reverse electron transfer
RNS	reactive nitrogen species
ROS	reactive oxygen species
Smac	second mitochondria-derived activator of caspases
SOD	superoxide dismutase
TNF	tumor necrosis factor
TNFR1	tumor necrosis factor receptor 1
TPP	triphenylphosphonium
TRAIL	tumor necrosis factor-related apoptosis-inducing ligand

1. INTRODUCTION

Normal cell functioning requires the occurrence of hundreds of chemical reactions, a lot of them being endergonic, which require the addition of energy to proceed. Endergonic reactions need to be coupled with other energetically favorable (exergonic) reactions. Cells rely on the existence of molecules that store energy in covalent bonds, such as adenosine triphosphate (ATP). A large number of reactions within cells depend on the energy that is liberated from the hydrolysis of the terminal pyrophosphate bond of ATP, yielding adenosine diphosphate (ADP) and inorganic phosphate. A continuous ATP production is crucial for most of cells, and conditions in which ATP generation is compromised are highly deleterious.

Cells use nutrients as source of energy, being carbohydrates and lipids the primary source for the production of ATP. The major products of glycolysis and the citric acid cycle are reduced forms of *nicotinamide adenine dinucleotide* (NADH) and *flavin adenine dinucleotide* ($FADH_2$). In addition, acetyl-CoA as a product of fatty acid beta-oxidation can also enter the citric acid cycle. NADH and $FADH_2$ are strong reducing agents (*i.e.* easily donate electrons), whereas molecular oxygen (O_2) is a potent oxidizing agent (*i.e.* easily gains electrons).

In consequence, the reaction between NADH (or $FADH_2$) and O_2 can release large amounts of energy. In order to effectively capture the released energy in the form of ATP, electrons are transferred sequentially through a series of stages, producing intermediate compounds ("electron carriers") with progressively lower reduction potential.

This process is known as ***oxidative phosphorylation***, occurring within the inner mitochondrial membrane through the coordination of an electron transport chain, the generation of a proton gradient and the action of the ATP synthase. Alternatively, ATP generation can take place in anaerobic conditions through fermentation, which is a highly inefficient and potentially harmful process able to produce lactic acidosis.

Mitochondrial function in critically ill patients can be impaired as a consequence of various mechanisms. In this chapter, the involvement of reactive oxygen species (ROS) and reactive nitrogen species (RNS) in the development of mitochondrial dysfunction is reviewed. Potential therapeutic implications are discussed.

2. Mitochondrial Physiology and Pathophysiology

Mitochondria are present in almost every eukaryotic cell. Their quantity and distribution are variable depending on the specific cell type and function. These organelles are delimited by an outer and an inner membrane. The inner membrane defines the mitochondrial matrix, and both membranes delimit the intermembrane space.

The outer membrane contains integral proteins called porins, which form channels that allow a free diffusion of ions and small molecules between the intermembrane space and the cytosol. The inner membrane is highly impermeable, permitting the maintenance of a proton gradient between the matrix and the intermembrane space.

The inner membrane has folds, or *cristae*, that increase its surface, and contains a number of transporters and the enzyme complexes that constitute the electron transport chain. A detailed review of mitochondrial physiology is not the purpose of this chapter, however, a general overview of oxidative phosphorylation is offered and some of the relevant cellular processes in which mitochondria participates are discussed. Participation of reactive species in these processes is reviewed.

Oxidative Phosphorylation

The final product of glycolysis is pyruvate. Pyruvate is transported to the mitochondrial matrix where it is used as substrate for acetil-CoA production, which enters the citric acid cycle yielding NADH and $FADH_2$. From these molecules hydride anion (H^-) is released, then splitting into a proton (H^+) and two electrons. Electrons move through the electron transport chain towards lower energy states, ultimately reacting with H^+ and O_2 to form water. As it is discussed later, the energy that is liberated from electrons is used for the maintenance of an electrochemical proton gradient, which in turn is taken advantage of by ATP synthase for ATP production.

The electron transfer chain consists in four multi-subunit complexes with different enzymatic activity: NADH-coenzyme Q reductase (complex I), succinate-coenzyme Q oxidoreductase (complex II), ubiquinol-cytochrome c oxidoreductase (complex III), and cytochrome c oxidase (complex IV). Also, two mobile molecules participate in oxidative phosphorylation: coenzyme Q (CoQ, also known as ubiquinone) and cytochrome c (Cyt-c). There are other alternative proteins having electron transfer activity in the inner mitochondrial membrane, but their contribution to the oxidative phosphorylation process is of less importance in animal cells.

Complex I catalyzes the transference of electrons from NADH to CoQ. The bovine enzyme consists in 46 subunits and has a molecular mass of approximately 1,000 KDa, being the largest of the four complexes. This enzyme has a dehydrogenase domain that binds NADH, a hydrogenase domain that reduces CoQ, and a transporter domain involved in proton pumping from the matrix to the intermembrane space. Electrons are transferred initially to flavin mononucleotide (FMN), and then to a series of iron-sulfur clusters until finally reducing CoQ. This process results in the translocation of 4 protons per NADH consumed.

Complex II participates in the citric acid cycle by catalyzing the oxidation of succinate to fumarate. It is a ubiquinone-reducing enzyme anchored to the membrane by two hydrophobic subunits. Following succinate oxidation, complex II transfers electrons through flavin adenine dinucleotide (FAD) and several iron-sulfur clusters to CoQ, this way contributing to the reduced-CoQ pool. Complex II does not participate in proton gradient creation.

Complex III (or cytochrome bc_1 complex) catalyzes the transfer of electrons from reduced CoQ to water-soluble Cyt-c. It has tree subunits with redox prosthetic groups: cytochrome b subunit, cytochrome c_1 subunit and an iron-sulfur protein. The activity of this enzyme results in proton translocation to the intermembrane space and reduction of Cyt-c.

Complex IV is a heme-copper oxygen reductase that catalyzes the oxidation of Cyt-c and the reduction of O_2 to water, a process that also results in proton translocation. This enzyme is potently inhibited by cyanide, carbon monoxide and nitric oxide ($NO^•$).

ATP synthase is also known as complex V. It is composed of a membrane extrinsic catalytic-F_1 sector and a transmembrane F_0 sector. The activity of this enzyme results in ATP synthesis from ADP and inorganic phosphate. The energy for ATP production is obtained from the proton electrochemical gradient that is generated by complexes I, III and IV. Translocation of protons produces a conformational change of the catalytic site, thus releasing ATP.

Sources of Reactive Species in Mitochondria

Mitochondria are a well-recognized site of ROS and RNS production. During electron transference, a number of electrons "leak" prematurely to oxygen, generating ROS. It is estimated that up to 1-2% of mitochondrial O_2 consumption is used for ROS generation. However, this estimation was done under artificial non-physiological conditions. In healthy tissues, mitochondrial ROS production might account for a lower fraction of the oxygen consumption.

Despite this consideration, mitochondria are a major source of superoxide ($O_2^{\bullet -}$) production through the one-electron reduction of O_2. Up to nine different enzymes are involved in mitochondrial ROS production including complexes I, II and III.

Experimental approaches using sub-mitochondrial particles have shown that complex I is a major site of mitochondrial ROS production [1]. Superoxide and oxygen peroxide (H_2O_2) generation occurs in complex I through a variety of processes still not fully understood. Superoxide arises from the reaction of fully reduced FMN with O_2 and the proportion of fully reduced FMN depends on the NADH/NAD$^+$ ratio [1]. Thus, any condition causing an increase of NADH can potentially lead to ROS formation.

Additionally, another process involved in complex I-ROS production is reverse electron transfer (RET). Under conditions of high electrochemical proton gradient and elevated levels of reduced CoQ, electron flux can revert from CoQ through complex I, a process that produces large amounts of $O_2^{\bullet -}$ and H_2O_2 [2].

Complex III is another known site of ROS production. Superoxide from complex III is released both to the mitochondrial matrix and to the intermembrane space. Considerable effort has been devoted to study the mechanism of $O_2^{\bullet -}$ production within complex III. It is accepted that $O_2^{\bullet -}$ arises from the reaction between O_2 and a ubisemiquinone (the partial oxidation product of reduced CoQ) [3]. Although in physiological conditions ROS generation in complex III is minimal compared to that in complex I, this could change under pathological conditions [2].

Nitric oxide is produced by a family of NADPH-dependent enzymes that are known as nitric oxide synthases (NOS). Mitochondria have their own NOS isoform (mtNOS) within the inner mitochondrial membrane and this way are able to produce NO$^\bullet$ [4]. In addition, in experimental models of sepsis the inducible NOS isoform (iNOS) has been identified in mitochondria [5]. As in other subcellular compartments, NO$^\bullet$ can react with $O_2^{\bullet -}$ and produce peroxynitrite (ONOO$^-$). Nitric oxide has many regulatory functions in mitochondria. Nitric oxide binds to cytochrome c oxidase (complex IV) and competes with O_2, this way inhibiting oxidative phosphorylation [6]. Additionally, ONOO$^-$ can inhibit complex I by producing nitrosylation and nitration modifications [7]. Through this mechanisms mtNOS activity could modulate mitochondrial O_2 consumption and uptake in different physiological and pathophysiological conditions, such as hypothyroidism [7]. In addition to the direct effects of NO$^\bullet$ and ONOO$^-$, these reactive species can promote ROS production indirectly by increasing the reduced forms of the electron transport chain components as a consequence of complex IV inhibition, and also by inhibiting electron transference in complex III, which in turn increases the levels of ubisemiquinone [8]. Moreover, reduction of complex IV affinity for O_2, such as induced by NO$^\bullet$, may locally increase O_2 availability for ROS production even in hypoxic conditions.

Accumulation of ROS or RNS within mitochondria can lead to mitochondrial dysfunction through the previously referred mechanisms and oxidative damage of lipids, proteins and DNA (for a detailed description of oxidative damage refer to chapter 1). In order to prevent this damage, mitochondria have an antioxidant defense system similar to that of the rest of the cell, involving enzymatic and non-enzymatic mechanisms.

This system includes the presence of α-tocopherol, glutathione (GSH), superoxide dismutase (SOD), catalase, peroxiredoxins and glutathione peroxidases [3]. Although there are some particularities to be noticed, for a specific review of the antioxidant defense system the reader is referred to chapter 1. Mitochondria lack of a GSH production system, but instead of that have a GSH uptake mechanism. It is also important to point out that mitochondria have their own specific SOD (MnSOD), which further supports the notion of a continuous $O_2^{\bullet-}$ production and the need for specific mitochondrial antioxidant defenses.

Mitochondria as an Oxygen Sensor

The rate of ROS production depends on the concentration of the participating enzyme, the proportion of the reduced form of the electron carrier and O_2 concentration. The latter is of particular importance because $O_2^{\bullet-}$ production increases along with the increase in mitochondrial O_2 concentration, which could explain in part the oxidative damage occurring in lungs exposed to high levels of O_2, as extrapolated from animal models.

The effect of a reduction in O_2 concentration is less straightforward. Several studies have shown an increase in mitochondrial ROS production in response to hypoxia [9]. Most of these studies focused on the function and activity of a hypoxia inducible factor-1 (HIF-1). Sensed changes in O_2 concentration can modulate the activity of HIF-1, a transcription factor that participates in adaptive responses to hypoxia, such as angiogenesis and erythropoiesis. This factor is a heterodimer composed by subunits HIF-1α and HIF-1β. HIF-1α expression is increased during hypoxia; however, the main regulatory mechanism is post-translational. Under normoxia, HIF-1α is hydroxylated in proline residues by prolyl hydroxylase using 2-oxoglutarate and O_2, which leads to ubiquitin labeling and degradation. During hypoxia, HIF-1α is no longer hydroxylated and in consequence does not undergo degradation. A functional electron transport chain is required for this response in hypoxia, but not for the stabilization of HIF-1α in anoxic conditions [10], which indicates that there is probably an alternative mechanism of O_2 sensing and HIF-1α stabilization.

It has been proposed that ROS may participate in the regulation of this factor. When using a model of hypoxia, cells depleted of mitochondrial DNA fail to produce ROS and activate HIF-1, an ability that is recovered through alternative mechanisms of ROS generation [11]. The effects of $NO^{\bullet}$ on HIF-1 activity are less clear. Nitric oxide is known to be an inhibitor of 2-oxoglutarate-dependent oxygenases.

Accordingly, there are studies that show activation of HIF-1 by $NO^{\bullet}$ donors [12]. However, these results are not in agreement with other studies reporting the contrary effect [13]. This discrepancy could be explained as a phenomenon in part due to the redistribution of O_2 in conditions of a $NO^{\bullet}$ inhibition of complex IV, this way preventing hypoxia sensing by prolyl hydroxylase. Furthermore, a dichotomic effect in HIF-1 activity has been attributed to $NO^{\bullet}$, depending on its concentration and the presence of a functional electron transport chain [14].

Overall, the current evidence supports the existence of probably more than one pathway for transcriptional activity regulation in response to changes in O_2 concentration. Mitochondria- produced reactive oxygen and nitrogen species are probably involved in this process, but the exact means by which this occurs remain to be determined. The mechanisms accounting for increased ROS production during hypoxia are also still not clear. Complex III arises as a possible important source of ROS during hypoxia, along with the previously referred effects of $NO^{\bullet}$-mediated complex IV inhibition and redistribution of O_2 towards sources of ROS within mitochondria.

Role of Mitochondria in Apoptosis

Apoptosis is the process of non-inflammatory and programmed cell death. Its occurrence is of vital importance for numerous physiological processes in multicellular organisms. The activation of apoptotic pathways leads ultimately to cell death through the activation of specific proteases called caspases. Apoptosis can be initiated through several mitochondrial independent and dependent pathways. Cellular apoptotic changes include DNA fragmentation, chromatin condensation, membrane blebbing, cytoskeletal scaffold proteins degradation, cell shrinkage and disassembly into membrane-enclosed vesicles. This process finishes with the removal of death cells by phagocytes, which does not involve an inflammatory response.

Apoptosis mechanisms have been classified in an extrinsic and an intrinsic mitochondria-associated pathway. Both pathways involve the activation of *initiator caspases,* which in turn activate the *effector caspases,* whose action leads to cell death. The extrinsic pathway initiates with the binding of a protein ligand to a surface transmembrane receptor (death receptor, DR). Several DRs and ligands have been characterized, but the best known are Fas-Fas ligand, tumor necrosis factor (TNF) receptor 1 (TNFR1), TNF-related apoptosis-inducing ligand (TRAIL) receptor 1 and TRAIL receptor 2. Death receptors have a cytoplasmic death domain (DD) that upon activation by its ligand initiates the recruitment of signaling molecules. Fas receptor activation results in recruiting of Fas-associated DD (FADD) protein and procaspase-8, leading to the formation of the death-inducing signaling complex (DISC) which in turn activates caspase-8. TNF-α binding to TNFR1 activates a similar pathway. The extent of caspase-8 activation will determine the following pathway. In cells where caspase-8 activation is strong, the type I apoptotic pathway is followed, with downstream activation of caspase-3 and other effector caspases such as caspase-6 and caspase-7. When caspase-8 activity is not strong enough for a direct activation of effector caspases, amplification of the death signal is achieved by following the type II-mitochondrial dependent (intrinsic) pathway, which will be reviewed in detail.

The mitochondrial apoptotic pathway was first identified as an alternative pathway that involved mitochondrial damage including structural changes, mitochondrial depolarization and release of Cyt-c. Releasing of Cyt-c and other molecules is crucial to proceed and occurs as a consequence of a process known as mitochondrial outer membrane permeabilization (MOMP). The occurrence of MOMP releases molecules that activate the caspase cascade and also compromises mitochondrial function, contributing to cell death. Two models are proposed for MOMP, the first one including the participation of BCL-2 family proteins in the formation of large pores within the outer mitochondrial membrane. The second (less characterized) mechanism involves the generation of a permeability transition pore in the inner mitochondrial membrane, leading to mitochondrial swelling and outer mitochondrial membrane rupture.

The BCL-2 (B-cell lymphoma-2) family consists of proteins that regulate apoptosis, including both antagonists and agonists. These proteins have classically been grouped in three classes. One class is composed of multi-domain apoptosis-inhibitor proteins (BCL-2, BCL-XL, BCL-W, MCL1, BCL-B and A1), whereas a second class includes apoptosis agonists (BAX, BAK and BOK). A third class is formed by proteins that share homology with the other two classes only through a short BH3 (Bcl-2 homology region 3) motif, the so called BH3-only proteins (BAD, BIK, BID, HRK, BIM, BMF, NOXA and PUMA). BAX and BAK are crucial for MOMP development and are usually inhibited by anti-apoptotic BCL-2 family members. BH3-only proteins can derepress BAX and BAK by inhibiting anti-apoptotic proteins or through its direct activation.

A number of processes can modulate apoptosis by modification of BH3-only proteins activation and by expression of BCL-2 family proteins, including growth factor deprivation, DNA damage, viral infections, radiation, toxins and others. The link between the extrinsic and intrinsic pathways occurs through these mechanisms. As referred previously, in type II cells caspase-8 activation is weak and amplification of the death signal through a mitochondria-dependent pathway is required. Caspase-8 cleaves BID (a BH3-only protein), generating an active fragment (tBID) that can directly activate BAX, leading to membrane permeabilization. Alteration of mitochondrial permeability allows the release of Cyt-c to the cytoplasm, along with other molecules such as apoptosis-inducing factor (AIF) and Smac/DIABLO (second mitochondria-derived activator of caspases/direct IAP binding protein with low isoionic point). Cytochrome c induces multimerization of apoptosis protease-activating factor (APAF-1) forming the apoptosome that activates caspase-9, which in turn activates effector caspase-3 and caspase-7. AIF is a flavoprotein with NADH oxidase activity that upon release from mitochondria translocates to the nucleus where it promotes chromatin condensation and DNA degradation. Inhibitors of apoptosis proteins (IAP) normally prevent the progression of this process by inhibiting caspase activation. Smac/DIABLO promotes apoptosis through the inhibition of IAP. Developing of MOMP can also compromise cell function through the bioenergetic derangement produced by loss of the proton electrochemical gradient and of Cyt-c for oxidative phosphorylation. Additionally, these conditions uncouple the electron transfer chain, thereby leading to ROS production.

Reactive oxygen species are known modulators of apoptosis. These reactive species increase in response to pro-apoptotic signals and are potent inducers of apoptosis. A detailed review is recommended for a deeper analysis of ROS participation in apoptosis [15]. The exact pathways by which ROS mediate apoptosis are still not fully clarified, although identified ROS-mediated processes include alteration of mitochondrial membrane permeability, mitochondrial DNA oxidative damage and caspase activity modulation.

3. Mitochondrial Dysfunction

Critically ill patients are exposed to a variety of conditions that can impair mitochondrial function. Any situation in which the oxygen delivery to mitochondria is impaired can potentially alter ATP production. Thus, common pathophysiological causes of shock, such as hypovolemia, reduced cardiac output and vascular tone impairment can impede appropriate mitochondrial functioning. This is also the case of conditions characterized by insufficient pulmonary oxygen exchange (e.g., pneumonia and acute respiratory distress syndrome) or other causes of low arterial O_2 content or transport ability, such as anemia and carbon monoxide poisoning. It is therefore not surprising that the goal of the therapeutic measures used in critically ill patients focused simply on improving O_2 delivery to the tissues. However, improving O_2 delivery in some cases has been shown to be ineffective or even detrimental. This phenomenon has been studied mainly in patients suffering from severe sepsis, but many of these mechanisms can also be occurring in other types of critically ill patients. Although contradictory evidence exists, there are many studies showing that in some cases of severe sepsis normal or even supranormal tissue O_2 tensions can be found, despite of which mitochondrial function can be compromised. It has been hypothesized that in these patients an impaired cellular O_2 utilization, rather than an altered O_2 delivery, is a more important feature, a condition that has been called *cytopathic hypoxia.* According to the current evidence, the impairment in O_2 utilization could be related to modulation and damage of key mitochondrial components, leading to what is known as mitochondrial dysfunction.

3.1. Evidence Supporting the Occurrence of Mitochondrial Dysfunction in Sepsis

Many advances have been achieved in the understanding of sepsis pathophysiology (see chapter 2: pathophysiology of sepsis and septic shock). Specifically, a large body of evidence supports a role of oxidative stress in this condition. Since mitochondria are a known source of ROS and mitochondrial dysfunction is a recognized feature of severe sepsis, an increasing attention is being paid to the role of oxidative stress in the dysfunction of this organelle and in sepsis progression towards multiple organ dysfunction syndrome (MODS) [16, 17].

Although most of the related research has been performed in sepsis models, mitochondrial dysfunction probably participates also in many non-infectious inflammatory critical conditions. Some of the, in our opinion, most representative evidence regarding the potential role of mitochondrial dysfunction in sepsis is discussed next. For a deeper understanding of the extensive literature on this subject, the reader is referred to a specific comprehensive review [18].

Mitochondrial dysfunction in sepsis has been evaluated in multiple animal models. In a model of cecal ligation and puncture (CLP) induced sepsis in mice, complex IV activity was evaluated in heart ventricle tissue, showing an early (6 h) competitive inhibition of cytochrome c oxidase, followed later (48 h) by a non-competitive inhibition, which associated also to a decrease in heme a,a_3 content [19]. However, in a rat model of endotoxemia that assessed myocardial function in an *ex vivo* design, early mitochondrial dysfunction (2 h) was not associated with mitochondrial damage, reduced complex IV activity or expression of apoptosis mediators [20].

These apparently contradictory results could be explained by the different timing of mitochondrial function evaluation. Furthermore, the results of the first referred study could be explained by an early inhibition of cytochrome c oxidase by $NO^{\bullet}$, through its extensively recognized capacity of competing with O_2. Later, oxidative damage of mitochondrial DNA could be participating in the impairment of electron transport chain components production, as discussed later.

In another model of CLP-induced sepsis in rats, mitochondrial function was shown to be impaired in the muscle after 6 days of sepsis. In addition, mitochondrial cytochromes concentration (a, b and c) was decreased in muscle, but not in the liver [21]. In contrast, a model of endotoxemia in pigs showed impaired mitochondrial function in liver after 24 h of endotoxin infusion, but not in kidney or skeletal muscle (quadriceps) [22]. In an endotoxemia rat model, reduced mitochondrial consumption of O_2 and also depletion of electron transport chain components in different subunits of complex I, III, IV and ATP synthase was observed in diaphragm muscle [23].

In an endotoxemia model performed in cats, injection of lipopolysaccharide (LPS) resulted in hepatic mitochondrial ultrastructural injury and dysfunction, along with electron transport chain uncoupling, even in absence of tissue hypoxia [24]. On the contrary, other studies have shown a paradoxical increase in liver mitochondrial function in rats after CLP-induced sepsis, associated with a reduction on hepatocyte O_2 consumption.

These results could be attributed to the selective mitochondrial isolation technique that was used, which could select a subset of more active mitochondria [25]. Similar animal models of endotoxemia have shown evidence of mitochondrial dysfunction in intestine, an organ that is known to be early compromised in sepsis, especially in conditions of hemodynamic instability.

In a rat model of endotoxemia, intestinal mucosal cells showed reduced mitochondrial function that was reverted by an iNOS inhibitor, supporting a role of $NO^{\bullet}$ in septic intestinal mitochondrial dysfunction [26]. Accordingly, endotoxic rats show less O_2 consumption in intestinal mucosa, an effect that is reverted by treatment with an iNOS inhibitor [27].

The pathophysiological mechanisms accounting for brain injury during sepsis are still unknown. Mitochondrial dysfunction has been considered a possible candidate. In a rat model of CLP-induced sepsis a decrease of mitochondrial complex I activity, but not of the other complexes, was observed in different brain structures: hippocampus, cerebellum, cortex and striatum [28].

In a similar CLP-induced sepsis model in mice, assessing of mitochondrial function in brain homogenates showed evidence of mitochondrial electron transport chain uncoupling according to an increased proportion of O_2 not being used for ATP production. Also, a reduced mitochondrial membrane potential, a decreased content of cytochromes and an inhibition of complex IV activity were observed. Interestingly, less H_2O_2 production was also seen, which the authors relate to the impaired electrochemical potential [29].

The participation of mitochondrial dysfunction in septic-organ damage has been less studied in human models, apart from indirect measurements of oxygen consumption [18]. Two recent studies investigated the presence of mitochondrial dysfunction in muscle tissue of patients with sepsis. Brealey *et al.* evaluated mitochondrial function in vastus lateralis muscle samples of critically ill septic patients, showing a reduction of ATP in patients who died, in relation to those who survived and controls [30].

In addition, complex I activity was inversely correlated to norepinephrine requirement and nitrite/nitrate concentrations, and positively correlated with ATP and reduced GSH concentrations. These findings further support the possibility of a role of mitochondrial dysfunction in severity progression and of $NO^{\bullet}$ in mitochondrial dysfunction.

Accordingly, Fredriksson et al. assessed mitochondrial complexes I and IV activity in intercostal and vastus lateralis muscle of septic patients with MODS [31]. Intercostal muscle showed less activity of complex I, while in vastus lateralis a reduced activity of complex IV was observed. Furthermore, vastus lateralis had lower concentration of ATP and higher concentration of lactate, which was not observed in intercostal muscle.

The authors conclude that these muscles respond differently to the septic insult through an unknown mechanism that could include the passive stretching of intercostal muscle during mechanical ventilation, that could result in improved blood flow, or an improved 'protection' of respiratory muscles.

3.2. Possible Mechanisms of Mitochondrial Dysfunction in Sepsis

As discussed in chapter 2, the inflammatory response in sepsis is associated with a large liberation of inflammatory mediators, one of them being TNF-α. This cytokine can induce cellular damage through apoptotic pathways that include caspase activation but also by MOMP-induced uncoupling of the mitochondrial electron transport chain. Apoptosis seems to be a prominent feature in septic cellular damage, since its inhibition through BCL-2 overexpression results in better survival in an animal model of sepsis [32].

TNF-α stimulation of sphingomyelinase produces ceramide, which is an important mediator of the apoptotic signaling pathway but also an independent stimulator of mitochondrial ROS production [33]. Ceramide co-localizes with BAX to liver mitochondria, being involved in mitochondrial membrane permeabilization [34] and in apoptosis [35]. Accordingly, ceramide has been proposed as a predictor of progression in sepsis, since the occurrence of MODS associates to high levels of peripheral mononuclear cells ceramide concentration [36].

Another proposed mechanism of indirect mitochondrial function impairment in sepsis is pyruvate dehydrogenase inhibition. In sepsis, pyruvate dehydrogenase activity has been shown to be reduced, a phenomenon that deviates pyruvate from entering the citric acid cycle to the production of lactic acid, contributing to mitochondrial dysfunction (due to reduced substrate offer), and to the hyperlactacidemia that is seen in these patients [37].

Oxidative stress is a known pathophysiologic event of severe sepsis. Besides mitochondrial function impairment, ROS can induce cellular damage through oxidative modifications of proteins, lipids and DNA. Indeed, besides their previously referred role in the regulation of apoptosis and oxidative phosphorylation impairment, ROS-mediated mitochondrial DNA damage can compromise the correct expression of genes encoding for electron transport chain enzymes.

As a consequence, electron transport uncoupling might occur, giving rise to further ROS production and mitochondrial DNA damage, in a cycle known as the *mitochondrial catastrophe hypothesis* [38].

This mechanism could be involved in the downregulation of electron transport chain components expression that has been observed in an animal model of sepsis [23]. In addition, increased mtNOS isoforms activity during sepsis leads to overproduction of $NO^{\bullet}$ and of $ONOO^{-}$ through the reaction with $O_2^{\bullet -}$ [39], with nitration of proteins and inhibition of oxidative phosphorylation, as discussed. Indeed, in an animal model, $ONOO^{-}$ could mediate mitochondrial dysfunction in muscle during sepsis [40]. However, a potential role in adaptation to sepsis has been attributed to $NO^{\bullet}$, since $ONOO^{-}$ can induce single-strand breaks in nuclear DNA, thereby activating poly (ADP-ribose) polymerase (PARP), an enzyme involved in DNA reparation.

Since PARP uses NAD^{+} as substrate, its over-activation can produce a depletion of NAD^{+}/NADH, leading to reduced oxidative phosphorylation activity through a decrease in complex I substrate, with less O_2 consumption and eventually lesser ROS production [41].

Although the exact mechanisms of mitochondrial dysfunction in sepsis are still not fully understood, it seems that oxidative stress plays a central role and is a final effector of many of these referred mitochondrial-damage pathways. The possible mechanisms accounting for mitochondrial dysfunction are summarized in figure 1.

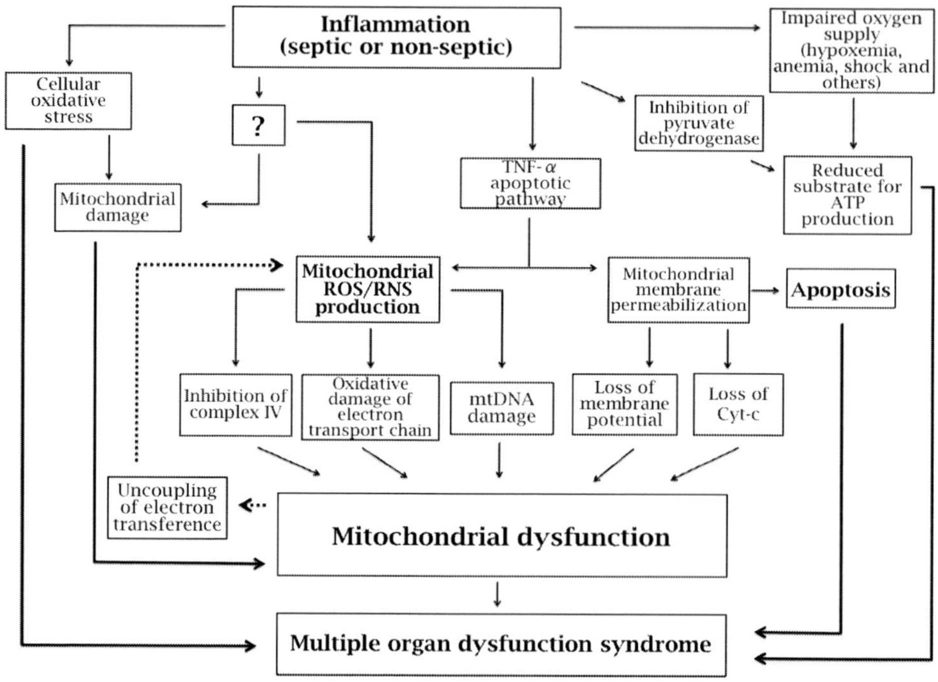

Figure 1. Possible mechanisms accounting for mitochondrial dysfunction. The dotted arrow depicts the production of ROS and RNS through electron transport chain uncoupling in mitochondrial dysfunction, configuring a self-sustaining and self-amplifying cycle. The question mark represents unknown mechanisms that can lead to mild mitochondrial damage or dysfunction, later being reinforced by the previously referred mechanism. ROS, reactive oxygen species; RNS, reactive nitrogen species; TNF-α, tumor necrosis factor alpha; ATP, adenosine triphosphate; Cyt-c, cytochrome c; mtDNA, mitochondrial DNA.

4.1. Mitochondria-Directed Antioxidant Based Therapies

Overall, the available evidence supports an important role of oxidative stress in sepsis. However, antioxidant-based therapeutic interventions have failed to show a considerable improvement in the clinical outcome of septic patients. Although this type of strategies is still being evaluated, the abundant evidence pointing to ROS-mediated mitochondrial dysfunction in sepsis suggests that antioxidant-based therapies directed specifically to mitochondria could be more successful. During the last years many researchers have focused in mitochondria-targeted antioxidant therapy with promising results.

A detailed review on this subject exceeds the scope of this chapter, so for this matter the reader is referred to comprehensive articles [17, 42]. Antioxidants can be targeted to mitochondria by using a specific carrier molecule, by administering an antioxidant that accumulates naturally within mitochondria or by modulating the activity of the endogenous antioxidant system. Other explored therapeutic strategies involve the supplementation with oxidative phosphorylation substrates and cofactors, such as L-carnitine, succinate, CoQ and Cyt-c [42]. Also, the use of mitochondrial membrane stabilizers such as cyclosporine A has been proposed [43]. Lipophilic cations can accumulate in mitochondria according to the negative mitochondrial membrane potential. One of these cations is triphenylphosphonium (TPP), which can be attached to CoQ and to tocopherol to form MitoQ and MitoVitE, respectively. This strategy has been evaluated in animal models of sepsis with promising results [44]. The compound TEMPOL is a ROS scavenger that can penetrate mitochondrial membranes. In an animal model of sepsis, TEMPOL attenuated organ damage and mitochondrial dysfunction [45]. Another potential mitochondria-directed therapy is the use of small positively charged peptides with ROS-scavenger capacity, which are known as 'SS peptides'. These peptides accumulate within mitochondria and can prevent oxidative damage in neurodegenerative disorders and ischemia-reperfusion injury models [46]. Additionally, α-lipoic acid is an organosulfur compound that is taken up and reduced within mitochondria to dihydrolipoate, which has ROS-scavenging properties. Treatment with α-lipoic acid attenuated mitochondrial dysfunction in a rat model of endotoxemia [47]. Finally, melatonin arises as a promising therapy for mitochondrial dysfunction. Melatonin is a lipophilic product of tryptophan that accumulates within mitochondria and has broad ROS and RNS scavenging capacity. In animal models of sepsis melatonin has been shown to reduce mtNOS expression and $NO^{\bullet}$ production [48], restore ATP production [49], reduce oxidative damage [50], and improve survival [51]. No large studies have been performed in humans, but favorable results have been obtained in a small series of melatonin treatment of septic newborns [52].

Conclusion

Mitochondrial dysfunction is a prominent pathophysiological feature of many diseases and critically ill conditions. In pathological conditions, mitochondrial production of reactive species can increase and overwhelm the antioxidant defense system, leading to mitochondrial oxidative stress. These insults can lead to loss of the membrane electrochemical potential, uncoupling of the electron transference and incapacity to properly restore damaged electron carriers, thus resulting in further reactive species production and further damage, constituting a self-sustaining and self-amplifying cycle. In addition, TNF-α, resulting from inflammatory process development, is able to activate apoptotic pathways and produce further mitochondrial dysfunction. Mitochondrial oxidative stress appears to be an inevitable consequence of all of these processes. Considering the large body of evidence sustaining a role of mitochondrial dysfunction in many diseases and the participation of reactive species in its genesis, a lot of attention is being paid to the designing of mitochondrial-directed antioxidant based therapies. This type of strategy has been explored in animal models with promising results, however, studies in humans are still lacking. This way, the potential use of mitochondria-directed antioxidants for these conditions in the clinical setting remains an open question.

References

[1] Hirst J, King MS, Pryde KR. The production of reactive oxygen species by complex I. *Biochem. Soc. Trans.* 2008; 36:976-980.

[2] Murphy MP. How mitochondria produce reactive oxygen species. *Biochem. J.* 2009; 417:1-13.

[3] Andreyev AY, Kushnareva YE, Starkov AA. Mitochondrial metabolism of reactive oxygen species. *Biochemistry (Mosc).* 2005; 70:200–214.

[4] Finocchietto PV, Franco MC, Holod S, Gonzalez AS, Converso DP, Antico Arciuch VG, Serra MP, Poderoso JJ, Carreras MC. Mitochondrial Nitric Oxide Synthase: A Masterpiece of Metabolic Adaptation, Cell Growth, Transformation, and Death. *Exp. Biol. Med. (Maywood).* 2009; 234:1020–1028.

[5] Lopez L, Escames G, Tapias V, Utrilla P, Leon J, Acuña-Castroviejo D. Identification of an inducible nitric oxide synthase in diaphragm mitochondria from septic mice: its relation with mitochondrial dysfunction and prevention by melatonin. *Int. J. Biochem. Cell Biol.* 2006; 38:267–278.

[6] Brown GC. Nitric oxide regulates mitochondrial respiration and cell functions by inhibiting cytochrome oxidase. *FEBS Lett.* 1995; 369:136–139.

[7] Franco MC, Antico Arciuch VG, Peralta JG, Galli S, Levisman D, López LM, Romorini L, Poderoso JJ, Carreras MC. Hypothyroid phenotype is contributed by mitochondrial complex I inactivation due to translocated neuronal nitric-oxide synthase. *J. Biol. Chem.* 2006; 281:4779–4786.

[8] Poderoso JJ, Carreras MC, Lisdero C, Riobó N, Schöpfer F, Boveris A. Nitric oxide inhibits electron transfer and increases superoxide radical production in rat heart mitochondria and submitochondrial particles. *Arch. Biochem. Biophys.* 1996; 328: 85–92.

[9] Hoffman DL, Salter JD, Brookes PS. Response of mitochondrial reactive oxygen species generation to steady-state oxygen tension: implications for hypoxic cell signaling. *Am. J. Physiol. Heart Circ. Physiol.* 2006; 292:H101–H108.

[10] Schroedl C, McClintock DS, Budinger GRS, Chandel NS. Hypoxic but not anoxic stabilization of HIF-1alpha requires mitochondrial reactive oxygen species. *Am. J. Physiol. Lung. Cell Mol. Physiol.* 2002; 283:L922–931.

[11] Chandel NS, Maltepe E, Goldwasser E, Mathieu CE, Simon MC, Schumacker PT. Mitochondrial reactive oxygen species trigger hypoxia-induced transcription. *Proc. Natl. Acad. Sci. U.S.A.* 1998; 95:11715–11720.

[12] Metzen E, Zhou J, Jelkmann W, Fandrey J, Brüne B. Nitric oxide impairs normoxic degradation of HIF-1alpha by inhibition of prolyl hydroxylases. *Mol. Biol. Cell.* 2003; 14:3470–3481.

[13] Hagen T, Taylor CT, Lam F, Moncada S. Redistribution of Intracellular Oxygen in Hypoxia by Nitric Oxide: Effect on HIF1alpha. *Science.* 2003; 302:1975–1978.

[14] Mateo J, García-Lecea M, Cadenas S, Hernández C, Moncada S. Regulation of hypoxia-inducible factor-1alpha by nitric oxide through mitochondria-dependent and -independent pathways. *Biochem. J.* 2003; 376:537–544.

[15] Circu ML, Aw TY. Reactive oxygen species, cellular redox systems, and apoptosis. *Free Radic. Biol. Med.* 2010; 48:749–762.

[16] Crouser ED. Mitochondrial dysfunction in septic shock and multiple organ dysfunction syndrome. *Mitochondrion.* 2004; 4:729–741.

[17] Galley HF. Oxidative stress and mitochondrial dysfunction in sepsis. *Br. J. Anaesth.* 2011; 107:57–64.

[18] Singer M. Mitochondrial function in sepsis: Acute phase versus multiple organ failure. *Crit. Care Med.* 2007; 35:S441–S448.

[19] Levy RJ, Vijayasarathy C, Raj NR, Avadhani NG, Deutschman CS. Competitive and Noncompetitive Inhibition of Myocardial Cytochrome C Oxidase in Sepsis. *Shock.* 2004; 21:110–114.

[20] Smeding L, van der Laarse WJ, van Veelen TA, Lamberts RR, Niessen HW, Kneyber MC, Johan Groeneveld AB, Plötz FB. Early Myocardial Dysfunction is Not Caused by Mitochondrial Abnormalities in a Rat Model of Peritonitis. *J. Surg. Res.* 2011 [Epub ahead of print].

[21] Tavakoli H, Mela L. Alterations of mitochondrial metabolism and protein concentrations in subacute septicemia. *Infect. Immun.* 1982; 38:536–541.

[22] Porta F, Takala J, Weikert C, Bracht H, Kolarova A, Lauterburg BH, Borotto E, Jakob SM. Effects of prolonged endotoxemia on liver, skeletal muscle and kidney mitochondrial function. *Crit. Care.* 2006; 10:R118.

[23] Callahan LA, Supinski GS. Downregulation of diaphragm electron transport chain and glycolytic enzyme gene expression in sepsis. *J. App. Physiol.* 2005; 99:1120–1126.

[24] Crouser ED, Julian MW, Blaho DV, Pfeiffer DR. Endotoxin-induced mitochondrial damage correlates with impaired respiratory activity. *Crit. Care Med.* 2002; 30: 276–284.

[25] Kantrow SP, Taylor DE, Carraway MS, Piantadosi CA. Oxidative metabolism in rat hepatocytes and mitochondria during sepsis. *Arch. Biochem. Biophys.* 1997; 345: 278–288.

[26] Unno N, Wang H, Menconi MJ, Tytgat SH, Larkin V, Smith M, Morin MJ, Chavez A, Hodin RA, Fink MP. Inhibition of inducible nitric oxide synthase ameliorates endotoxin-induced gut mucosal barrier dysfunction in rats. *Gastroenterology* 1997; 113:1246–1257.

[27] King CJ, Tytgat S, Delude RL, Fink MP. Ileal mucosal oxygen consumption is decreased in endotoxemic rats but is restored toward normal by treatment with aminoguanidine. *Crit. Care Med.* 1999; 27:2518–2524.

[28] Comim CM, Rezin GT, Scaini G, Di-Pietro PB, Cardoso MR, Petronilho FC, Ritter C, Streck EL, Quevedo J, Dal-Pizzol F. Mitochondrial respiratory chain and creatine kinase activities in rat brain after sepsis induced by cecal ligation and perforation. *Mitochondrion.* 2008; 8:313–318.

[29] d'Avila JDCP, Santiago APSA, Amâncio RT, Galina A, Oliveira MF, Bozza FA. Sepsis induces brain mitochondrial dysfunction. *Crit. Care Med.* 2008; 36:1925–1932.

[30] Brealey D, Brand M, Hargreaves I, Heales S, Land J, Smolenski R, Davies NA, Cooper CE, Singer M. Association between mitochondrial dysfunction and severity and outcome of septic shock. *Lancet*. 2002; 360:219–223.

[31] Fredriksson K, Hammarqvist F, Strigard K, Hultenby K, Ljungqvist O, Wernerman J, Rooyackers O. Derangements in mitochondrial metabolism in intercostal and leg muscle of critically ill patients with sepsis-induced multiple organ failure. *Am. J. Physiol. Endocrinol. Metab*. 2006; 291:E1044–E1050.

[32] Coopersmith CM, Chang KC, Swanson PE, Tinsley KW, Stromberg PE, Buchman TG, Karl IE, Hotchkiss RS. Overexpression of Bcl-2 in the intestinal epithelium improves survival in septic mice. *Crit. Care Med*. 2002; 30:195–201.

[33] García-Ruiz C, Colell A, Marí M, Morales A, Fernández-Checa JC. Direct effect of ceramide on the mitochondrial electron transport chain leads to generation of reactive oxygen species. Role of mitochondrial glutathione. *J. Biol. Chem*. 1997; 272:11369–11377.

[34] Crouser ED, Julian MW, Huff JE, Joshi MS, Bauer JA, Gadd ME, Wewers MD, Pfeiffer DR. Abnormal permeability of inner and outer mitochondrial membranes contributes independently to mitochondrial dysfunction in the liver during acute endotoxemia. *Crit. Care Med*. 2004; 32:478–488.

[35] Haefen von C, Wieder T, Gillissen B, Stärck L, Graupner V, Dörken B, Daniel PT. Ceramide induces mitochondrial activation and apoptosis via a Bax-dependent pathway in human carcinoma cells. *Oncogene*. 2002; 21:4009–4019.

[36] Delogu G, Famularo G, Amati F, Signore L, Antonucci A, Trinchieri V, Di Marzio L, Cifone MG. Ceramide concentrations in septic patients: a possible marker of multiple organ dysfunction syndrome. *Crit. Care Med*. 1999; 27:2413–2417.

[37] Vary TC. Sepsis-induced alterations in pyruvate dehydrogenase complex activity in rat skeletal muscle: effects on plasma lactate. *Shock*. 1996; 6:89–94.

[38] Fariss MW, Chan CB, Patel M, Van Houten B, Orrenius S. Role of mitochondria in toxic oxidative stress. *Mol. Interv*. 2005; 5:94–111.

[39] Boveris A, Alvarez S, Navarro A. The role of mitochondrial nitric oxide synthase in inflammation and septic shock. *Free Radic. Biol. Med*. 2002; 33:1186–1193.

[40] Boczkowski J, Lisdero CL, Lanone S, Samb A, Carreras MC, Boveris A, Aubier M, Poderoso JJ. Endogenous peroxynitrite mediates mitochondrial dysfunction in rat diaphragm during endotoxemia. *FASEB J*. 1999; 13:1637–1646.

[41] Khan AU, Delude RL, Han YY, Sappington PL, Han X, Carcillo JA, Fink MP. Liposomal NAD(+) prevents diminished O(2) consumption by immunostimulated Caco-2 cells. *Am. J. Physiol. Lung Cell Mol. Physiol*. 2002; 282:L1082–L1091.

[42] Dare AJ, Phillips ARJ, Hickey AJR, Mittal A, Loveday B, Thompson N, Windsor JA. A systematic review of experimental treatments for mitochondrial dysfunction in sepsis and multiple organ dysfunction syndrome. *Free Radic. Biol. Med*. 2009; 47:1517–1525.

[43] Larche J, Lancel S, Hassoun SM, Favory R, Decoster B, Marchetti P, Chopin C, Neviere R. Inhibition of mitochondrial permeability transition prevents sepsis-induced myocardial dysfunction and mortality. *J. Am. Coll Cardiol*. 2006; 48:377–385.

[44] Lowes DA, Thottakam BMV, Webster NR, Murphy MP, Galley HF. The mitochondria-targeted antioxidant MitoQ protects against organ damage in a lipopolysaccharide–peptidoglycan model of sepsis. *Free Radic. Biol. Med*. 2008; 45:1559–1565.

[45] Cuzzocrea S, McDonald MC, Mazzon E, Filipe HM, Centorrino T, Lepore V, Terranova ML, Ciccolo A, Caputi AP, Thiemermann C. Beneficial effects of tempol, a membrane-permeable radical scavenger, on the multiple organ failure induced by zymosan in the rat. *Crit. Care Med.* 2001; 29:102–111.

[46] Szeto HH. Mitochondria-targeted peptide antioxidants: novel neuroprotective agents. *AAPS J.* 2006; 8:E521–E531.

[47] Vanasco V, Cimolai MC, Evelson P, Alvarez S. The oxidative stress and the mitochondrial dysfunction caused by endotoxemia are prevented by α-lipoic acid. *Free Radic. Res.* 2008; 42:815–823.

[48] Escames G, Leon J, Macías M, Khaldy H, Acuña-Castroviejo D. Melatonin counteracts lipopolysaccharide-induced expression and activity of mitochondrial nitric oxide synthase in rats. *FASEB J.* 2003; 17:932–934.

[49] Escames G, López LC, Ortiz F, López A, García JA, Ros E, Acuña-Castroviejo D. Attenuation of cardiac mitochondrial dysfunction by melatonin in septic mice. *FEBS J.* 2007; 274:2135–2147.

[50] Şener G, Toklu H, Kapucu C, Ercan F, Erkanli G, Kaçmaz A, Tilki M, Yeğen BC. Melatonin Protects Against Oxidative Organ Injury in a Rat Model of Sepsis. *Surg. Today.* 2004; 35:52–59.

[51] Reynolds F, Dauchy R, Blask D, Dietz PA, Lynch D, Zuckerman R. The pineal gland hormone melatonin improves survival in a rat model of sepsis/shock induced by zymosan A. *Surgery.* 2003; 134:474–479.

[52] Gitto E, Karbownik M, Reiter RJ, Tan DX, Cuzzocrea S, Chiurazzi P, Cordaro S, Corona G, Trimarchi G, Barberi I. Effects of melatonin treatment in septic newborns. *Pediatr. Res.* 2001; 50:756–760.

In: Oxidative Stress and the Critically Ill Patient
Editors: Ramón Rodrigo and Bettina von Dessauer

ISBN: 978-1-62081-576-2

Chapter V

ENDOTHELIAL DYSFUNCTION

Emilia M. Sanhueza Reinoso
Pathophysiology Program-ICBM
Faculty of Medicine, University of Chile, Chile

ABSTRACT

The functional state of endothelium can be described as three types of conditions: 1) *Basal* physiological condition where endothelium maintain a balance in vascular tone that could be adapted to maintain the blood flow according the tissue metabolic requirements also preventing thrombosis and regulating the normal fluid distribution between intravascular and interstitial space and allowing the innate immune system to protect the organism. 2) An *Activated* physiological state, where the endothelial cells became stimulated by different mediators or agents that allow it to acquire a new endothelial function which is going to be beneficial for the host, i.e. the defense response to an antigen or micro organism or to repair a tissue damage, among others, and 3) A *Dysfunctional* state, where the endothelium failure to adequately perform its homeostatic function thereby the principal alterations are the deregulated vascular tone (increased or decreased), usually associated to a predominantly protrombotic activity, which also can be associated to a deterioration in the control of liquid and molecules movement through the vascular wall. Significant injury damages the endothelial cell and the subsequent dysfunctional state usually contributes to a vicious circle where both the endothelium and the entire organism are progressively to be damaged.

ABBREVIATIONS

ADMA	asymmetric dimity-L-arginine
DDAH	dimethylarginine dimethyaminohydrolase
AGII	angiotensin II
CGRP	calcitonin gene-related peptide
CNP	C-type natriuretic peptide

CO	carbon monoxide
EDHF	endothelial derived hyperpolarizing factor
EDCF	endothelial derived contracting factor
$EET_{(S)}$	epoxyeicosatrienoic acids
ET-1	endothelin -1
$HETE_{(S)}$	hydroxyeicosatetraenoic acids
H_2O_2	hydrogen peroxide
H_2S	hydrogen sulfide
NO	nitric oxide
NOS	nitric oxide sinthase
NPY	neuropeptide Y
OS	oxidative stress
PGE_2	prostaglandin E2
$PGF_{2\alpha}$	prostaglandin F2 α
PGI_2	prostacyclin
PGJ_2	J series prostaglandine
PPARY	peroxisome proliferator activated receptor-gamma
RNS	reactive species derived from nitrogen
ROS	reactive species derived from oxygen
SO_2	sulfur dioxide
TxA_2	tromboxane A_2
VIP	vasoactive intestinal peptide

2. Introduction

The vascular tree represent a very important mass of the body, traditionally it is separated in arterial, venous capillary and lymphatic vessels. All of them have specific function and are present in all of the different organs. Their structure and vascular composition is different, however, all of them have endothelium as their inside component.

In general endothelium is described as an organ that controls: 1) the vascular tone and blood flow by a local balance between vasodilators (paracrine release of diffusible vasodilator mediators, such as nitric oxide, prostacyclin and vasopressors endothelin-1 among others); 2) the coagulation to keep blood in a fluid state by preventing thrombosis; 3) the exchange of fluid and macromolecules between the blood and the tissues; and 4) the local balance between pro- and anti-inflammatory mediators.

The endothelium is constantly detecting and responding to a wide variety of mechanical and chemical stimuli that trigger its functional and physical changes. Endothelial cells respond to hormones and chemicals that are present in the blood plasma levels which are actively changing according to the physiological or pathological conditions of the organism. The change in endothelial cell function also results in change in the interaction with other cells. In addition, the endothelium actively participates in the metabolism of substances that are important for activity in other cells.

Patients in critical health condition usually have endothelial cells damage where the oxidative stress (OS) represents one of the most important injury conditioners. However the endothelium not only is a target for OS but it also in a dysfunctional condition contributes to generate more reactive species derived from oxygen (ROS) or nitrogen (RNS) (see chapter 1), these reactive molecules can damage and jeopardized the antioxidant capacity of the entire organism.

The condition best known that produces a severe endothelial dysfunctional state is sepsis, where the systemic inflammatory response which at the beginning could be beneficial for the organism, promptly became in a deleterious mechanism, due to the massive production of inflammatory cytokines. In other clinical conditions associated with sterile inflammation, similar damage may occur due to activation of inflammatory cytokines by leucocytes that produce increased ROS production that damage endothelial function.

The endothelium is an important organ that in critical health conditions suffers damage by different mechanisms; one of them is OS that conduces to a dysfunctional state of the endothelium. The abnormal function of these cells could contribute to aggravate the clinical condition of the patient by a progressively damage of different organs as to configure a multiorganic failure with high risk of death due a diverse complications (see chapter 6).

The endothelial tissue produces a great variety of vasoactive substances; it is considered the most important regulator of the arteriolar vascular resistance in normal condition. Furthermore, its modified or dysfunctional condition plays a central role in the pathophysiology of different diseases, included frequent health problems as hypertension, atheromatosis and diabetes mellitus, which can coexist with other pathological condition in the very ill patients particularly in senescent adults.

Patients of critical care unit could have a wide variety of diseases that compromise to a critical level their general health condition, most of them have severe infections with sepsis, or systemic inflammation by necrosis as occurs with severe burns or polytraumatism, others have a final condition of an acute or terminal cardiovascular, respiratory or renal disease, or a terminal state of a malignancy with or not the complication of the antineoplasic therapy, among others.

All individuals of different ages, have a certain risk of either acute or chronic, serious deterioration in their health status by transforming into a critically ill patient. The diseases or pathological conditions that precipitate it could be very different, moreover some patients have a basal condition that aggravate them to face an over imposed aggression to their health basal condition, as occurs in patients with damage of the endothelial function as mentioned above were a basal OS could contributes to a lesser capacity to tolerate a new pathological condition.

The unbalance between oxidative and antioxidant mechanisms, could to predispose them to have more risk when they are in critical condition, since due to a progression of their disease or to a superimposed event, that conduce them to an increase in the reactive species production or a deterioration in their antioxidant capacity. This could be due to a homeostasis imbalance where hypoxic, metabolic, ischemic-reperfusion phenomena and particularly inflammatory mechanisms (of diverse origin) that contribute to a further increase in reactive species with deleterious effect on diverse cells. Endothelial cells are particularly exposed to it, due to its direct relation with diverse components and solutes present in circulating fluids, which can stimulate it with an over activation or damage of these cells or aggravating a previous dysfunctional state, when this occurs, the incapacity of the endothelial cell to maintain its normal function could be deleterious for others cells of different organs.

A critical health condition could develop a progressive compromise that can produce a multiple organic failure with high risk of death. The way by which occurs, direct or indirectly involves a reduction of the systemic oxygen delivery and/or the difficulty to use the oxygen at the cellular level usually in a context of a systemic inflammatory condition.

The inflammatory response has two characteristics that produce antagonist effects in health: a) a major role as initial host defense, particularly against infections and b) to be a response that in generally is imprecise and can cause collateral damage in tissues. Furthermore is necessary to consider that the stimulus for the inflammatory response could be infectious or not (see Chapter 3). There have been major advances in the understanding of how microbes can trigger this response, but lesser is the information about the sterile inflammation.

Sterile inflammation is induced by dead cells or irritant particles, could be very diverse in it origin respect of type of dead cellule or particle that induced it, however the innate immune system may recognize them in similar ways and stimulate the inflammatory response via common pathways. [1].

In this chapter general aspects of endothelium and its relation with pathological condition are reviewed, particularly its role in critical health condition and its relation with OS.

3. General Characteristics of Endothelium

The endothelium consist in a monolayer of endothelial cells, constitutes the inner cellular lining of the blood vessels (arteries, veins and capillaries) and also the lymphatic system, and therefore is in direct contact with the blood/lymph and the circulating cells. The total volume of the endothelial cells of the human body is comparable to that of the liver.[2]

The endothelium forms part of the intima of the vessels along with the basal lamina to which it is anchored. The basal lamina has 80-nm, is an important component of the blood vessels because it permits structural organization to wall, where the endothelial cells are lined in its internal side to the vascular lumen and in the other side of the basal lamina are muscle cells or pericytes. The basal lamina is in great part produced by the endothelial cells, which can synthesize virtually all the proteins that constituting it and also produce the relevant enzymes involved in its remodeling, such as matrix metalloproteinases that degrade this extracellular matrix, an important action for the plasticity of the blood vessels and for angiogenesis [2]. However, vascular endothelial cells are not all alike, exists important morphologic, physiologic and phenotypic variations between endothelial cells in the different parts of the arterial tree as well as between arteries and veins [3, 4].

In some territories the endothelial cells are associated with a basement membrane that is characterized by the presence of large fenestrations of 100 - to 200-nm. This occurs in the sinusoidal vascular beds in the liver, mainly, but also in the spleen and bone marrow. The structural heterogeneity of endothelial cells is also given by differences in form and by the diversity of the structural components of the endocytic pathway, such as clathrin coated pits or via caveolae transcytosis, as in the different levels of expression of various intercellular junctions. Furthermore, there are also differences in the composition of the glycocalyx, and the endothelial surface layer associated, these structures are important to influence the transport of water and solutes through the endothelium [5].

Endothelial cells and hematopoietic cells arise from the mesoderm by the differentiation of the same precursor cells, the hemangioblast. Hemangioblasts give rise to angioblasts or endothelial progenitor cells, which in turn differentiate into endothelial cells of arteries, veins and capillaries, each cell type being identified by a specific expression pattern of gene markers. Epigenetic induced heritable changes, histone methylation and acetylation, occur in the early phase of differentiation, while micro-environmental changes, which are not transmitted during mitosis, occur predominantly in the late phase of differentiation, i.e., organ-specific differentiation of the endothelial cells. However, other cell lineages, such as adipose lineage cells or neural stem cells, can transdifferentiate into endothelial cells. The remarkable plasticity of the endothelial cells could be seen as its principal property. One can make the assumption that each one of the total endothelial cells included in our body is phenotypically distinct since, everyone has to sense and adapt to the needs of the various neighboring cells and to many different microenvironments [2].

In general in many aspects the morphology and physiology are closely interdependent. The endothelium morphology varies across the vascular tree but in general, the endothelial cells have the characteristic to be thin and slightly elongated. Its dimension has been described in the range of 50–70 μm long, 10–30 μm wide and 0.1–10 μm thick. They are oriented in the fluid flow direction through the vascular vessels so it offer a lesser friction resistance to blood flow by minimizing the shear stress, particularly in the arteriolar territory. It have been calculated that this single layer is constituted by approximately 10 to 60 × 10^{13} endothelial cells in the human body. Endothelium occupies a surface (blood/endothelium interface) measuring approximately 300 to 1000 m^2 [2]. These morphological data indicate that endothelial cells are a privileged site for exchange of many substances and gases, both that circulate by the vascular tree and captured by cells and others that are delivered by it to the circulation.

4. Endothelium Physiology

Despite many years of research dedicated to the physiology of the cardiovascular system [6] has only been in recent decades that has been described the important role played by the endothelium (Figure 1). The endothelium has been recognized as the principal regulator of the vascular tone, vascular permeability and leukocyte mobilization into the tissues, in health and pathological conditions. The historical concept about the endothelium was coined in 1865 by Wilhelm His, a Swiss anatomist. Initially the endothelium was, preventing the egress of figure elements from the blood, but allowing gases, nutrients and metabolic product to diffuse through it, but after in the last four decades, it was recognized that the endothelium produces substances that can influence the vascular tone and the activity of the platelets, as occurred with the discovery of the production of prostacyclin by endothelial cells. Then came the era of nitric oxide and endothelin, both contribute to reinforce the importance of this noble tissue that actively participates, in the efficient oxygenation of the different territories. Furthermore, a great interest in research about endothelium properties has allowed a better knowledge, about its physiological and pathophysiological characteristic and how these are important to human health.

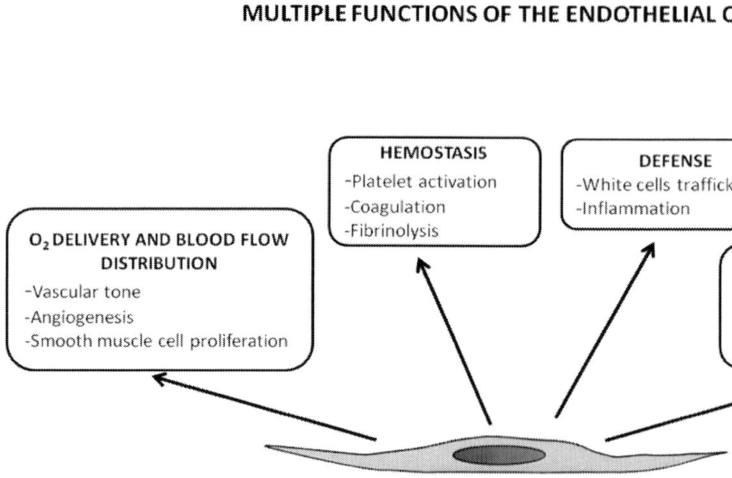

Figure 1. Multiple functions of endothelial cells.

Today we could consider as a transcendental and revolutionary, the discovery of nitric oxide production by the endothelium that also was recognized by the Nobel Prize in Physiology or Medicine in 1998 given to Furchgott R, Ignarro l and Murad F, by their discovery about the nitric oxide as a signaling molecule in the cardiovascular system.

Endothelial cells can develop various functions that are carried out some in general by all of them, and other that are specific for cellular subgroups belonging to different organs and vascular beds. At the present, the endothelium is considerate an important tissue almost it could be considered as an organ due to its significant and specific functions, it has been recognized that endothelium is a pivotal actor in the control of blood fluidity, platelet aggregation and vascular tone, regulates immunological and inflammatory responses, and also participates as a metabolizing and endocrine organ [2].

In response to various substances (released by autonomic and sensory nerves or platelets), circulating hormones, autacoids, cytokines, and drugs, as well as to physical and chemical stimuli (i.e., changes in pressure, shear stress, and pH), endothelial cells synthesize and release various factors that modulate angiogenesis, inflammatory responses, hemostasis, as well as vascular tone and permeability [7].

4.1. Endothelium as a Sensor of Mechanical Forces

The endothelium suffers the mechanical forces that are present into blood vessels as a constant mechanical loading from blood pressure and flow which cause internal stresses (endothelial shear stress and circumferential wall stress, respectively). The mechanical forces not only cause morphological changes of endothelium and blood vessel wall, but also trigger biochemical and biological events.

The physiologic stresses and strains (stretch) exert vasoprotective roles via NO and provide a homeostatic oxidative balance. A perturbation of tissue stresses and strains can disturb biochemical homeostasis and lead to vascular remodeling and possible dysfunction (e.g. altered vasorelaxation, tone, stiffness, etc.). These distinct biological endpoints are caused by some common biochemical pathways [8].

The heart induces a pulsatile blood pressure whilst the blood flow circulates throughout the vasculature. The blood flow produces a frictional force (wall shear stress) on the endothelial cells that is opposed by tension and deformation in the endothelium, while the circumferential distension of blood pressure, is opposed by circumferential stress and strain (stretch) of the different components of the vessel wall (intima, media and adventitia). These flow and pressure loads and the resulting internal stresses with deformation of the fibers and cells of the vessel wall, triggering the releasing of biochemical reactants that contribute to maintain physiological function of blood vessels.

Under physiological conditions, the endothelium is in a state of homeostasis, with balance in the response produced against various physical and chemical stimuli. A disturbance of this equilibrium in which mechanical stimuli are too high or low can lead to physiological adaptation or, conversely cause a disease of the vascular wall. The most important physiological conditions of changes in blood pressure and blood flow are seen in: pregnancy, exercise, growth and development among others.

In the case of pathological conditions changes in blood pressure may be due to hypertension, or blood flow and/or decreased vascular resistance that tend to produce hypotension, all conditions that are usually present in critically ill patients. In addition, frequent pathologies with physical and chemical alterations in the body, can change not only the blood vessel function but also change their morphology, as occurs in diabetes, hypercholesterolemia, and smoking, which may modify the properties of the vessels and the ability to deform or stretch in response to pressure within the normal range (normotensive) or hypertension status, favoring the development of morbidity and co-morbidity. In both conditions, there is an increased mechanical pressure and circumferential flow with pressure induced strain, but in hypertension moreover, there is an structural change due to remodeling that reduce the vascular lumen.

The mechanisms involved in blood vessel's ability to sense physical changes and modify their activity involves the participation of a wide variety of receptors, integrins, and extracellular matrix components. The vessel diameter has a great importance in determining the flow-mediated vasodilation, since an inverse relationship between baseline artery diameter and flow-mediated vasodilation has been identified using reactive hyperemia to create a shear stress stimulus in human conduit arteries. The response to shear stress is not uniform across differently sized vessels; the impact of baseline diameter on flow-mediated vasodilation is distinct within the radial artery and brachial artery. In the brachial artery, handgrip exercise-induced flow-mediated vasodilation may be useful in comparing the endothelial function of groups with significantly different baseline diameters, addressing an important limitation that is associated with reactive hyperemia flow-mediated vasodilation tests [9].

Chronic hypertension induces an adaptive remodeling with increased wall thickness, which contributes to increase arteriolar vascular resistance. The increased circumferential stretch due to pressure-overload can enhance endothelial permeability and vascular tone. Furthermore an increase in circumferential stretch can also enhance superoxide production in both endothelium and smooth muscle cells. The possible origin of the superoxide overproduction, include: upregulated NADPH oxidase, mitochondrial oxidant and xanthine oxidase [8].

4.2. Endothelium and Vascular Tone

The endothelium controls the vascular tone by releasing various relaxing and contracting factors (Figure 2) that influence the activity of the underlying vascular smooth muscle cells, and by interacting directly with the vascular smooth muscle cells.

Endothelial cells controls vascular tone, and thereby blood flow, by synthesizing and releasing relaxing and contracting factors such as NO, metabolites of arachidonic acid via the cyclooxygenases, lipoxygenases and cytochrome P450 pathways, various peptides (Endothelin-1, urotensin, C type Natriuretic Peptide, adrenomedullin, etc.), adenosine, purines, ROS and so on. Additionally, endothelial cell produce ectoenzymes that participate in the generation of vasoactive hormones such as angiotensin II.

In arterial and venous vessels the endothelial cells are separated from the smooth muscle only by the basal lamina that is derived in great part from the endothelium, so, there is a tight connection between the endothelial and smooth muscle cell function. The vascular resistance is in great part dependent from the endothelium activity that controls the arteriolar vascular tone. The endothelial cell both directly or indirectly could change the vascular tone since for producing substances that diffusing across the basal lamina and act in a paracrin effect, or indirectly through the conversion of circulating precursors that are converted to its active form by endothelial ectoenzymes for finally constitutes vasoactive substances that are recognized by the muscle cell receptors. In basal physiologic conditions the vasoactive agents produced by endothelium are in equilibrium but it could change according to body requirements or pathological conditions.

The vasoactive function of endothelium was reviewed and published recently in a very complete analysis by Michel Félétau [(2)].

Among vasoactive substances produced by endothelium, is relevant the production of vasodilators, where NO could be considered today's as the most important both in physiological and pathological conditions. There is considerable literature on the role of wall shear stress in flow-mediated vasodilation. NO generated from endothelial NO synthase (eNOS) is the critical biochemical that mediates the response to shear stress. Endothelium-derived NO is a paracrine factor that controls vascular tone, inhibits platelet function, prevents adhesion of leukocytes, and reduces proliferation of the intima. NO is the most important as powerful vasodilator, but it also plays important biological roles in the gastrointestinal, respiratory, nervous and immune systems.

There are three nitric oxide syntase (NOS) isoforms that produce NO from L-arginine. The most important for the endothelium is the endothelial NOS (eNOS, NOS 3) present as a constitutively form in endothelial cells. The other two isoforms are neural NOS, also constitutive (nNOS, NOS-1) that participates in neurotransmition and the inducible isoform (iNOS, NOS-2), present in macrophages that are stimulated by lipopolisacarides (LPS) and interferon γ, as part of the inflammatory stimuli and also when these cells have bactericidal activity or destroy neoplasic cell.

However the NOS expression of the different isoforms is not tissue specific since they were also described in others cells: nNOS not only is present in perivascular nerves, also it can be detected in endothelial cell and smooth muscle cell, iNOS is also present in the cardiovascular system, it has been detected in the blood vessel wall this includes endothelial and smooth muscle cells as well as fibroblasts, leukocytes and mast cells, and eNOS is the preponderant isoform in healthy endothelial cells and is predominantly.

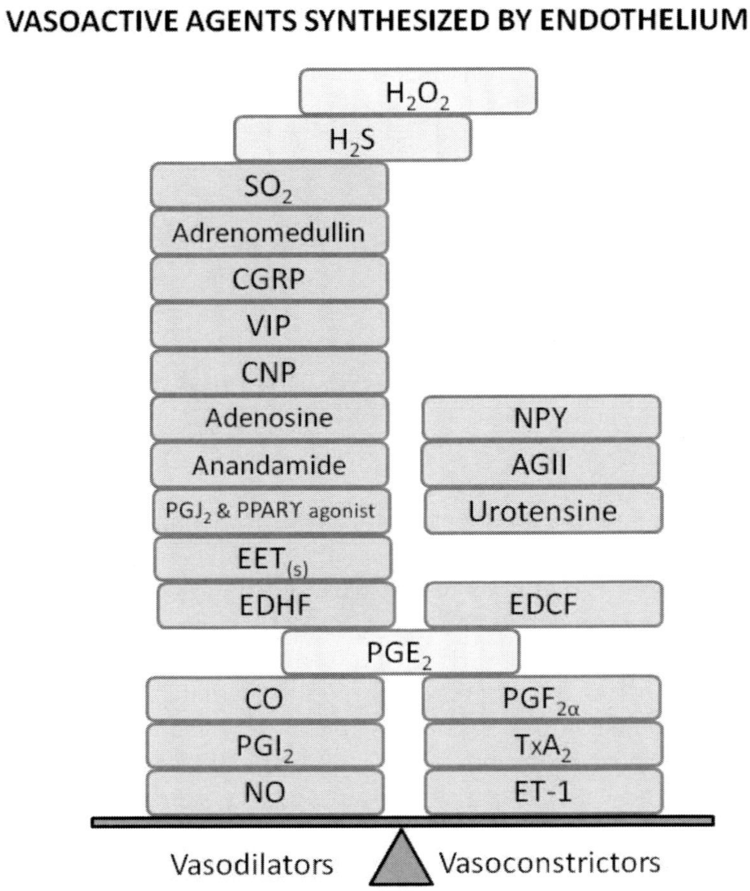

Figure 2. Vasoactive agents synthesized by the endothelium: Endothelium produces both vasodilators and vasoconstrictors factors. Under physiological conditions a dynamic equilibrium exists between them, which allows blood flow is consistent with what the body requires. The figure shows the principal action of agents, however some of them have both action, on depending of doses, specific organ and tissue receptors. Angiotensin II (AGII), calcitonin gene-related peptide (CGRP), C-type natriuretic peptide (CNP), carbon monoxide (CO), endothelial derived hyperpolarizing factor (EDHF), endothelial derived contracting factor (EDCF), epoxyeicosatrienoic acids ($EET_{(S)}$), endothelin-1 (ET-1), hydroxyeicosatetraenoic acids ($HETE_{(S)}$), hydrogen peroxide (H_2O_2), hydrogen sulfide (H_2S), nitric oxide (NO), neuropeptide Y (NPY), prostaglandin E_2 (PGE_2) , prostaglandin $F_{2\alpha}$ ($PGF_{2\alpha}$), Prostacyclin (PGI_2), J series prostaglandine (PGJ_2), peroxisome proliferator activated receptor-gamma (PPARY), sulfur dioxide (SO_2), tromboxane A_2 (TxA_2) and vasoactive intestinal peptide (VIP).

The conversion of l-arginine to NO by eNOS involves two steps:1) The NADPH-dependent hydroxylation of l-arginine to NG-hydroxy-arginine, a reaction requiring calcium-calmodulin, which is accelerated by the presence of BH_4. 2) Generation of NO, with the stoichiometric formation of l-citrulline is also calcium-calmodulin-dependent, requires O_2 and NADPH and is also accelerated by BH_4.

Other essential characteristic of the three NOS, apart from their functional independent domains, is that the NO-synthase activity requires dimerization. The heme and a tetra coordinated zinc ion held by four thiols (two from each monomer), play an essential role in the formation of the homodimer and BH_4 stabilizes the dimer once formed.

The synthesis of NO could be affected during oxidative stress condition because the zinc thiolate center and BH_4 are subject to attack by peroxynitrite, which disrupts and releases the zinc ion, and oxidizes the thiols. Upon thiol reduction, eNOS dimers dissociate into monomers and become uncoupled; this is an important mechanism for the alteration in endothelial function due to oxidative stress that produce a reduction in the capacity of endothelial cell to generate NO.

Since NO is a gaseous free radical with a high biological reactivity, its synthesis has to be tightly controlled in order to be delivered at the right time, the right place and in the right amount. The transcription of eNOS is regulated by various physical, chemical and pharmacological stimuli.

The endothelial cell-restricted expression of eNOS is also under the control of an epigenetic mechanism of gene regulation involving DNA methylation and a specific endothelial histone code. The transcription of eNOS is enhanced, for instance, by laminar and oscillatory shear stress, hydrogen peroxide, inhibition of histone deacetylase, micro-RNA, statins and, possibly, estrogens.

In response to laminar flow, the transcription of eNOS is coordinated with the regulation of the expression of many other genes that not only control vascular tone since they contribute to an atheroprotective, anti-thrombotic and anti-inflammatory phenotype. The half-life of eNOS mRNA has been reported to be as long as 10 to 35 hours, indicating that post-transcriptional regulation of the transcripts half-life could be a more rapid and efficient strategy than to regulate eNOS transcription. The post-transcriptional regulation (mRNA processing and polyadenylation, mRNA export from the nucleus and mRNA degradation) is heavily controlled by various different stimuli, some of those also regulate eNOS transcription. eNOS is subjected to several overlapping post-translational regulatory modifications, including lipidation, phosphorylations, S-nitrosylations, acetylation and protein–protein interactions. The activation of eNOS also requires the calcium-dependent binding of calmodulin, and the amount of eNOS protein can only partially predict overall enzymatic activity.

In endothelial cells, eNOS is predominantly located in the plasma membrane and in the Golgi system. The sub-cellular location of eNOS is critical for its state of activation and multiple levels of regulation are responsible for the trafficking of the enzyme. A process involving the enzymatic acylation of eNOS residues is responsible for this targeting of eNOS to membrane structures in caveolaeas and Golgi. The association of eNOS with caveolin-1 inhibits its activity. Additionally, eNOS activity is regulated by serine, threonine and tyrosine phosphorylations.

Furthermore, the trafficking of eNOS involves various types of proteins such as actin cytoskeleton, NOSIP (eNOS interacting protein), NOSTRIN (eNOS trafficking inducer protein), Gab1 (growth factor receptor-bound protein-associated binding protein-1), PECAM-1 (platelet–endothelial cell adhesion molecule-1) or dynamin. These various eNOS-associated proteins can be also associated with various kinases and phosphatases, and their own post-translational phosphorylations and S- nitrosylations play an important regulatory role. Finally, the degradation of eNOS determines its availability and must be regulated. Unfortunately, very little is known at present on these processes [2].

Others vasodilators known are Prostacyclin (PGI_2), Endothelial derived hiperpolarizating factor (EDHF), Carbon monoxide (CO), Adenosin diphosphatase (ADPasa), that depending of metabolic condition can be or not more active. Vasocontrictors produced by endothelial cell are Tromboxan (TxA2), and the potent vasoconstrictor Endothelin among others that are important to maintain vascular tone. Furthermore some agents have both actions vasodilatation and vasoconstriction on depending their concentration, the type of vessels and the receptors present on it.

4.3. Endothelium and Hemostasis

The normal hemostasis allows both the free circulation of the blood flowing through the heart, arteries, capillaries and veins, by maintaining blood in fluid condition and also prevents an important blood loss due a vascular damage by clot formation changing its physical properties in a localized region.

The blood flow is in contact with healthy endothelial cells that contribute for it remains in fluid state. The luminal surface of quiescent endothelial cells is anticoagulant and non-thrombogenic. The platelets and leukocytes do not adhere to it and the coagulation system remains inactivated. By contrast, the macromolecules of the basal lamina, synthesized by the endothelial cells, are strongly thrombogenic, and activated endothelial cells promote thrombus formation. The endothelial cells, therefore, regulate the equilibrium between thrombosis, hemostasis and thrombo resistance [2].

When a disruption or activation of the endothelium occurs, this quickly transformed in an area where it actively facilitates clotting, activating platelets and also inhibits fibrinolytic activity to potentiate fibrin formation. The anti and procoagulant activity of the endothelium is not uniform throughout the vascular tree, the heterogeneity depends on environmental and genetic factors, so that endothelial cells express in different form the von Willebrand factor (vWF), the plasminogen activator factor and the tissue factor. Exposure to different hemodynamic forces and humoral and cellular mediators contribute to the diverse phenotype of the endothelial cells through the circulatory system.

The disruption of the endothelium continuity allows that the subendothelial matrix and collagen fibers are exposed directly to the blood flow. The circulating platelets adhere to these structures and starting the hemostatic process. The initial platelet recruitment depends of the vWF associated to the vascular wall, it predominantly synthesized by the endothelial cells.

The vWF appears to play a major role in thrombus formation, especially when the blood flow is elevated (high shear rate), it is a multimeric protein, is stored in the endothelial cells in one of their characteristic ultrastructural features, the Weibel–Palade bodies. When the endothelium is activated, vWF is released into the circulation, where it stabilizes factor VIII (FVIII) and is associated with collagen VI in the subendothelium. At sites of vascular injury, vWF acts as a bridge between the tissues and the platelet via the GPIb/IX/V glycoprotein receptor. Additionally, endothelial cells synthesize the platelet-activating factor (PAF) that promotes the activation of platelets, and their adhesion to the own endothelial cells.

When platelets are activated, in a second phase more platelets are recruited, initiating their aggregation and morphological changes with degranulation of the activated platelets. They release ADP, ATP, thromboxane A2, serotonin, vWF and fibrinogen with further activation of neighboring platelets, amplifying the aggregation process and also producing vascular smooth muscle contraction facilitating the formation of the hemostatic plug, due to a reduction in blood flow velocity.

Neighboring and healthy endothelial cells, in response to most of these mediators liberated from the activated platelets, normally could releasing prostacyclin and NO, in order to limit the aggregation and thrombosis as local phenomena. However, in some pathological circumstances, endothelial cells can also contribute to the amplification of the thrombotic phenomenon, and in response to ADP, ATP or serotonin, endothelial cells can release arachidonic acid metabolites such as thromboxane A2, and, in response to thrombin, following the activation of protease-activated receptors, they release vWF, and also occurs up-regulation of the expression of tissue factor (TF), that contributes to the activation of the extrinsic via of coagulation cascade with a risk of severe trombosis.

In physiological conditions the principal anticoagulant properties of endothelial cells are: 1) Heparan-sulphate expressed on the endothelial surface, its accelerates the interaction between antithrombin and its target enzymes, among which factor Xa and thrombin (IIa), 2) Trombomodulin and endothelial protein C receptor are also membrane proteins and are involved in protein C activation, 3) Tissue factor pathway inhibitor liberated into the blood combining with factor Xa, and after binds to and neutralizes the TF/VIIa complex on cell surfaces and 4) Protein S also released to the blood, is the cofactor of activated protein C which degrades factors Va and VIIIa [10].

Also the normal endothelium has antitrombotic activity related to: 1) Degradation by ectonucleotidases of ADP, necessary for platelet aggregation, 2) Prevention of platelet adhesion and aggregation by: a) Prostaciclin derived from araquidonic acid by action of cicloxygenase, b) Nitric oxide produced from L-Arginine by eNOS c) Carbon Monoxide derived from hem group by hemoxygenase (HO-1) during the biliverdin syntesis. The last three agents have a vasodilator activity that also contributes to a lesser trombotic activity.

4.4. Endothelium and Fluid Distribution

The endothelial-endothelial cell interactions allow to form the endothelium as a monolayer that controls the permeability of the vascular wall by the coefficient of permeability, the hydrostatic and oncotic pressures at both sides of the endothelium (intravascular and interstitial), are the forces which determining interchange of fluid through the vascular wall, but the permeability of the wall (particularly of endothelium) plays a key role for the efficiency of that physical forces.

The permeability is different in the diverse vessels of the microvascular unit of the tissue and also heterogeneous between the different organs, where capillary structure has particular characteristics that influence their relative coefficient of permeability.

Moreover, NO cascade and eNOS as mentioned above, are best known for their role in endothelium-mediated relaxation of vascular smooth muscle, but also the activation of eNOS by certain inflammatory stimuli and enhanced NO release have also been shown to promote increased microvascular permeability.

However, it is not entirely clear why activation of eNOS by certain vasodilatory agents, like acetylcholine, does not affect microvascular permeability, whereas activation of eNOS by other inflammatory agents that increase permeability, like platelet-activating factor, does not cause vasodilation. [11]

Vascular endothelial growth factors (VEGFs) are key regulators of permeability. Studies have shown that in vivo and in vitro VEGF-mediated permeability differs in its time course, but has common involvement of many specific signaling pathways, in particular VEGF receptor-2 activation, calcium influx through transient receptor potential channels, activation of phospholipase C gamma and downstream activation of nitric oxide synthase. Pathways downstream of endothelial nitric oxide synthase appear to involve the guanylyl cyclase-mediated activation of the Rho-Rac pathway and subsequent involvement of junctional signaling proteins such as vascular endothelial cadherin and the tight junctional proteins zona occludens and occludin linked to the actin cytoskeleton.

The signaling appears to be coordinated through spatial organization of the cascade. Many proteins have been identified to be involved in the regulation of vascular permeability by VEGF, but the mechanisms that control the permeability are dependent on the experimental system, and still not fully understood [12]

4.5. Endothelium and Inflammatory Response

The endothelium controls the migration of activates leukocytes through the vessel wall, diverse stimulus change the functional state of the endothelial cell to transforming it in and activated cell that express adherence molecules (such as VCAM 1), for the migration of leukocyte by a diapedesis movement through the intercellular space or transcellular way. Studies with TNFα show that endothelium has a very active role in the migration of leucocytes with changes as a local softening of the endothelial cytoskeleton right underneath an invading leukocyte [13].

Endothelium plays a critical role in orchestrating the host response to sepsis and it is the target of the pathogen and its products and of a myriad of host mediators, thereby the intensity on the inflammatory response (see chapter 3) in great part depends of the functional state of endothelial cells.

5. Pathophysiology of Endothelial Dysfunction

5.1. The Origin of Endothelial Dysfunction

In normal conditions, endothelial cells become activated according to organism needs, i.e., stopping a hemorrhage and repairing the local injured vascular tissue, or to permit leucocytes migration as part of defense mechanisms to front an infection.

The increasing knowledge about the diverse and important endothelial functions, opening some years ago the concept of Endothelial Dysfunction (ED), that configures an abnormal state of endothelial cells that constitute a pathological condition, which is involved in diverse diseases, encompassing multiple potential defects of these cells. However it is principally related to an imbalance in production of vasoactive agents and in the hemostatic mechanisms, which predispose toward hypertension, and a procoagulating state, with high risk of atherothrombosis, arterial thrombosis (stroke, visceral and peripheral artery occlusive diseases), venous thrombosis, intravascular coagulation and thrombotic microangiopathies. The abnormal function of endothelium contributes to their development and perpetuation.

Pathophysiologically, ED is described as a paradoxical response of the vasculature to acetylcholine, reacting with constriction instead of relaxation. Normally, acetylcholine triggers the specific endothelium-derived release of·NO, leading to a reduction in vascular smooth muscle tone that results in vasodilatation and reduction in vascular resistance.

The ED seems part of the natural ageing, studies in animal models and humans have proven that the bioavailability of NO is continuously diminished and, moreover in parallel there is an increase in endothelium-derived $\cdot O_2-$, related it with an oxidative stress condition [14]

ED could be also related to an increase of H_2O_2, studies with H_2O_2 induce premature senescent-like phenotype of human umbilical vein endothelial cells, associated to galactosidase activity, also the cells are enlarged, flattened cell morphology and sustained growth arrest, that could be due to a decreased activity of superoxide dismutase secondary to a down-regulated protein expression [15].

Vascular OS with an increased production of ROS contributes to mechanisms of vascular dysfunction. OS is mainly caused by an imbalance between the activity of endogenous pro-oxidative enzymes (such as NADPH oxidase, xanthine oxidase, or the mitochondrial respiratory chain) and anti-oxidative enzymes (such as superoxide dismutase, glutathione peroxidase, heme oxygenase, thioredoxin peroxidase/peroxiredoxin, catalase, and paraoxonase) in favor of the former. Also, small molecular weight antioxidants may play a role in the defense against OS.

Increased ROS concentrations reduce the amount of bioactive NO by chemical inactivation to form toxic peroxynitrite. Peroxynitrite-in turn-can "uncouple" endothelial NO synthase to become a dysfunctional superoxide-generating enzyme that contributes to vascular OS, both OS and ED can promote atherogenesis [16]

ROS have been extensively appointed as deleterious agents for the cell, however the studies shows initially controversial results that were clarifying to accept that ROS are also relevant for the normal cell function [17]. In physiological condition the production of ROS results in very low basal levels, but with a major physiological role in several aspects of intracellular signaling and regulation that are necessary for: a) redox regulated production of NO; b) ROS production by phagocytic NAD(P)H oxidase (oxidative burst); c) ROS production by NAD(P)H oxidases in non phagocytic cells; d) regulation of vascular tone and other regulatory functions of NO•; e) ROS production as a sensor for changes of oxygen concentration; f) redox regulation of cell adhesion; g) redox regulation of immune responses; h) ROS-induced apoptosis and other mechanisms [18].

An imbalance between the generation of ROS and the antioxidant defense systems results in an oxidative stress, due a condition that promotes an increase in generation of ROS, or a decrease in antioxidant protective mechanisms or both. By far the dominant alteration is the increased generation of ROS due to alterations in metabolism either in mitochondrial organelle or in fatty acids or carbohydrates substrates.

Endothelial mitochondria, the major site of ATP generation, modulate the intracellular dynamics of ROS, which, in turn, control endothelial function. Both hypoxia and hyperoxia may favor the overproduction of ROS leading to oxidative stress, mitochondrial damage and endothelial dysfunction. The EC hypoxic response is mediated by the hypoxia master regulator HIF-1alpha [19].

ROS have been described as involved endothelial dysfunction observed in hypertension and others clinical conditions that compromise the vascular wall such as diabetes mellitus and atherosclerosis [20].

ROS and RNS play a key role in the modulation of the smooth muscle tone in vascular system; they can mediate the action of many vasoactive agents such as Nitric oxide Angiotensin II, Endothelin and urotensine-II. In physiological conditions there is a low intracellular concentration of ROS that contributes to maintain the vascular function and integrity. However in pathophysiological conditions there are increased ROS levels that promote the vascular dysfunction and a progressive remodeling due to oxidative damage.

ED is a key alteration for genesis and progress of hypertension, in this condition there is a decreased NO synthesis and an increased production of superoxide anion and hydrogen peroxide, thereby the vascular tone tends to increase due to the lesser vasodilator action of NO. Moreover, the increase in ROS is a consequence and also a cause of ED, thereby it represents a vicious circle for the progress of vascular damage in hypertension. Furthermore, this pathological condition is aggravated by a decreased bioavailability of endogenous antioxidants observed in human hypertension.

ROS function as intracellular second messenger to increase intracellular calcium concentration that results in vasoconstriction. Studies on ageing in animal models and humans have proven that the bioavailability of •NO is continuously diminished and, in parallel, endothelium-derived •O2− increases [21]

Superoxide is a highly efficient scavenger for •NO, causing formation of the very reactive and deleterious ONOO−. At high concentrations (micromolar range), peroxynitrite oxidizes unspecifically any biological macromolecule, such as DNA, proteins and lipids. At lower concentrations (nanomolar), it interferes with important vascular signalling pathways, such as •NO and prostaglandin signalling, calcium homeostasis, mitogen activated protein kinase cascade, nuclear factor κB(NFκB) and activator protein 1. Thus an increase in •O2− and the subsequent peroxynitrite formation reduces the bioavailability of •NO and leads to endothelial dysfunction, one of the major causes for the progression of vascular disease and senescence.

The distribution of 3-nitrotyrosine residues, as end-product of the reaction of ONOO− with biological compounds, shows the most significant accumulation of nitrotyrosine in the mitochondria, suggesting primarily a mitochondrial source of •O2−, other potential sources could be the subunits of the NADPH oxidase, xanthine oxidase, and an uncoupled eNOS. Both upregulation of eNOS and reduced levels of enzyme expression have been observed with increasing age, also increase both in expression and in activity of eNOS support the concept that eNOS may, as an oxidase, become part of a redox system that increases electron transfer to molecular oxygen.

ROS have an established role in inflammation and host defense, as they kill intracellular bacteria and have been shown to activate the NLRP3 inflammasome. ROS generated by mitochondrial respiration are important for normal lipopolysaccharide (LPS)-driven production of several proinflammatory cytokines. A variety of antioxidants dampen LPS-induced MAPK phosphorylation and inflammatory cytokine production. However, gp91phox and p22phox reduced nicotinamide adenine dinucleotide phosphate (NADPH) oxidase subunits are dispensable for inflammatory cytokine production, indicating that NADPH oxidases are not the source of proinflammatory ROS. Pharmacological blockade of mitochondrial ROS efficiently reduces inflammatory cytokine production after LPS stimulation in healthy controls, these suggest that mitochondrial ROS may be novel therapeutic target in inflammatory diseases [22]

Cardiovascular diseases as hypertension and atheromatosis associated with the ED state, are important health problems that contribute to the progression and complication of other pathologies, such as chronic kidney disease (CKD). Patients with CKD have an increased risk of cardiovascular disease related mortality. ED is a primary event in the development of atherosclerosis and hypertension and likely contributes to the elevated cardiovascular risk in CKD due a compromise of the peripheral vasculature of patients with both severe and moderate CKD.

Mechanisms include OS, L-arginine deficiency, and elevated plasma levels of asymmetric dimethyl-L-arginine (ADMA), that produces a decrease en NO synthesis due an interference with the NOS activity. Interventions designed to restore vascular function in patients with CKD have shown mixed results. Evidence from cell culture studies suggest that the accumulation of uremic toxins inhibits L-arginine transport and reduces nitric oxide production. Studies suggest that endothelial dysfunction may become less reversible with advancing kidney disease [23].

Obesity is another chronic disease with multifactorial origin that can be defined as an increase in the accumulation of body fat. Adipose tissue is not only a triglyceride storage organ, white adipose tissue produce adipokines, among them there are some with inflammatory functions, such as Interleukin-6 (IL-6); others, such as leptin regulates food intake, therefore exerting a direct effect on weight control. However, these adipokines induce the production of ROS, generating OS.

Since adipose tissue is the organ that secretes adipokines, it is considered an independent factor for the generation of systemic OS. The mechanisms by which obesity produces OS are: a) the mitochondrial and peroxisomal oxidation of fatty acids, which can produce ROS in oxidation reactions and b) an over-consumption of oxygen, which generates free radicals in the mitochondrial respiratory chain that is coupled with oxidative phosphorylation in mitochondria.

Furthermore lipid-rich diets that are frequently associated to obesity are also capable of increasing ROS because they can alter oxygen metabolism. Moreover the repercussion of obesity on health and oxidative stress is aggravated due to that the increase of adipose tissue, is associated to a decrease in the activity of antioxidant enzymes such as superoxide dismutase (SOD), catalase (CAT), and glutathione peroxidase (GPx), that were found to be significantly diminished.

The high ROS production and the decrease in antioxidant capacity leads to various abnormalities in obesity, among which there is an endothelial dysfunction, which is characterized by a reduction in the bioavailability of vasodilators, particularly NO, and an increase in endothelium-derived contractile factors, favoring atherosclerotic disease [24].

Since obesity is a frequently health problem that constitutes a high cardiovascular risk factor and considering it association to others pathologies as hypertension, atheromatosis and diabetes mellitus that also have an OS and ED condition, it could be expected an increasing number of obese patients in critical care unit, and their evolution in a critical health condition could be more difficult due to their initial high OS.

5.2. Endothelial Dysfunction and Oxidative Stress in Critically Ill Patients

In many critically ill conditions there is a loss of vascular tone control with a progressive compromise of the hemodynamic condition of the patient, which evolves to a generalized hypoperfusion state due to a systemic inflammatory response. The deficient delivery of oxygen plus nutrients to the different organs and the incapacity of a sufficient wash out of the metabolic wastes of the cells, promotes a progressive damage of the metabolic state of different organ cells which determine organ dysfunction. The generalized hypoperfusion state that precedes the functional and organic damage occurs by diverse pathophysiological mechanisms. The most characteristic is the diminished vascular resistance due the action of the inflammatory mediators or cytokines that are produced as part of the inflammatory process associated to the septic or sterile conditions, which can determine directly or indirectly a marked reduction in the smooth muscular vascular tone that results in an altered blood distribution. Moreover, it has been reported that the endothelial cells suffer structural changes, with cellular detachment and denudation mediated by TNF-α and also LPS that could directly activate receptors on the endothelial surface as part of the inflammatory response of these pathologic condition, that could stimulates apoptosis as a programmed cell death mechanism, which contributes to aggravate the clinical condition by the progressive development of multiorganic failure.

However, the decrease in the oxygen delivery is not the only mechanism to determine a hypoxic condition, also there is a difficulty of the cell to use the oxygen due in part to the mitochondrial dysfunction (see chapter 4) that also compromise de endothelial cells.

Both the hypoxic systemic or cellular conditions and the changes in the homeostatic state due a metabolic or respiratory pathological condition, promotes in very critically ill patients, a deregulation in their redox balance that predisposes to an OS. In that situation the endothelium is directly exposes to the systemic and local conditions that contribute to the generation of free radicals and a lesser efficiency of the antioxidant mechanisms.

Free radicals originated as ROS and RNS (see chapter 1), have several potentially important effects on endothelial function that are also implicated in both physiological regulation and disease pathophysiologic mechanisms. In a hypoperfusion condition as occurs in shock, it is more probable an imbalance between the production of ROS and their effective removal by non-enzymatic and enzymatic antioxidants systems, these contribute to induce or increase a preexistent ED that aggravates the hemodynamic condition due to: alteration in vascular tone regulation, increase of endothelial cell adhesion properties (especially to leukocytes and platelets) and vascular wall permeability, and a change in the endothelial functional characteristics to a pro-coagulant state, that is clue in the most critical condition.

Increasing evidence supports the idea that the principal cause of ED during sepsis is cell injury, it has been very difficult to study endothelial cell in vitro without prevent the lost of their natural characteristics as occurs in vivo. Mitochondria plays a crucial role in the development of critical condition particularly in association with sepsis, ROS and RNS contribute to mitochondrial dysfunction by a range of mechanisms and induce both necrotic and apoptotic cell death (see chapter 4). Stimulation of endothelial cells with LPS leads to a decrease in mitochondrial oxygen consumption that is related to a specific inhibition at Complex I, enhanced ROS production and an altered redox state due to a decreased GSH content. There is a mitochondrial dysfunction, oxidative stress and/or GSH depletion in LPS-treated human umbilical vein endothelial cells (HUVEC) and HUVEC stimulated with plasma from patients with sepsis.

HUVEC cells exposed to 21% *vs* 1% O_2 present more marked expression of NOS-2 that seemed to return to nearly basal levels at 24 h in both oxygen conditions. Stimulation with LPS leads to a decrease in mitochondrial oxygen. The role of oxidative stress in mitochondrial dysfunction has been explored with the use of mitochondria-specific antioxidants, Mitoquinona (MQ), mitochondria-targeted ubiquinone and GSH-releasing molecule (GEE), a molecule of ubiquitous intracellular distribution which also reaches the mitochondria. Importantly, GSH, the most abundant cellular redox-active and antioxidant molecule, is not synthesized in the mitochondria, and its presence in this compartment is fully dependent on its synthesis in the cytosol by the ATP-requiring enzymes γ-glutamylcysteine ligase and GSH synthetase, upon which it is transported into mitochondria. Then, it is logical to postulate that early oxidative stress in the mitochondria can affect intramitochondrial GSH levels prior to those in the other cellular compartments. [25]

In addition, mitochondrial antioxidants are of benefit in managing mitochondrial dysfunction and oxidative damage during sepsis. The results provide insights for the potential therapeutic use of mitochondrial antioxidants, such as GEE and MQ, and redox-active compounds during conditions of septic shock [25].

Despite recent advances in biomedical research, sepsis remains an important medical challenge (see chapter 2). An estimated 750,000 cases of severe sepsis are diagnosed each year in the United States alone [26]. Severe sepsis is a major cause of morbidity and mortality, claiming between 36000 and 64000 lives annually in the UK, with a mortality rate of 35%. [27]

Septic shock and septic vascular dysfunction are characterized by systemic hypotension, persistent vasodilatation, hyporesponsiveness to vasoconstrictors, and impairment of endothelium-dependent vasodilator response, the last is the principal characteristic of ED. Moreover the endothelium in septic conditions and in systemic inflammatory response also has a protrombotic state, as part of the ED, which contributes to the development of a disseminated intravascular coagulation (DIC), and thereby to the severity of the clinical condition. The most common and dramatic clinical feature is sepsis associated to DIC, moreover the widespread thrombosis in the microcirculation of different organs may importantly contribute to solitary or multiple organ dysfunction (MODS) (see chapter 6). The development of MODS is a major determinant of mortality in sepsis.

DIC is classically associated with Gram negative bacterial infections but it can occur with a similar incidence in Gram positive sepsis. However, systemic infections with other micro-organisms, such as viruses, Rickettsiae and even parasites (e.g. Plasmodium falciparum) may also result in DIC. The pathophysiology of sepsis-associated DIC is extremely complex, the key event is the systemic inflammatory response to the infectious agent. The causative micro-organisms express unique cellular constituents not found in vertebrate animals, now referred to as pathogen-associated molecular patterns (PAMPs), or microbial- associated molecular patterns (for example endotoxin or lipopolysaccharide, LPS). Moreover, during infection, inflammation or stress, host cell-derived factors are generated as "danger signals" (alarmins) which, together with PAMPs, are referred to as danger-associated molecular patterns (DAMPs). These elements are recognized via specific receptors called pattern recognition receptors (PRRs), among which the Toll-like receptors (TLRs) and the complement receptors, by immune and other host cells (monocytes-macrophages, platelets and endothelial cells among others), with the subsequent activation of specific intracellular signal-transduction pathways reactions. Inflammation can also results in activated cells that amplify the inflammatory eventually results in the synthesis of a number of proteins including proinflammatory cytokines. The latter, together with other mediators generated by the inflammatory cascade, including those derived from complement activation, act in concert with the micro-organisms and/or their products to trigger the coagulation pathways, DIC and organ dysfunction. Interestingly, enzymes generated during the clotting cascade can also interact with specific cellular receptors thus eliciting cell responses reactions. Inflammation can also result in cell apoptosis or necrosis and recent evidence indicates that products released from dead cells, such as nuclear proteins, are able to propagate further inflammation, coagulation, to cause cell death and organ failure.

In these conditions the key event underlying sepsis complication is the overwhelming inflammatory host response to the infectious agent leading to the over expression of inflammatory mediators. These host response, together with the microorganism and its derivatives, predispose to an haemostatic abnormalities ranging from subclinical activation of blood coagulation (hypercoagulability), which may contribute to localized venous thromboembolism, to DIC, characterized by massive thrombin formation and widespread microvascular thrombosis, partly responsible of the MODS, and subsequent consumption of platelets and coagulation proteins causing, in most severe cases, bleeding manifestations.

The endothelial dysfunction plays a key role in CID development, in this state there is a: 1) Up-regulation of procoagulant molecules, primarily tissue factor (TF), which is produced mainly by stimulated monocytes-macrophages and by specific cells in target tissues; 2) Impairment of physiological anticoagulant pathways (antithrombin, protein C pathway, tissue factor pathway inhibitor), and 3) Suppression of fibrinolysis due to increased plasminogen activator inhibitor-1 (PAI-1) by endothelial cells and likely also to thrombin-mediated activation of thrombin-activatable fibrinolysis inhibitor (TAFI).

The inflammatory response can be seen amplified by the involvement of hemostasis factors that have enzymatic activity that not only lead to microvascular thrombosis but can also directly or indirectly elicit cellular responses as cell apoptosis or necrosis. The products released from dead cells, such as nuclear proteins (particularly extracellular histones), are able to propagate further inflammation, coagulation, cell death and MODS. These insights into the pathogenetic mechanisms of DIC and MODS may have important implications for the development of new therapeutic agents that could be potentially useful particularly for the management of severe sepsis [10].

One of the well-established mechanisms for the vascular dysfunction is the activation of nuclear factor (NF)-kB patways. Bacterial pathogens and their products, such as LPS, activate NF-kB, which causes iNOS expression, leading to an excessive production of NO, that causes vasodilatation, vascular hiporeactivity, and hypotension by activating soluble guanylyl cyclase-dependent mechanism. Also NF-kB activation mediates the expression of numerous cytokines, which lead to further activation of NF-kB, amplifying, and perpetuating the inflammatory response. Furthermore, LPS and cytokines as TNF-α, down-regulate endothelial eNOS expression, which contributes to the development of ED.

Studies show that the constitutive NF-kB blockade did not inhibit LPS-induced tissue factor expression in the heart, kidney, or liver. However, this blockade prevented LPS induced downregulation of endothelial protein C receptor and thrombomodulin protein expression, inhibited TNF-a converting enzyme activity, ameliorated protein C levels, and reduced PAI-1 gene expression. Using transgenic mice that conditionally over expressed the NF-kB inhibitor I-kBa, results in a selective inhibition of endothelial NF-kB caused significantly less hypotension and no impairments in vasoconstriction and endothelium-dependent vasodilatory responses upon LPS challenge. Transgenic mice with selective endothelial NF-kB blockade also reduced aortic inducible NOS expression, decreased plasma and aortic levels of nitrite/nitrate, increased aortic endothelial NOS expression and reduced aortic TNF-a expression, thus mitigating the cascade of events that leads to septic vascular dysfunction [28].

In sepsis the resultant vascular dysfunction is associated to raised plasma asymmetric dimethyl-L-arginine (ADMA) concentrations that can be a strong predictor of death in patients with sepsis and thus may be useful as a prognostic marker. Impaired endothelial and microvascular function due to decreased endothelial NO production may be a mechanism linking ADMA with organ dysfunction and mortality. The dimethylaminohydrolase-(DDAH)-ADMA axis is a potential therapeutic target and may be important in individual tailoring of therapy. Agents which compete with ADMA for NOS (such as L-arginine) or which potentiate DDAH activity should be further investigated in sepsis [29].

Moreover the difficulty to cover the diverse requirements of tissues in sepsis, is aggravated by the coexistence of a myocardial dysfunction (see chapter 13) that occurs through multiple pathophysiologic mechanisms, which are increasingly shown to be interrelated. The Mitochondrial dysfunction and the TLR-4/NF-kB signal transduction pathways are likely the most promising areas of research for the development of new therapeutic agents. New drugs against sepsis and septic cardiomyopathy will not only ameliorate morbidity/mortality but also improve cost containment as intensive care is shortened [30].

Acute systemic inflammatory and procoagulant response in sepsis, not only produce ED since it also result in structural and functional alterations in the endothelium. An activation of number of cytokines, especially TNF-α, are released by lipopolysacharide (LPS)-activated inflammatory cells. During the onset of an endotoxin response this cells are important for host immune defense and resolution of the inflammatory response as they interact with invading pathogens. In response to these pathologic processes, endothelial cells undergo structural and functional changes including cellular detachment and denudation, altered vasomotor tone, and programmed cell death, which can lead to microvascular injury of organs and a decrease in capillary perfusion, an important element in the development of multiorgan failure in sepsis. These alterations often yield further activation of other myeloid-derived cells and/or endothelium. In the last decade, the concept of postnatal vasculogenesis has been revolutionized to include angiogenesis by mature endothelial cells and vasculogenesis by endothelial progenitor cells. These cells are recruited from the bone marrow to areas of endothelial injury, at which point they differentiate and promote revascularization of the endothelium, which has been shown to have significant prognostic and therapeutic implications in a variety of ischemic vascular disorders.

This relative new concept also it has been applied to the mechanisms that are involved in the vascular dysfunction during sepsis and was described that there is a reconstitution of the endothelial layer that occurs via migration and proliferation of surrounding mature endothelial cells. However, differentiated endothelial cells have low proliferative potential and their ability to repair damaged endothelium is limited. Endothelial protein C receptor (EPCR), primarily expressed on hematopoietic leukocytes and non hematopoietic endothelium, binds protein C and increases the rate of protein C activation on the endothelium. Circulating endothelial progenitor cells may be an important mechanism of vascular repair, and thus shows significant promise for prognostic and therapeutic strategies in critical illness, namely sepsis and sepsis-related organ dysfunction [31].

Recently, several clinical studies documented mobilization of endothelial progenitor cells (EPCs) during endotoxemia, with the probability of patients' survival correlating with the rise in circulating EPCs. This fact combined with endotoxemia-induced vascular injury led to hypothesize that the developing functional EPC incompetence could impede vascular repair and that adoptive transfer of EPCs could improve hemodynamics in endotoxemia.

In experimental models with LPS injection, EPCs isolated from endotoxemic mice exhibited impaired clonogenic potential and LPS exerted Toll-like receptor 4-mediated cytotoxic effects toward EPCs, which was mitigated by embedding them in hyaluronic acid (HA) hydrogels. Adoptive transfer of EPCs in LPS-injected mice improved control of blood pressure and reduced hepatocellular and renal dysfunction. Specifically, EPC treatment was associated with the restoration of renal microcirculation and improved renal function. These findings establish major therapeutic benefits of adoptive transfer of EPCs, especially when embedded in HA hydrogels, in mice with LPS-induced endotoxemia, and they argue that hemodynamic and renal abnormalities of endotoxemia are in significant part due to developing incompetence of endogenous EPCs [32].

The capacity of endothelium to contribute to the vascular repair is in part due to the vascular endothelial growth factor (VEGF) activity. Yang et al. studied in patients with septic shock due to pneumonia, and patients with pneumonia without organ dysfunction, and their major findings were that circulating levels of soluble vascular endothelial cell growth factor receptor-1 (sVEGFR-1) and urokinase-type plasminogen activator (uPA) were associated with organ dysfunction and mortality, however vascular VEGF levels had no such predictive power. The study serves not only to provide evidence in support of new diagnostic biomarker targets in sepsis, but also to augment the growing evidence of an important role of the endothelium in sepsis in general, and the VEGF signaling axis in particular [33, 34].

Conclusion

The endothelium is a heterogeneous and dynamic organ, distributed along the body, in direct relation with the diverse circulating elements and substances present on its vascular luminal face, and also with the basal lamina and the subjacent tissues of the vascular wall. Through a big area for interchanges and interactions, the endothelium promotes homeostasis in physiologic conditions by sensing and transducing signals between blood and tissue, to coordinate the blood flow regulation, and to maintaining an anti trombogenic surface, also it controls the traffic of hematopoietic cells. The endothelium responds rapidly to diverse stimuli such as shear stress, coagulation proteins, growth factors, cytokines and microbial components among others. When the endothelium is perturbed by one of this stimulus, it changes to an "activated" state that is beneficial for the organism because in general it defends to face microorganism agents and for repair tissue injury, usually this response is localized. However under some circumstances endothelial responses are detrimental to the host as occurs in ED. The most characteristic of them is the severe sepsis in which the endothelial activation has the characteristic of exaggerated, sustained, systemic and finally progressively deleterious for the organism.

The translation of research data about endothelium studies into clinical practice is very difficult due the heterogeneity among species (animals *vs.* humans), tissues/organs (e.g., lungs *vs.* gut), and vessel segments (macrovessels *vs.* microvessels). However it is necessary to incorporate new therapeutic strategies that allow improving the evolution and prognosis of critical patients where endothelium plays a clue role as a target of many types of factors that both are exogenous (i.e. pathogens and their products, toxic agents) and endogenous (i.e. cytokines, metabolic components) which activate the endothelium, to coordinate the host response, but the endothelium from a patient in a critical condition could be overwhelmed in its regulator capacity and becoming in a dysfunctional state that ultimately is detrimental to the organism. Clinical conditions with severe hemodynamic compromise are usually heterogeneous and change with time, therefore it requires acute evaluation of the therapeutic regimen and the patient characteristics and clinical condition [35, 36].

The attenuation of the endothelial OS state is clue for the patient prognosis, in this sense there is a promissory future by the actual development of both OS biomarkers for clinical diagnosis and the antioxidant therapies (see chapters 11 and 12). However, other therapies that could be very effective to replace the injured cells to cut the deleterious circle of damaged and dysfunctional endothelium seems to need more time to be incorporated.

References

[1] Rock KL, Latz E, Ontiveros F, Kono H. The sterile inflammatory response. *Annu. Rev. Immunol.* 2010;28:321-42.

[2] Félétou M. The Endothelium, Part I: Multiple Functions of the Endothelial Cells--Focus on Endothelium-Derived Vasoactive Mediators. *Integrated Systems Physiology: from Molecule to Function to Disease.* San Rafael (CA): Morgan and Claypool Life Sciences;. 2011.

[3] Aird WC. Phenotypic heterogeneity of the endothelium: I. Structure, function, and mechanisms. *Circ. Res.* 2007,100:158-73.

[4] Aird WC. Phenotypic heterogeneity of the endothelium: II. Representative vascular beds. *Circ. Res.* 2007;100:174-90.

[5] Tarbell JM. Shear stress and the endothelial transport barrier. *Cardiovasc. Res.* 2010;87(2):320-30.

[6] Aird WC. Discovery of the cardiovascular system: from Galen to William Harvey. *J Thromb Haemost* 2011;9 Suppl 1:118-29.

[7] Félétou M, Vanhoutte PM. Endothelial dysfunction: a multifaceted disorder (The Wiggers Award Lecture). *Am. J. Physiol. Heart Circ. Physiol.* 2006;291:H985-1002.

[8] Lu D, Kassab GS. Role of shear stress and stretch in vascular mechanobiology. *J R Soc Interface* 2011:1379-1385.

[9] Jazuli F, Pyke KE. The impact of baseline artery diameter on flow-mediated vasodilation: a comparison of brachial and radial artery responses to matched levels of shear stress. *Am. J. Physiol. Heart Circ. Physiol.* 2011;301:H1667-77.

[10] Semeraro N, Ammollo CT, Semeraro F, Colucci M. Sepsis-associated disseminated intravascular coagulation and thromboembolic disease. *Mediterr. J. Hematol. Infect. Dis.* 2010;2:e2010024.

[11] Durán WN, Breslin JW, Sánchez F a. The NO cascade, eNOS location, and microvascular permeability. *Cardiovasc Res* 2010;87:254-61.

[12] Bates DO. Vascular endothelial growth factors and vascular permeability. *Cardiovasc. Res.* 2010;87:262-71.

[13] Stock C, Riethmuller C. Endothelial activation drives lateral migration and diapedesis of leukocytes. *Cell Immunol* 2011;271:180-3.

[14] van der Loo B, Schildknecht S, Zee R, Bachschmid MM. Signalling processes in endothelial ageing in relation to chronic oxidative stress and their potential therapeutic implications in humans. *Exp. Physiol.* 2009;94:305-10.

[15] Liu D-H, Chen Y-M, Liu Y, Hao B-S, Zhou B, Wu L, Wang M, Chen L, Wu W-K, Qian X-X. Rb1 protects endothelial cells from hydrogen peroxide-induced cell senescence by modulating redox status. *Biol. Pharm. Bull.* 2011;34:1072-7.

[16] Förstermann U. Nitric oxide and oxidative stress in vascular disease. *Pflügers Archiv* 2010;459:923-39.

[17] Dröge W. Free radicals in the physiological control of cell function. *Physiol. Rev.* 2002;82:47-95.

[18] Valko M, Leibfritz D, Moncol J, Cronin MTD, Mazur M, Telser J. Free radicals and antioxidants in normal physiological functions and human disease. *Int. J. Biochem. Cell Biol.* 2007;39:44-84.

[19] Ferrero E, Fulgenzi A, Belloni D, Foglieni C, Ferrero ME. Cellfood™ improves respiratory metabolism of endothelial cells and inhibits hypoxia-induced reactive oxygen species (ros) generation. *J. Physiol. Pharmacol.* 2011;62:287-293.

[20] Rodrigo R. Hypertension in: Oxidative Stress and Antioxidants: Their role in Human Disease. Ed Nova Biomedical Books New York 2009; Chap2:25-62.

[21] van der Loo B, Labugger R, Skepper JN, Bachschmid M, Kilo J, Powell JM, Palacios-Callender M, Erusalimsky JD, Quaschning T, Malinski T, Gygi D, Ullrich V, Lüscher TF. Enhanced peroxynitrite formation is associated with vascular aging. *J. Exp. Med.* 2000;192:1731-44.

[22] Bulua AC, Simon A, Maddipati R, Pelletier M, Park H, Kim KY, Sack MN, Kastner DL, Siegel RM. Mitochondrial reactive oxygen species promote production of proinflammatory cytokines and are elevated in TNFR1-associated periodic syndrome (TRAPS). *J. Exp. Med.* 2011;208:519-33.

[23] Martens CR, Edwards DG. Peripheral vascular dysfunction in chronic kidney disease. *Cardiol. Res. Pract.* 2011;2011:1-9.

[24] Fernández-Sánchez A, Madrigal-Santillán E, Bautista M, Esquivel-Soto J, Morales-González A, Esquivel-Chirino C, Durante-Montiel I, Sánchez-Rivera G, Valadez-Vega C, Morales-González J a. Inflammation, oxidative stress, and obesity. *Int. J. Mol. Sci.* 2011;12:3117-3132.

[25] Apostolova N, Garcia-Bou R, Hernandez-Mijares A, Herance R, Rocha M, Victor VM. Mitochondrial Antioxidants Alleviate Oxidative and Nitrosative Stress in a Cellular Model of Sepsis. *Pharm. Res.* 2011;28:2910-2919.

[26] Angus DC, Linde-Zwirble WT, Lidicker J, Clermont G, Carcillo J, Pinsky MR. Epidemiology of severe sepsis in the United States: analysis of incidence, outcome, and associated costs of care. *Crit. Care Med.* 2001;29:1303-10.

[27] Daniels R. Surviving the first hours in sepsis: getting the basics right (an intensivist's perspective). *J. Antimicrob. Chemother.* 2011;66 Suppl 2:ii11-23.

[28] Ding J, Song D, Ye X, Liu SF. A pivotal role of endothelial-specific NF-kappaB signaling in the pathogenesis of septic shock and septic vascular dysfunction. *J. Immunol.* 2009;183:4031-4038.

[29] Davis JS, Darcy CJ, Yeo TW, Jones C, McNeil YR, Stephens DP, Celermajer DS, Anstey NM. Asymmetric dimethylarginine, endothelial nitric oxide bioavailability and mortality in sepsis. *PLoS One* 2011;6:e17260.

[30] Balija TM, Lowry SF. Lipopolysaccharide and sepsis-associated myocardial dysfunction. *Curr. Opin. Infect. Dis.* 2011;24:248-253.

[31] Cribbs SK, Martin GS, Rojas M. Monitoring of endothelial dysfunction in critically ill patients: the role of endothelial progenitor cells. *Curr. Opin. Crit. Care* 2008;14: 354-360.

[32] Ghaly T, Rabadi MM, Weber M, Rabadi SM, Bank M, Grom JM, Fallon JT, Goligorsky MS, Ratliff BB. Hydrogel-embedded endothelial progenitor cells evade LPS and mitigate endotoxemia. *Am. J. Physiol. Renal. Physiol.* 2011;301:F802-F812.

[33] Yang K-Y, Liu K-T, Chen Y-C, Chen C-S, Lee Y-C, Perng R-P, Feng J-Y. Plasma soluble vascular endothelial growth factor receptor-1 levels predict outcomes of pneumonia-related septic shock patients: a prospective observational study. *Crit. Care* 2011;15:R11.

[34] Shapiro NI, Aird WC. Sepsis and the broken endothelium. *Crit. Care* 2011;15:135.

[35] Ceneviva G, Paschall JA, Maffei F, Carcillo JA. Hemodynamic support in fluid-refractory pediatric septic shock; *Pediatrics.* 1998;102:1-6.

[36] Aneja R, Carcillo J. Differences between adult and pediatric septic shock. *Minerva. Anestesiol.* 2011;77:986-992.

In: Oxidative Stress and the Critically Ill Patient
Editors: Ramón Rodrigo and Bettina von Dessauer
ISBN: 978-1-62081-576-2

Chapter VI

PATHOPHYSIOLOGY OF MULTIPLE ORGAN DYSFUNCTION SYNDROME IN SEPSIS

***Diego Saa Lic*[1] *and Ramón Rodrigo*[*2]**
[1]Renal Pathophysiology Laboratory, Molecular and Clinical Pharmacology Program,
Institute of Biomedical Sciences,
Faculty of Medicine, University of Chile, Chile
[2]Molecular and Clinical Pharmacology Program
Institute of Biomedical Sciences, Faculty of Medicine,
University of Chile, Chile

ABSTRACT

Multiple Organ Dysfunction Syndrome (MODS) accounts for a leading risk of morbidity and mortality among intensive care unit patients (ICU) patients. It results from progressive functional impairment of different organs in an acutely ill patient. In Sepsis, complex interactions between multiple immunomodulating mediators, various cell populations activated by the initial septic insult and the increased oxidative stress could cause the development of organ dysfunction, through chaotic, uncontrolled inflammatory cascades. Nevertheless, in conjunction with the injurious effects of these pathophysiological events, recent insights into MODS pathophysiology understanding have arisen, providing new approaches to this pathology, considering that it might represent an adaptive response in response to an overwhelming injury to avoid irreversible end-stage organ damage.

Keywords: MODS – Sepsis – Oxidative Stress – ROS/RNS

[*] Corresponding author. Address: Reyes Lavalle 3415, Depto. 71, Las Condes, Santiago, Región Metropolitana, Chile

ABBREVIATIONS

α-KDH	α-ketonic acid dehydrogenase
ACCP	American College of Chest Physicians
AKI	Acute kidney injury
AKIN	Acute kidney injury network
ALI	Acute lung injury
ARDS	Acute respiratory distress syndrome
AP-1	Activator protein-1
ATS	American Thoracic Society
BAL	Bronchoalveolar lavage fluid
Casp-3	Caspase-3
CBF	Cerebral blood flow
CLR	Calcitonin receptor-like
CNS	Central nervous system
CSF	Cerebral spinal fluid
CO	Cardiac output
COX-2	Ciclooxygenase-2
DIC	Disseminated intravascular coagulation
EC	Endothelial cells
EEG	Electroencephalogram
EF	Ejection fraction
ESICM	European Society of Intensive Care Medicine
FiO_2	Inspirated O_2 fraction
GFR	Glomerular filtration ratio
GI	Gastrointestinal
GSH	Reduced Glutathione
GSSG	Oxidized Glutathiondimmers
HDL	High density lipoprotein
HMBG-1	High morbility group protein box-1
HIV	Human Immunodeficiency virus
ICAM-1	Intercellular adhesion molecule-1
ICU	Intensive care unit
IFN- γ	Interferon-γ
IL-1, -4, -6, -8, -10, -13	Interleukin-1, -4, -6, -8, -10, -13
IL-1 β	Interleukine-1β
IL-1Ra	Interleukin-1 receptor antagonist
iNOS	Induced Nitric oxide synthase
KBR	Ketone body ratio
L-NAME	L-NG-Nitroarginine-methyl-ester
LPS	Lipopolysacharide
MAP	Mean arterial pressure
MDA	Malondialdehyde
MMDS	Mitochondrial and Microcirculatory distress syndrome
MODS	Multiple organ dysfunction syndrome

MUST	Multiple urgent sepsis therapies
$NAD^+/NADH+H^+$	Oxidized Nicotinamide adenine dinucleotide to reduced nicotinamide adenine dinucleotide
NF-κB	Nuclear factor kappa B
NMDA	N-methyl-D-aspartate receptor
NO	Nitric oxide
NOD	Nucleotide-binding oligomerization domain-containing protein
$ONOO^-$	Peroxinitrite anion
PAMP	Pathogen-associated molecular pattern
PaO_2	Arterial O_2 pressure
PARP	*Poly (ADP-ribose) polymerase*
PCT	Procalcitonin
PCWP	Pulmonary capillary wedge pressure
PRR	Pattern recognition receptor
RBF	Renal blood flow
RLR	Retinoic acid inducible gene I-like receptor family
RNS	Reactive nitrogen species
ROS	Reactive oxygen species
ROS/RNS	Reactive oxygen and nitrogen species
SCCM	Society of Critical Care Medicine
SE	Septic encephalopathy
SIS	Surgical Infection Society
SIRS	Systemic inflammatory response syndrome
SOAP	Sepsis Occurrence in Acutely Ill Patients study
SVR	Systemic vascular resistance
TBARS	Thiobarbituric acid reactive substances
TF	Tissue factor
TFPI	Tissue factor plasmatic inhibitor
TGF-β	Transforming growth factor-B
TLR	Toll-like receptor
TNF-α	Tumor necrosis factor-a
TRAP	Total radical-trapping antioxidant parameter

2. Introduction: An Overview of MODS Reality

The current term of Multiple Organ Dysfunction Syndrome (MODS) was defined in the early 1990's by The American College of Chest Physicians (ACCP) and the Society of Critical Care Medicine (SCCM) in a Consensus Conference where they established definitions for adult septic patients [1]. Despite recent review of these definitions by different entities such as the European Society of Intensive Care Medicine (ESICM), the American Thoracic Society (ATS) and the Surgical Infection Society (SIS), they remain largely accepted and unchanged [2]. In this Consensus Conference, the terms Systemic inflammatory response syndrome (SIRS), sepsis, severe sepsis and septic shock were defined [1,2], and also, the old term "septicaemia,", was recommended to be eliminated [1], since it straddles the definitions of sepsis, severe sepsis, and septic shock [3]. Finally, the Multiple Organ Dysfunction Syndrome (MODS) was defined as the presence of multiple altered organ function in an acutely ill patient, such that homeostasis cannot be maintained without intervention, thereby describing a pattern of multiple and progressive symptoms and signs that are thought to be pathogenetically related [1].

2.1. Multiple Organ Dysfunction Syndrome or Multiple Organ Failure?

Several terms have been introduced in time to describe this evolving process of an otherwise unexplained progressive physiologic failure of several interdependent organ systems in critically ill patients, including: *progressive* or *sequential organ failure, multiple organ failure* and *multiple systems organ failure*. Nevertheless, this terminology has been considered to be inadequate to accurately describe this syndrome, since they are based on the concept of organ *failure*, a dichotomous event that is either present or absent; rather than organ *dysfunction*, a concept representing a continuum of physiologic derangements. In summary, this terminology proposes a dynamically changing concept, a continuum of change over time, rather than static criteria of organ function absence [1].

2.2. Primary and Secondary MODS

Etiologically, MODS can be described in terms of two different, but not exclusive entities. Primary MODS is defined as the direct result of a well-defined insult, in which organ dysfunction occurs early and can be directly attributable to the initial insult, and the abnormally excessive host inflammatory response is not as evident as in secondary MODS. Conversely, secondary MODS develops after a negative evolution of a primary severe disease, not in direct response to an initial insult, but as a consequence of a host response, representing a life-threatening event in SIRS/Sepsis [1].

3. Epidemiology of MODS: Why Should MODS Be Considered as an Important Health Care Issue?

Using the PAHO/CENDES method of Priorization in Health Planning [4], it can be stated that MODS should be considered an important Health Care issue.

3.1. Magnitude, Transcendence and Tendencies of MODS: Prevalence, Incidence and Morbid-mortality

The increasing incidence and prevalence of morbidity and mortality of MODS has paralleled improvements in the life-support technologies available to patients admitted to an ICU [1], becoming the leading cause of morbid-mortality for patients admitted to an ICU, and developing in about 15% of all ICU admissions [5]. In addition, the incidence of sepsis in large epidemiological studies of up to 6 million people give an incidence of 3 per 1000 population per year or about 750000 cases a year in the United States [3] showing that the incidence of sepsis, severe sepsis and septic shock is increasing year by year. Although mortality is decreasing, it remains unacceptably high [5,6]. Similarly, The SOAP study, a observational, prospective and multicentre study, conducted in European countries showed a marked difference in the frequency of sepsis between countries, and higher frequencies of sepsis were mirrored by higher mortality rates [6,7]. Also, the assessment of key organ systems shows that increasing severity of organ dysfunction and the number of involved organ systems correlates with increasing mortality, which rises from 25-30% for severe sepsis up to 40-70% for septic shock in adults [3], as shown by the SOAP study where patients with no organ dysfunction on admission had mortality rates of 6% whereas those with four or more organ failures had mortality rates of 65% [7–9]. Numerous factors are thought to contribute to this increasing incidence, including advancing age, immunosuppression due to aggressive cancer therapy and the increased prevalence of HIV and multidrug-resistant infections due to indiscriminate use of broad spectrum antibiotics [5,6]. On the other hand, reductions in mortality have not been attributed to sepsis-specific knowledge or interventions, but rather to earlier and more general improvements in acute and intensive hospital care [5]. Additionally, it has been found that comorbidities influence the risk and outcome of sepsis and those cumulative comorbidities are associated with greater organ dysfunction [5]. In this context, it has been found that a major threat to survival was not the underlying illness or even a single complication thereof, but rather a process of an otherwise unexplained progressive physiologic failure of several interdependent organ systems in critically ill patients, termed MODS [1]. Thus, the development and persistence of MODS in the context of sepsis, is the major contributor to death in most instances [5].

3.2. The Economic Burden of MODS: Budget, Expenses and Costs

The concept of Burden-of-illness consists in the direct and indirect costs related to a specific disease. Direct costs are those resulting directly from health interventions and are divided into medical and non-medical costs [10]. Direct medical costs associated with severe sepsis primarily consist of hospital personnel, accounting for 45-60% of the total ICU budget, while variable costs including drugs, other consumables, laboratory and diagnostic services, amounted to 30% of total costs, demonstrating why caring for septic patients has been shown to be 6-fold than caring for ICU patients without sepsis [11].

According to data from the US, each septic patient consumes, during hospitalization, about US$ 25,000, corresponding to approximately $17 billion annually [12], which may increase with severity of illness and outcome [13,14]. Thus, it can be concluded that an effective reduction in costs for a patient with severe sepsis in the ICU, could be achieved either by shortening length of stay or by reducing drug consumption [10]. In parallel, indirect or social costs have also been estimated as being excessively elevated, and have been estimated as 2–3 times the direct costs [10]. These costs, account for the productivity loss associated with absenteeism, due to temporary unfitness for work, premature retirement, or premature death [10,15].

Finally, Schmid et al. [16] estimated the burden of illness in Germany, ranging from €3,647 to €7,874 million per year. Productivity loss due to mortality represented the largest portion (56%), followed by direct costs (28%), productivity loss due to permanent morbidity (12%), and due to temporary morbidity (4%).

3.3. Vulnerability and Cost-Effectiveness of Current Treatments

Prevention of sepsis depends on defining the risk group and the availability of appropriate and on-time interventions. For example, invasive pneumococcal disease in agammaglobulinaemic patients has declined since the advent of intravenous gammaglobulin and vaccination is available. Thus, bacteremia with pneumococci seems to be reduced in the vaccinated population [3].

Evatuating the costs and cost-effectiveness of integrated protocols using the Surviving Sepsis Campaign guidelines [17], Shorr et al. [18] evaluated the economic impact of an evidence-based sepsis protocol in their institutions. In addition to increased survival rates, the median total hospital costs were significantly lower with use of the protocol, mainly because of shorter length of stay. Hence, the implementation of a sepsis management protocol was able both to improve mortality rate and to substantially save money.

Similarly, Tamor et al [19] evaluated the impact of the Multiple Urgent Sepsis Therapies (MUST) protocol, based on early goal-directed therapy [20]. They reported an association between adoption of this integrated sepsis protocol and increased in-patient survival at a moderate increase in treatment costs, due to increased ICU length of stay.

Finally, a recent systematic review was carried out to identify critical care interventions that are cost-effective [21]. The authors concluded that only drotrecogin alfa (activated) -a recombinant human activated protein C- for patients with sepsis, mechanical ventilation, and early admission to the ICU itself had acceptable cost-effectiveness ratios. Conversely, unfavorable was the use of drotrecogin alfa (activated) in septic patients with low risk (APACHE<25), mechanical ventilation in patients over 40 years with stroke, and admission to the ICU for patients with hematologic malignancies.

4. Pathophysiological Mechanisms Involved in MODS

4.1. Natural History of Sepsis-Induced MODS

Sepsis originates from a breach of integrity of the host barriers, either physical (skin and mucous membranes) or immunological and direct penetration of the pathogen into the bloodstream. Loss of integrity of the external barrier by trauma, urinary catheters, intravenous cannulas or an endotracheal tube or loss of integrity of the internal barrier in the gastrointestinal tract and hepatobiliary system [3], allows the development of an inflammatory response against an infectious agent (bacteria, virus, parasite or fungi) through the release of pro and anti-inflammatory mediators. The eliciting pathogen can be recognized by the Host Innate Immune System through evolution-conserved molecules, known as PRR

(Pattern recognition receptors, i.e. TLR, NOD, RLR, CLR) which can interact with specific pathogen-associated molecular patterns (PAMP) located on structural molecules on the bacterial cell wall (Lipopolysaccharide, Lipoteichoic acid, Peptidoglycan), specific bacterial proteins (Flagellin) or bacterial, viral and fungi Nucleic acids, initiating the organism's defense response. The interaction between the Lypopolysaccharide (LPS) and Toll-like receptor-4 (TLR-4, the more characteristic PRR) initiates a proinflammatory molecular cascade, which activates different transcription factors such as NF-κB (Nuclear factor kappa-light chain enhancer of activated B cells) and AP-1 (activator protein-1), which further induce the expression of proinflammatory mediators. Hence, the expression of cytokines, chemokines, adhesion molecules and other inflammatory-induced enzymes (COX-2, iNOS) becomes up-regulated. In addition, the ischemic and hypoxic state of tissue in the context of severe sepsis or septic shock, further promote the activation of proinflammatory mediators, due to effective volume loss, disseminated intravascular coagulation and vasoplegia [22].

The vasoplegia can be explained in terms of elevated levels of NO and opening of ATP-dependent K^+-channels (K^+_{ATP}-channels) due to decreased intracellular ATP concentration, which leads to closure of Ca^{+2}-channels, thus relaxing the vascular tone [23]. Therefore, the early institution of effective volume substitution and catecholamine therapy can both optimize the tissue oxygen delivery reducing the mortality as shown by Rivers et al. [20], and also control the inflammatory response by reducing the expression of proinflammatory biomarkers such as TNF-α, ICAM-1, IL-8, IL-1Ra and Casp-3 [22].

4.2. Role of ROS/RNS in the Pathophysiology of Sepsis-Induced MODS

Sepsis is associated with oxidative stress, as manifested by the increased activity of Xanthine oxidase and iNOS, and the elevated levels of reactive oxygen species (ROS), nitric oxide (NO) and peroxynitrite ($ONOO^-$) in plasma, resulting in both structural defects and dysfunctions of cellular processes. The increased production of ROS and reactive nitrogen species (RNS) is offset by a decreased antioxidant capacity. Thus, the plasma total radical-trapping antioxidant parameter (TRAP) which depends upon levels of uric acid, sulfhydryl (SH) groups of proteins, unconjugated bilirubin, vitamin C and vitamin E as well as other yet unidentified antioxidant factors are reduced, while the concentrations of lipid peroxides, nitrotyrosine and thiobarbituric acid reactive substances (TBARS), including malondialdehyde (MDA) and 4-hydroxynonenal are increased.

Also, they present reduced levels of α-tocopherol, selenium, vitamin A, β-carotene, lycopene and ascorbic acid. In fact, elevated levels of lipid peroxidation products, and lower plasma selenium and ascorbic acid levels have been associated with higher incidence of MODS and worse prognosis. Finally, within the cellular compartment the reduced glutathione (GSH) decreases and increases the concentration of oxidized Glutathione dimers (GSSG), leading to a decreased GSH/GSSG ratio [22,24].

4.3 .Cellular dysfunction: Roles of Microcirculatory and Mitochondrial dysfunction

Thus, considering the impairment of Macrocirculation in context of severe Sepsis and Septic shock, changes due to oxidative stress in the Microcirculation might take place. These changes are characterized by the presence of initial arteriolar vasoconstriction, the opening of arteriovenous shunts and capillary occlusion by activated leukocytes. In addition, the impaired capillary barrier function leads to loss of fluid from the intravascular into the interstitial space, generating a positive fluid balance. The impaired microcirculation and the extension of the diffusion route, thus contribute to organ hypoperfusion and injury. Furthermore, in recent years besides the disruption of substrate supply, cellular oxygen utilization disorders caused by inflammatory mediators and increased oxidative stress have been identified [22]. This interaction has been termed Mitochondrial and Microcirculatory distress syndrome (MMDS) and could account for the cellular hypoxia and explain its dysfunction in sepsis [25]. Further mechanisms of both Mitochondrial and Endothelial dysfunction can be found in Chapters 4 and 5, respectively.

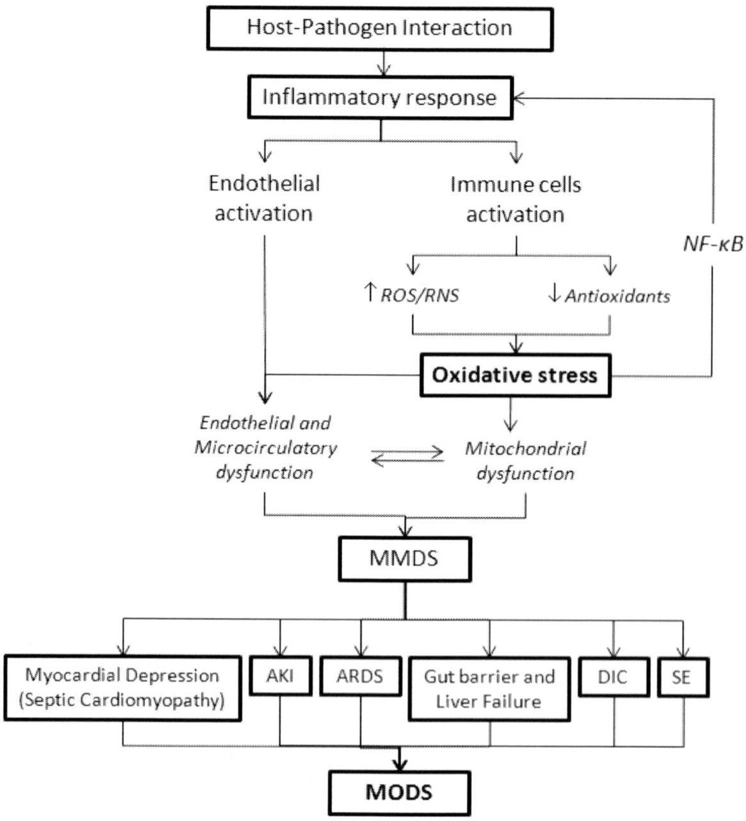

Figure 6.1. Pathophysiological mechanisms in sepsis-induced multiple organ dysfunction syndrome (MODS). Scheme highlighting the role of oxidative stress in microcirculatory and mitochondrial dysfunction leading toward organ-specific hypoxia and dysfunction. AKI: Acute kidney injury; ARDS: Acute respiratory distress syndrome; DIC: Disseminated intravscular coagulation; MMDS: Mitochondrial and microcirculatory distress syndrome; NF-κB: Nuclear factor-kappa B; ROS/RNS: reactive oxygen species and reactive nitrogen species; SE: Septic encephalopathy.

Finally, a possible integrated mechanistic vision the pathophysiological processes involved in MODS development is available in Figure 6.1.

5. Mechanisms of Specific Organ Dysfunction

It has been described that the main organs involved in MODS are the Cardiovascular system, the Brain, the Kidney, the Gastrointestinal tract, the Lung, the Liver and the Blood and the mortality of dysfunction of cardiovascular system ranked the highest [9].

5.1. Circulatory Dysfunction: Myocardial Depression (Septic Cardiomyopathy)

Myocardial depression or septic cardiomyopathy is a major contributor to morbi-mortality. It presents as a contractile dysfunction with biventricular dilatation, reversible decrease in the ejection fraction (EF), diminished blood pressure response to IV fluids, and blunted ability to adapt and augment cardiac output (CO) according to requirements, despite increased levels of circulating catecholamines. Commonly, the pathophysiologic alterations have been described biphasically; an early hyperdynamic ("warm") shock with increased CO, decreased systemic vascular resistance (SVR) and warm, perfused skin, followed by a hypodinamic ("cold") shock, where SVR is increased to compensate a decreased CO, leading to tissue hypoperfusion, cold and pale skin, and eventual MODS.

The exact trigger of septic cardiomyopathy is still unknown, but it is present even in early hyperdinamic shock, as manifested when septic stroke work indices are compared with non-septic patients. Thus, lower indices have been found in septic patients, correlating with a right- and downward shift in the Frank-Starling curve, leading to left ventricle dilatation.

Inflammatory mediators, such as TNF-α, IL-1β and IL-6, and their respective intracellular molecular signal transduction cascades have been under investigation, in order to determine a role in altered cardiac contractility, based on interactions in Ca^{+2} homeostasis, ATP-consuming reactions and mitochondrial function [26]. For further details, please see Chapters: Pathophysiology of sepsis and septic shock, and myocardial depression.

5.2. Respiratory Dysfunction: Acute Lung Injury (ALI) and Acute Respiratory Distress Syndrome (ARDS)

The definitions from the American-European Consensus Conference on ARDS the terms acute lung injury (ALI) and acute respiratory distress syndrome (ARDS) were established, and consists in an acute syndrome of non-cardiogenic pulmonary edema due to inflammation and increased permeability that is associated with respiratory distress signs and symptoms such as dyspnea, severe hypoxemia and decreased lung compliance with diffuse bilateral pulmonary infiltrates on chest radiograph. Thus, the exclusion of left atrial hypertension as the primary cause of hypoxemia is critical to this definition and the measurement of pulmonary capillary wedge pressure may be necessary (PCWP<18 mmHg). The distinction between ALI and ARDS is the degree of hypoxemia, defined for adults by the PaO_2/FiO_2 ratio; ALI is defined by a ratio less than 300 mm Hg, while a ratio less than 200 mm Hg is consistent with ARDS [27]. The mortality rates of ARDS are reported to be 30–60%, but a decrease of mortality has been documented using lung protective ventilation with low tidal volumes [28].

In sepsis-induced ARDS, the injured lung is believed to go through three phases: exudative, proliferative, and fibrotic. In the initial exudative phase, the key pathophysiological damaging mechanism rest on endothelial activation, which is central for lung endothelium injury and can occur by several mechanisms, although neutrophil-dependent lung injury is probably the final pathway. In sepsis, neutrophils accumulate in the vasculature and become activated, leading to degranulation and the release of several toxic mediators including: proteases, ROS, cytokines, and procoagulant molecules, which result in increased vascular permeability and a sustained loss of normal endothelial barrier function. Furthermore, recent evidence suggests a role of neutrophil-sequestrated platelets in lung endothelial injury, because they can interact with neutrophils and monocytes, which are sources of proinflammatory cytokines. However, the molecular pathways that link platelet- and neutrophil-mediated injury are incompletely understood. Thus, neutrophils integrate signals received from the endothelium and platelets, which can cause vascular injury. Additionally, some inflammatory mediators act directly on the lung endothelium, resulting in increased expression of chemokines and cell-surface leukocyte-adhesion molecules. As a result, leukocyte adhesion to the endothelium leads to inflammatory lung injury and further accumulation of other leukocytes in the lung. Once neutrophils have traversed the epithelium and enter the air spaces, they adhere to the apical surface, where they may phagocytize and kill bacteria. Under physiologic conditions, neutrophils can cross the paracellular space and reseal epithelial intercellular junctions, thereby maintaining an intact epithelial barrier and dry air spaces. However, under pathologic conditions, a large number of activated neutrophils can damage the alveolar epithelium, probably by the release of toxic intracellular molecules that induce dissolution of tight junctions and promote apoptosis and necrosis of alveolar epithelial type I and type II cells. These toxic mediators include proteases such as elastase and matrix metalloproteinases, cationic peptides such as defensins, and ROS, which via indirect proinflammatory effects can cause epithelial injury through either apoptotic or necrotic pathways. Consequently, the alveolar protein-rich and neutrophil-containing edema irreversibly damages type I cells and the denuded space is replaced by the deposition of proteins, fibrin, and cellular debris producing hyaline membranes, while injury to the surfactant-producing type II cells contributes to alveolar collapse, thus decreasing the lung compliance and developing a diffuse restrictive ventilatory pattern accompanied by atelectasis. Due to this, right-left shunts are produced and local mismatch of ventilation/perfusion ratio develops, increasing the vascular pulmonary resistance and leading to a pronounced hypoxemia. Also, it must be noted that due to decreased compliance in conjunction with a profound state of hypoxemia, respiratory muscles increase their anaerobic metabolism, which later will lead to muscle fatigue and hypoventilation. Resolution of alveolar edema requires transport of NaCl across the apical and basolateral membranes of alveolar epithelial type I and II cells into the lymphatics or the microcirculation, thereby generating a osmotic gradient for water reabsorption. Na^+ is reabsorbed apically by an epithelium sodium channel and basolaterally by the active Na^+/K^+-ATPase, while Chloride is reabsorbed by paracellular or by an unknown transcellular route. However, in ALI/ARDS the alveolar epithelium edema removing capacity is markedly impaired due to inflammatory, oxidative and toxin-mediated damage to ion channels. Thus, for lung recovery, the inflammatory injury must cease, which might be mediated by lipid mediators such as lipoxins and resolvins, IL-10 and T regulatory cells ($CD4^{+}CD25^{+}Foxp3^{+}$) in part by up-regulating TGF-β. In the proliferative phase, type II cells proliferate with some epithelial cell regeneration, fibroblastic reaction, and remodeling. Finally in the late phase some patients progress to an irreversible fibrotic phase with changes in the lung tissue involving collagen deposition in alveolar, vascular, and interstitial beds with development of microcysts [27,29,30]. Further information regarding treatment strategies and clinical management, are discussed in Chapter: 9.

5.3. Kidney Dysfunction: Acute Kidney Injury (AKI)

According to the Acute Kidney Injury Network (AKIN), AKI may be defined as an abrupt (within 48 h.) decrease in kidney function as measured by an absolute increase in serum creatinine ≥0.3 mg/dl (26.5 μmol/l), a 50% increase in serum creatinine or a reduction in urinary output <0.5 ml/kg/h (within 6 h.). AKI presents in approximately 25-30% of adult patients in the ICU and less frequently in infants and children, and its mortality rates have been reported to be from 30-70% even with advances in renal replacement therapy, thus arising as an independent risk factor for mortality. [31]

Sepsis-induced AKI can be characterized by a vasomotor nephropathy with disturbances in renal microcirculation, activation of proinflammatory mediators and activation of renal cell apoptosis, resulting in kidney failure and imbalances in body water and electrolyte homeostasis. Current understanding of the pathophysiology of sepsis-induced AKI has suffered a paradigm shift from renal vasoconstriction, ischemia, and acute tubular necrosis to heterogeneous vasodilatation, hyperemia, and acute tubular apoptosis, because the concept of renal vasoconstriction and ischemia is valid for low-flow states (i.e. cardiogenic or hypovolemic shock), while in hyperdynamic states such as sepsis there is a reduced perfusion to microvascular beds despite an elevated renal blood flow (RBF). Thus, the cardiac output (CO) is the only statistically significant predictor of RBF, and the sepsis-induced AKI probably occurs in a setting of normal or even elevated RBF. The decrease in the glomerular filtration rate (GFR) may be explained in terms of hemodynamic derangements within the glomerulus, where a disproportionate vasodilatation of the efferent arterioles as compared with the afferent arterioles takes place, thus reducing the GFR, causing oliguria and reducing solute clearance. In addition to the intraglomerular hemodynamic derangements, tubular dysfunction also plays a role in reducing the GFR. Proinflammatory cytokines such as TNF-α, released by endotoxin-stimulated mesangial cells can induce tubular cell apoptosis, thus reducing the tubular transport capacity and down-regulating the expression of transport systems. This diminished tubular transport capacity increases the concentration of NaCl in the tubular lumen, which in turn may further decrease the GFR by means of the tubule-glomerular feedback activation, adenosine release in the Macula densa and activation of Adenosine A_1-Receptors in the afferent arterioles leading to vasoconstriction [23,31]. Finally, nephrotoxic effects in the context of Sepsis can also be seen, and are mediated through Factor XII activation of the alternative pathway of the Complement cascade, which further damages the kidney through Granulocytes-released lisozyme, hidrolase, proteolytic enzymes and ROS [23].

Other common conditions in sepsis and MODS that can increase the onset of sepsis-induced AKI are hyperglicemia and DIC. Hyperglycemia treatment with intensive insulin therapy (IIT) can attenuate the ischemic and endotoxemic AKI by increasing the HDL, as demonstrated in experimental models. It also can reduce the expression of iNOS, ICAM-1, TNF-α, IL-6, the release of ROS/RNS and the infiltration of inflammatory cells, which lead to renal tubular injury. However, tight glucose control strategies are being reevaluated, since the incidence of hypoglycemia has increased [32]. On the other hand, activated protein C has anti-inflammatory, antithrombotic and profibrinolytic properties, which reduces the expression of inflammatory cytokines, apoptosis, acute tubular necrosis and mortality in severe sepsis [31].

5.4. Gastrointestinal and Liver Dysfunction

The gastrointestinal tract (GI) is covered by a single layer columnar epithelium and interepithelial tight junctions, which reside at the apical region of the paracellular space, thus polarizing the cell into apical and basolateral regions and regulating passive diffusion of solutes and macromolecules. The primary function of the GI tract is to absorb nutrients. It also acts as a barrier serving as the first line of defense against a hostile environment within the intestinal lumen, due to mechanisms that reduce the ability of pathogens and their toxins to invade the mucosa, and mechanisms that ensure rapid repair of defects in the epithelial monolayer. Therefore, the GI tract functions as a barrier that allows passive diffusion across the barrier of selected solutes that are beneficial to the host, while preventing the passage of antigens, bacterial toxins, and pathogens. Once the epithelial barrier is disrupted, epithelial repair mechanisms rapidly reform a continuous epithelial monolayer to prevent absorption of bacterial toxins, but require to reform tight junctions to document the barrier function. The most sensitive measure of mucosal barrier function is transepithelial electrical resistance (TER), reflecting the resistance to ion currents across traverse tissue. There are two routes ions may passively cross the epithelium: transcellular and paracellular. In the small intestine, apical epithelial membranes have a resistance to passive flow of ions 1.5–3 log units greater than that of epithelial monolayer as a whole. Thus measurements of TER largely reflect the paracellular resistance, which has been calculated to account for 75–94% of the total passive ion flow and is determined by the tight junction integrity. Another method of measuring the paracellular pathway resistance is by using a variety of probes that selectively traverse epithelium via the paracellular space, such as mannitol (mucosa-to-serosa flux or blood-to-lumen clearance)[33]. However, non-invasive assessment of claudins could provide information on paracellular gut barrier integrity. Claudin-3 seems to be a suitable candidate marker for early non-invasive detection of intestinal tight junction integrity loss due to its small size, abundant endogenous intestinal expression and paracellular localization, showing a strong relation between intestinal tight junction loss and urinary claudin-3 levels in rat models and clinical settings [34].

In sepsis, vasodilatation and redistribution of regional blood flow occur, prioritizing certain organs above others. According to animal and human studies, gastrointestinal mucosal blood flow is impaired during septic shock and microcirculatory perfusion deficits have been associated with gut injury and a decrease in gut barrier function, possibly causing augmentation of systemic inflammation and distant organ dysfunction [35]. Therefore, in septic shock with low GI perfusion, mucosal injury can be mediated by ischemia/reperfusion injury episodes, with elevated levels of xanthine oxidase and subsequent increases in neutrophil infiltration, or by increases in luminal bile salt concentration, which increase mucosal permeability and alter electrolyte transport. The cytotoxic mechanisms of bile salts are poorly understood, but it is thought that bile salts increase fragility of membrane vesicles through amphipathic solubilization of lipid membranes, thus increasing influx of extracellular Ca^{+2} and H^+ into enterocytes and generating ROS by activation of phospholipase and the metabolism of arachidonic acid, hence further promoting inflammation. Morphologic alterations show villus contraction and epithelial sloughing from the tip towards the crypt [33]. All of these changes lead to inflammatory mediator production and drainage to mesenteric lymphatics and the systemic circulation, thus promoting systemic inflammation. Furthermore, in cellular culture models resembling sepsis, the incubation of intestine epithelium cells with TNF-α, IL-1β and IFN-γ leads to an increase in anaerobic glycolysis and ATP conversion, and a decrease in $NAD^+/NADH+H^+$ ratio, due to protein and nucleic acid synthesis driven by the cytokine stimulation, which is further reinforced under hypoxic conditions. In this model, other substances have proven to prevent the O_2-consumption decay as effectively as a PARP-inhibitor, which accelerates de decay of peroxynitrite, acting as scavengers for Superoxide anions and NO, manifesting the important role of peroxynitrite-mediated DNA damage. However, in cytokine-stimulated enterocytes the substitution of NAD^+ in liposomal form leads to normalization of cellular O_2 consumption, reduction in gut barrier function and anti-inflammatory effects by reducing further activation of NF-κB and iNOS [22].

In summary, increased permeability could be a potential cause or sequel of the perpetuation of severe inflammatory activity in infectious states, thus leading to distant organ failure.

The connection between intestinal inflammation and liver disease is not clearly established and should be investigated. The liver probably plays an essential role in the maintenance of the pathophysiological cascade that can lead to MODS. In contrast, the diagnostic and therapeutic options are very limited. Clinical diagnosis features hyperbilirubinemia (5-10 mg/dl), changes in plasma proteins and decreased synthesis of clotting factors. In addition to the functional changes, increases in transaminases often discordant to bilirubin, show damage to the liver cell. It is also not frequent in infants and children in the context of sepsis. A frequent cause of death in adults is hepatic encephalopathy associated with cerebral edema. A common complication of sepsis regardless of gram-negative or gram-positive agents is cholestasis that can be induced by TNF-α, IL-6 and NO by inhibiting the canalicular excretion of conjugated bilirubin and showing in the liver biopsy mild portal inflammation.

Additionally, in experimental conditions, hepatocytes show an inhibition of mitochondrial function by proinflammatory mediators, such as TNF-α, and endotoxin. The reduction of mitochondrial function with LPS was more pronounced when substrates to complexes I and IV were applied, rather than those for complex II. In addition, co-culture systems of LPS-treated hepatocytes and Kupffer cells NOS-inhibitors (L-NAME, aminoguanidine) diminished the reduction in mitochondrial function, arguing in favor for a role of NO, which increases in a time-dependent manner in hepatocytes treated with IL-1β. In parallel, there was a decrease in cellular ATP content and a strong reduction of the ratio of acetoacetate/β-hydroxybutyrate (ketone body ratio, KBR), which is directly proportional to mitochondrial $NAD^+/NADH+H^+$ ratio. In this context, it was also observed a correlation of increased plasma Nitrate/Nitrite levels with strongly decreased KBR [22].

5.5. Neurologic Dysfunction: Septic Encephalopathy (SE)

The septic encephalopathy (SE) is characterized by an acute, reversible and generalized detriment in cerebral functions, manifested by changes in the Vigilance, without the presence of direct brain infection. It appears in 23% of septic patients and elevates mortality when associated with hypoxic-ischemic encephalopathy.

Pathophysiologically, in SE the O_2-consumption and cerebral blood flow (CBF) are reduced in one third compared to non-septic controls. This CBF reduction is however not correlated to changes in the mean arterial pressure (MAP). In addition, reactivity to CO_2 of vascular smooth muscle remains preserved, at least in the early phase. Considering that the Brain function is glucose-supply dependent as energy source, a hypocapnic hyperventilation should be avoided by all means, since hypocapnia produces vasoconstriction, which aggravates the reduced CBF, thus increasing the risk of cerebral hypoxia. However, NO act as a vasodilator and can cause hypotension in the course of sepsis with reduction of vascular resistance and impaired autoregulation. Also, excessive levels of NO seem to be neurotoxic because of mitochondrial respiratory chain function impairment and energy depletion.

Additionally, early in the course of septic shock, a significantly elevated branched-chain/aromatic aminoacid ratio can be found, which correlates to elevated procalcitonin (PCT) and IL-6 levels. Also it has been demonstrated that TNF-α and IL-1 can be uptaken through active transport systems into the CNS, where they further activate astrocytes and microglia to release cytokines. In a rat animal model endotoxin, TNF-α, IL-1α or β mediated the activation of α-ketonic acid dehydrogenase (α-KDH), an enzyme that limits the oxidation of branched chain amino acids in muscles, and could contribute to its accelerated degradation in sepsis. Pretreatment with cortisone prevented the endotoxin-mediated activation of α-KDH. Also, patients who died had higher levels of aromatic amino acids as compare to the survivors, and those aromatic aminoacid levels correlated significantly to the APACHE-II score. Elevated levels of Phenylalanine can be found in cerebral spinal fluid (CSF) from septic patients, while in hepatic encephalopathy all aromatic amino acids can be found. Metabolites from L-Tryptophan, Quinolinic acid, kynurenic acid and L-kynurenine, whose production is enhanced by TNF-α and IFN-γ, work as excitatory neurotransmitters on the NMDA receptor, thereby activating NOS and other calcium-dependent enzymes, increasing the ROS production and leading to DNA damage, cell energy depletion and inducing cell death. Nevertheless, in sepsis there is a receptor activation cascade rather than an isolated activation of NMDA receptors, thus finding decreased concentrations of Noradrenalin, Dopamin and Serotonin. Through this activation/inhibition imbalance of different transmitter systems, different symptoms such as agitation or hallucinations arise.

In addition, there may be a link between the neurotoxicity induced by monoamines and binding of monoamines to the serotonin-binding proteins, providing the latter an oxidative step that could be promoted by superoxide radicals and inhibited by radical scavengers.

Finally, leukocyte accumulations in the brain do not occur in the course of sepsis in general, however, inflammatory mediators such as TNF-α and IFN-γ can cross the blood-brain barrier, increasing the permeability of endothelial cells by stimulating pinocytosis with no apparent effect on intercellular cell junctions. The intracerebral injection of IL-1 or IL-2 in the rabbit and rat can also induce EEG abnormalities and sleep-like effects as seen in septic encephalopathy [36].

5.6. Hematological Disorders Associated with MODS

Sepsis is almost invariably associated with haemostatic disorders ranging from isolated thrombocytopenia and/or subclinical activation of blood coagulation (hypercoagulability), to acute disseminated intravascular coagulation (DIC). DIC is defined as a sustained systemic clotting activation with massive thrombin and fibrin formation and subsequent consumption of platelets and coagulation factors, leading both to thrombosis and hemorrhages. DIC is classically associated with Gram negative bacterial infections but it can occur in Gram positive sepsis, viral, rickettsial and even parasitic infections.

The pathophysiological mechanisms by which the pathogen can drive fibrin formation and deposition, can be explained by simultaneously acting pathways that include direct pathogen-haemostatic system interaction and release on inflammatory mediators, whereby up-regulate procoagulant pathways, down-regulate physiological anticoagulants and suppress fibrinolysis.

The aberrant in vivo expression of tissue factor (TF) plays a pivotal role in the activation of blood coagulation in the setting of sepsis and endotoxemia, because TF expression is increased in many organs and cell types. The main source of TF appear to be activated monocytes- macrophages acting as the main triggers of blood coagulation during sepsis or endotoxemia, but it also can be reinforced by up-regulation in multiple extravascular cell types, namely lung (alveolar epithelial and alveolar type II cells and in bronchoalveolar lavage fluid, BAL), kidney (tubular and/or glomerular epithelial cells) and brain (astrocytes). Moreover, the well known increase in vascular permeability and vascular damage occurring during severe inflammation will allow the exposure of normal extravascular TF to blood, thus increasing coagulation activation. Endothelial cells (ECs) and mononuclear phagocytes can be induced to synthesize TF by microorganisms, LPS, peptidoglycan, lipotheicoic acid, proinflammaory cytokines and chemokines, and HMBG-1, while classical anti-inflammatory cytokines, namely IL-4, IL-10, IL-13 are able to inhibit TF synthesis.

Finally, TF expression by human platelets and polymorphonuclear leukocytes remains controversial. Released inflammatory mediators via endothelial dysfunction impair both physiological anticoagulant mechanisms (antithrombin III, activated protein C and TFPI) and fibrinolysis, thus leading to microcirculatory thrombosis and ischemia that contribute to parenchimal cell injury and multiple organ dysfunction along with inflammatory cells-mediated toxic effects. HMGB-1 is released from apoptotic/necrotic cells into circulation, amplifying inflammation and coagulation. However, TF inhibitors and antithrombin III concentrates have not been able to significantly reduce mortality on septic patients, as activated protein C has and is the only drug that reduces mortality in high risk septic patients [37]. Finally, diagnosis of DIC is based on platelet count, prothrombin time, activated partial thromboplastin time, fibrinogen concentration, and a fibrin-related marker, such as D- dimer.

6. New Hypothesis for Understanding MODS

Singer et al. recently proposed that facing the context of an impending injury, such as severe infection, major trauma, surgery, pancreatitis, major burns and other critical illnesses, a biphasic inflammatory, immune, hormonal and metabolic response is produced. In the early phase, a increase in mitochondrial and metabolic activity takes place, due to elevated adrenocorticotropic hormone and cortisol, glucagon, cathecolamines and growth hormone. However, in the late phase of sustained inflammation, changes in endocrine profile tend to decrease energy production, O_2 consumption, metabolic rate and normal cellular processes, leading to multiple organ dysfunction. Thus, this perceived organ failure could be instead a functional adaptation of the organism to extreme conditions in an attempt to prevent end-stage organ damage, since reduced cellular metabolism could increase cellular survival chances in the event of recovery. Evidence supporting this hypothesis is based on the fact that the histological appearances of the failed organs are often normal, with minimum or no apoptosis or necrosis, and organ dysfunction could be triggered by mitochondrial dysfunction, induced by acute-phase hormones and inflammatory mediators [38].

Another interesting discussion arising from this paradigm is the suitability of the therapeutical strategies aimed to correct the different organ or system dysfunctions toward normality. This maybe questioned due to the shift of homeostatic setpoints for different variables, leading to a new state of homeostasis.

Conclusion

Sepsis is a common disorder that arises from a severe infection and the overwhelming host inflammatory response unleashed. It should be considered as an important health care issue due to its increasingly expensive medical and non-medical costs and the elevated morbi-mortality rates, especially those associated with MODS development. Sepsis and MODS improving management and outcome has been related to earlier clinical interventions and technological improvements in health care and protocols, rather than better understanding of the underlying pathophysiological mechanisms. Therefore, the objective of the clinical management is to prevent MODS either by improving early detection protocols, on-time expert management or by any other means necessary. Current approaches to organ dysfunction have been focusing on the role of Oxidative stress and ROS/RNS in determining specific dysfunctions in cellular processes and their relationship with distant organ dysfunction and clinical features. However, a gap still exists between basic science knowledge and clinical behavior. Hopefully, new insights into MODS pathophysiology could account for better understanding and new target-directed therapeutic strategies to prevent and treat this condition.

REFERENCES

[1] Bone RC, Balk RA, Cerra FB, Dellinger RP, Fein AM, Knaus WA, Schein RM, Sibbald WJ. Definitions for sepsis and organ failure and guidelines for the use of innovative therapies in sepsis. The ACCP/SCCM Consensus Conference Committee. American College of Chest Physicians/Society of Critical Care Medicine. *Chest* 1992; 101:1644-1655.

[2] Levy MM, Fink MP, Marshall JC, Abraham E, Angus D, Cook D, Cohen J, Opal SM, Vincent JL, Ramsay G; International Sepsis Definitions Conference . 2001 SCCM/ESICM/ACCP/ATS/SIS International Sepsis Definitions Conference. *Intensive Care Med.* 2003; 29:530-8.

[3] Lever A, Mackenzie I. Sepsis: definition, epidemiology, and diagnosis. *Br. Med. J.* 2007; 335:879-883.

[4] Hilleboe H, Barkhuus A, Thomas W, editors. The PAHO-CENDES Method. In: Approaches to National Health Planning. *World Heath Organization,* 1972: 52-68.

[5] Esper AM, Martin GS. Extending international sepsis epidemiology: the impact of organ dysfunction. Crit Care (London, England) 2009; 13:120.

[6] Qureshi K, Rajah A. Septic Shock: A Review Article. *BJMP* 2008; 1:7-12.

[7] Vincent JL, Sakr Y, Sprung CL, Ranieri VM, Reinhart K, Gerlach H, Moreno R, Carlet J, Le Gall JR PD. Sepsis in European intensive care units: results of the SOAP study. *Crit Care Med.* 2006; 34:344-353.

[8] Barie PS HL. Epidemiology of multiple organ dysfunction syndrome in critical surgical illness. *Surg. Infect.* (Larchmt) 2000; 1:173-185.

[9] Zhang SW, Wang H, Su Q, Wang BE, Wang C YC. [Clinical epidemiology of 1,087 patients with multiple organ dysfunction syndrome]. Zhongguo Wei Zhong Bing Ji Jiu Yi Xue 2007; 19:2-6.

[10] Silva E, Araujo DV. Economic and Social Burden of Severe Sepsis. In: Vincent J-L, ed. Yearbook of Intensive Care and Emergency Medicine. *Springer-Verlag Berlin Heidelberg,* 2009: 129-140.

[11] Edbrooke D, Hibbert C, Kingsley J, Smith S, Bright N, Quinn J. The patient- related cost of care for sepsis patients in a United Kingdom adult general intensive care unit. *Crit. Care Med.* 1999; 27:1760-1767.

[12] Angus D, Linde-Zwirble W, Lidicker J, Clermont G, Carcillo J, Pinsky M. Epidemiology of severe sepsis in the United States: Analysis of incidence, outcome, and associated costs of care. *Crit. Care Med.* 2001; 29:1303-1310.

[13] Braun L, Riedel A, Cooper L. Severe sepsis in managed care: analysis of incidence, one-year mortality, and associated costs of care. *J. Manag. Care Pharm.* 2004; 10: 521-530.

[14] Brun-Buisson C, Roudot-Thoraval F, Girou E, Grenier-Sennelier C, Durand-Zaleski I. The costs of septic syndromes in the intensive care unit and influence of hospital-acquired sepsis. *Intensive Care Med.* 2003; 29:1464-1471.

[15] Moerer O, Schmid A, Hofmann M, Herklotz A, Reinhart K, Werdan K, Schneider H, Burchardi H. Direct costs of severe sepsis in three German intensive care units based on retrospective electronic patient record analysis of resource use. *Intensive Care Med.* 2002; 28:1440-1446.

[16] Schmid A, Burchardi H, Clouth J, Schneider H. Burden of illness imposed by severe sepsis in Germany. *Eur. J. Health Econ.* 3: 77–82 2002; 3:77-82.

[17] Dellinger RP, Levy MM, Carlet JM, Bion J, Parker MM, Jaeschke R, Reinhart K, Angus DC, Brun-Buisson C, Beale R, Calandra T, Dhainaut JF, Gerlach H, Harvey M, Marini JJ, Marshall J, Ranieri M, Ramsay G, Sevransky J, Thompson BT, Townsend S, Vender JS, Zimmerman JL, Vincent JL Surviving Sepsis Campaign: international guidelines for management of severe sepsis and septic shock: 2008. *Critical care medicine* 2008; 36:296-327.

[18] Shorr A, Micek S, Jackson WJ, Kollef M. Economic implications of an evidence- based sepsis protocol: can we improve outcomes and lower costs? *Crit. Care Med.* 35: 1257–1262 2007; 35:1257-1262.

[19] Talmor D, Greenberg D, Howell M, Lisbon A, Novack V, Shapiro N. The costs and cost-effectiveness of an integrated sepsis treatment protocol. *Crit. Care Med.* 2008; 36:1168-1174.

[20] Rivers E, Nguyen B, Havstad S, Ressler J, Muzzin A, Knoblich B, Peterson E, Tomlanovich M; Early Goal-Directed Therapy Collaborative Group. Early goal-directed Therapy in the Treatment of Severe Sepsis and Septic Shock. *N. Engl. J. Med.* 2001; 345:1368-1377.

[21] Talmor D, Shapiro N, Greenberg D, Stone P, Neumann P. When is critical care medicine cost-effective? A systematic review of the cost-effectiveness literature. *Crit. Care Med.* 2006; 34:2738-2747.

[22] Wendel M, Heller a R, Koch T. [Pathomechanisms of organ failure. Mitochondrial dysfunction in sepsis]. *Der Anaesthesist* 2009; 58:343-52.

[23] Schmidt C, Steinke T, Moritz S, Graf BM, Bucher M. [Acute renal failure and sepsis□: Just an organ dysfunction due to septic multiorgan failure?]. *Der Anaesthesist* 2010; 59:682-99.

[24] Crimi E, Sica V, Williams-Ignarro S, Zhang H, Slutsky AS, Ignarro LJ, Napoli C. The role of oxidative stress in adult critical care. *Free Radic. Biol. Med.* 2006; 40:398-406.

[25] Balestra GM, Legrand M, Ince C. Microcirculation and mitochondria in sepsis: getting out of breath. Current opinion in anaesthesiology 2009; 22:184-90. 26.

[26] Flynn A, Chokkalingam Mani B, Mather PJ. Sepsis-induced cardiomyopathy: a review of pathophysiologic mechanisms. *Heart Fail Rev.* 2010; 15:605-611.

[27] Udobi K, Childs E, Touijer K. Acute respiratory distress syndrome. *Am. Fam. Physician* 2003; 67:315-322.

[28] Kurahashi K. Therapeutic strategy for acute respiratory distress syndrome: recent understanding of the pathophysiology of the disease. *Journal of anesthesia* 2011; 25:155-6.

[29] Rensing H, Bauer M. Multiorganversagen. *Der Anaesthesist* 2001; 50:819-841.

[30] Matthay M, Zemans R. The Acute Respiratory Distress Syndrome: Pathogenesis and Treatment. *Annu. Rev. Pathol.* 2011; 28:147-163.

[31] White LE, Chaudhary R, Moore LJ, Moore F a, Hassoun HT. Surgical sepsis and organ crosstalk: the role of the kidney. *Journal of surgical research* 2011; 167:306-15.

[32] NICE-SUGAR Study Investigators T. Intensive versus Conventional Glucose Control in Critically IIll Patients. *New Engl. J. Med.* 2009; 360:1283-1297.

[33] Blikslager AT, Moeser AJ, Gookin JL, Jones SL, Odle J. Restoration of barrier function in injured intestinal mucosa. *Physiol. Rev.* 2007; 87:545-564.

[34] Grootjans J, Thuijls G, Verdam F, Derikx JP, Lenaerts K, Buurman W a. Non-invasive assessment of barrier integrity and function of the human gut. *World J. Gastrointest Surg*. 2010; 2:61-69.

[35] van Haren F, Sleigh J, Pickkers P, Van der Hoeven J. Gastrointestinal perfusion in septic shock. Anaesth Intensive Care 2007; 35:679-694.

[36] Eggers V, Schilling a, Kox WJ, Spies C. [Septic encephalopathy. Diagnosis und therapy]. *Der Anaesthesist* 2003; 52:294-303.

[37] Semeraro N, Ammollo CT, Semeraro F, Colucci M. Sepsis-associated disseminated intravascular coagulation and thromboembolic disease. Mediterr J Hematol Infect Dis. 2010;2:e2010024.

[38] Singer M, De Santis V, Vitale D, Jeffcoate W. Multiorgan failure is an adaptive, endocrine-mediated, metabolic response to overwhelming systemic inflammation. *Lancet* 2004; 364:545-8.

In: Oxidative Stress and the Critically Ill Patient
Editors: Ramón Rodrigo and Bettina von Dessauer
ISBN: 978-1-62081-576-2

Chapter VII

NUTRITION IN THE CRITICALLY ILL HOSPITALIZED PATIENT

Bettina von Dessauer
Director of the Pediatric Intensive Care Unit, Doctor Roberto del Río Children´s Hospital, Santiago de Chile, Ass Prof. of Pediatrics, University of Chile

1. ABSTRACT

Adequate nutrition is essential and part of the basic support for any hospitalized patient, particularly in critical illness. Acute malnutrition in underfed hospitalized patients is frequent in spite of the knowledge about the central role of adequate nutrition in any disease state. Incidence is even higher in the critically ill patient. Difficulties in the establishment of individual needs increase the risk of under or over-nutrition. Enhanced demands, fast changing needs, lack of adequate tools to determine specific nutritional needs, and inadequate supply could play a role in the inflammatory response, the systemic metabolic stress response (SMSR), speed of tissue repair and further complications.

The magnitude of the SMSR depends on the releasing factors and is highest in clinical situations such as acute respiratory distress syndrome (ARDS), septic shock, trauma, burning and after major surgery. As an adaptive response it facilitates energy for the metabolic processes. Provision of the required nutrients depends on preexistent individual storage of nutrients, which is age-dependent in an inverse related manner, and also from the external programmed pathology-specific supply. Oxidative stress (OS) may be a consequence of the previously related phenomena when non-stopped and prolonged over time. Antioxidants from different sources may be insufficient to counterbalance the oxidative process. Details of supplementation are still lacking in the literature to be applied with practical clinical purposes.

Sepsis and septic shock is associated with high morbidity and mortality. Early specific nutritional support may be crucial in stabilizing the patient and avoiding further derangement due to SMSR and OS.

Surgery is a major insult to the organism, independent of the specific site also triggering a SMSR in a multifactorial way. Contributing factors are the perioperative stress, including the pre-, intra- and post-operative period.

Greatly burned and trauma patients react similarly with peculiarities according to the accident and multiple factors including age, pre-existing disease and nutritional status.

The inflammatory response, OS and cell destruction influence tissue repair and delay the healing process. This, together with insufficient goal-directed nutrition and eventually insufficient specific antioxidants, enhances the risk of a negative clinical outcome.

A first approach for clinical purposes would be to determine the optimal amount of macro- and micronutrients, which could have a positive effect preventing or modulating the inflammatory, immunologic, and metabolic processes.

Abbreviations

ALI	Acute lung injury
ARDS	Acute respiratory distress syndrome
EN	Enteral Nutrition
FR	Free radicals
ICU	Intensive Care Unit
IFO_2	Inspired Fraction of O_2
MODS	Multiple organ dysfunction syndrome
OS	Oxidative Stress
ROS	Reactive oxygen species
REE	Resting energy expenditure
RNS	Reactive nitrogen species
RQ	Respiratory Quotient
SIRS	Systemic inflammatory response syndrome
SMSR	Systemic metabolic stress response

2. Introduction and Epidemiology

Adequate nutrition is essential and part of the basic support of any patient, more in the critically ill. Early physiologic stabilization and avoidance of further derangement is the overall goal [1]. Incidence of malnutrition in patients hospitalized in an ICU (intensive care unit) varies from 20-60% in different studies. The risk is higher in more severe patients, requiring longer than the median ICU stay of 4-5 days. Malnutrition in hospitalized patients influences the outcome. Prolonged hospital stay, higher incidence of infectious and non-infectious complications, and increased global hospital costs are included [2,3].

Not enough has changed in clinical practice since the first studies were published decades ago alerting about the risk of a worse outcome in malnourished critically ill patients. Benefits of early nutrition include reduction of ICU-stays, earlier control of SMSR, a lesser and shorter period of catabolism, earlier anabolism, improved tissue reconstruction and a faster wound healing. The use of the enteral route is the preferred one and as soon as possible, so contributing to a sooner stabilization [4].

Motility disorders of the gastrointestinal tract are observed with higher incidence in adults than in children. In infants and children enteral tolerance may be reduced in shock and due to the use of specific drugs altering splanchnic perfusion and bowel movement, including vasoactive drugs, morphine and muscle relaxants [5]. Also physicians have to be aware of gastroparesia in greatly burned patients, more often than with other patient groups.

If the intestines cannot be used, or only partially, then additional parenteral nutrition is a valid alternative for providing nutritional requirements. Every patient can be nourished, at least on a low initial and then progressive schedule.

Hypo-alimentation has been correlated with a difficult weaning process from the ventilator, increased morbimortality and prolonged ICU stay. Hyperalimentation is associated with increased thermogenesis, oxygen consumption, respiratory breathing work, liver steatosis and hyperglycemia, among other consequences [6].

Until now it has been difficult to establish an optimal nutritional support with balanced nutrients for the particular patient. Requirements change quickly in the critically ill, unstable patient. No precise diagnostic tool is available to the clinician for a continuous assessment.

Former predictive equations for the calculation of nutritional needs can only be a guide today; they were formulated in the past, for healthy individuals and in another medical context. The modern, technology-based vital support in ICU-patients influences and may reduce the energy requirements when correctly applied. Mechanical ventilation, vasoactive drugs, heavy sedation, paralysis, hypothermia and other usual procedures in the ICU reduce the patient's own physiologic work and may influence the resting energy expenditure (REE). Requirements for exercise and growth are minimized in these conditions.

There are differences in the amount and quality of nutrients required in the acutely unstable and the later stabilized patients. In the former, in the catabolic ebb and early flow phase, needs are fewer than in the latter, the anabolic recovery phase. Calorimetry evidenced in pediatric ventilated patients that the Schofield equation (primary for healthy children) overestimated REE. Hypometabolism was more frequent than hypermetabolism, against the generally accepted expectation. Many factors may influence this result [7]. The REE is not yet easy to determine. It changes quickly in critical care settings, so that isolated values of indirect calorimetry are not enough to program an accurate specific support.

In Canadian adult ICUs a trial evidenced that 39.7% of the patients never received nutrition during their stay. Enteral feeding was initiated at an average of 1.6 days after the admission and only in 10% during day 1. Only 58% of the prescribed nutrition was really delivered during the first 12 days of ICU stay [8]. General guidelines were developed to improve this medical behavior. The diversity of requirements led to the search for personalized regimens based on genetic profiles, called nutrigenomics and nutrigenetics.

Neither the amount, nor how and what kind of preparations to feed were until now protocolled in clinical settings, with endpoints still lacking. Supplements are not clear, including the role of immune-nutrition.

A significant number of children are admitted to the ICU with previous malnutrition, as a consequence of a pre-existent chronic disease, prolonged fasting or under-nutrition during the previous hospitalization outside the ICU. The same situation is seen in adults.

The critically ill patient has a stress response responding to the primary insult. Secondary malnutrition is multifactorial due to increased demands, failure in the estimation of real detailed nutritional needs, and/or inadequate delivery [2].

The SMSR is part of the physiologic reaction to any severe disease. Increases of insulin, glucagon, cortisol, catecholamine and pro-inflammatory cytokines are counter-regulated, between other mechanisms, by elevated insulin and growth hormone resistance with the aim of providing more energy substrate. The systemic inflammatory response syndrome (SIRS), due to infection or to non-infectious stimuli such as trauma, surgery, pancreatitis or ischemia, is a common triggering cause of morbidity and mortality in patients admitted to the ICU. In critically ill patients, this accounts for 10% to 50% of all deaths.

Oxidative stress (OS) is a risk after the development of SIRS of any cause. It is derived from an imbalance between the amount of free radical production and the antioxidant defense system. In critical illness, overwhelming inflammatory mediator response to infective or non-infective stimuli results in excessive production of free radicals (FR), oxidative (ROS) and nitrosative (RNS) ones. Antioxidants are in charge of the counter-reaction detoxifying them, pretending to maintain the balance between production and destruction, so they have a crucial role in the occurrence of OS and have to be provided as part of a goal-directed pharmaco-nutrition when endogenous reserves are insufficient, a situation expected to occur in the critically ill patient [9].

Sepsis and septic shock are clinical conditions requiring, worldwide, a great amount of resources and health organization systems for early detection and treatment, with the aimpretending to achieve a better outcome. In spite of a decreasing mortality, the problem remained similar in the last decade due to an increasing incidence. Guidelines helped as an initial strategy, but were not always able to be observed in time. Around the world, the diagnosis of the primary disease leading to sepsis and septic shock is not the same, so neither are the consequences. Local adaptations of protocols and guidelines are necessary. Prevention and treatment of the underlying conditions, including chronic diseases or malnutrition, mostly in developing countries, are keystones and have to be included in the schedule of the initial management of the patient. The intent of a detention of the pathophysiologic phenomena triggering OS and finally MODS (Multiple Organ Dysfunction Syndrome) is essential. Restoring the intravascular space with liberal fluid loading, a corner stone in the emphasis over the last years, without taking into account the whole physiologic derangement in the critically ill child, has been proven to be deleterious in some patients. Expectable primary or secondary myocardial dysfunction is now increasingly top of mind in the resuscitation of septic shock and other conditions seen in the ICU and is related to a better outcome when early managed.

These considerations are important given the relationship between the amount of calories and the requirement of fluids for their adequate metabolism, and, also, because severely malnourished people, especially infants, do not tolerate a quick replacement of huge amounts of intravenous fluids lacking nutrients as a consequence of a, while in rest, hidden myocardial dysfunction.

Adequate nutrition is not only meant to maintain lean body mass and organ function, but is also important to modulate the inflammatory and immune response avoiding OS. For this purpose starvation and fasting periods have to be minimized or avoided. It is well recognized that adequate nutrition in critical patients improves outcome, maintaining immune competence of the patient, and reduces complications. Pharmaco-nutrition, with supplementation of special nutrients, has proven to be helpful in the immunomodulation and in improving outcome [10]. It is still not common practice to use them or to find them included in massively available commercial formulas.

Surgery and the perioperative period are more important triggers of catabolism than simple starvation. It is a major insult to the whole organism, independent of the specific site of the procedure, and may be the initiator of a SMSR, in a multifactorial way. Involved factors are preoperative stress as a consequence of major trauma, accidental burning, delayed diagnosis of an infectious focus, intraoperative hemorrhage or hypovolemic shock, prolonged operative time with hypothermia, and different episodes or complications in the postoperative period. Greatly burned and trauma patients react similarly with peculiarities according to the accident and individual factors including age, severity of the accident, involved body surface, pre-existing disease and nutritional status.

Fasting may be present in the perioperative period, changing metabolic pathways as an adaptation to obtain enough calories for basic metabolic energy supply. A re-feeding syndrome may take place in severe cases of prolonged malnourishment when a wrong, too quick nutritional recovery is planned. Activated, alternative metabolic pathways to obtain glucose include muscle breakdown and fatty acid oxidation. Simultaneous depletion, due to loss and lack of enough support of electrolytes, micronutrients and trace elements, including reduced intracellular stores, impede a normal organ function [11].

The inflammatory response, oxidative stress and cell destruction influence the speed of tissue repair and the healing process. An insufficient goal-directed nutrition, and eventually insufficient specific micronutrient support including different antioxidants, enhance the risk of a general negative outcome.

This chapter is meant to try to revalue in the mind of the clinicians a relationship between an appropriate early, ideally tailor-made nutrition, and an improved outcome of critically ill patients. The goal is to avoid further metabolic derangement, including the risk of SIRS, OS, and finally, MODS, due to insufficient emphasis on the nutritional support between other modifiable factors.

3. Pathophysiology

3.1 Nutrition

Nutrition is a basic physiologic function determined to maintain people's health and ability to confront their daily oscillating energy needs. Total and specific requirements differ between individuals, depending on age, weight, height, exercise load, environmental changes, external injury and disease states. Nutrients are utilized for basic metabolism, dynamic specific action, exercise, growth, and development in children. Water is essential, must be maintained in balance with the supply of nutrients (more in infants, which have a higher total body water content compared with adults) and is related to the caloric consumption and metabolism [3].

Protein requirements are increased in infancy when growth occurs. An equilibrated supply of essential and non-essential aminoacids is crucial to avoid a negative nitrogen balance. Carbohydrates stored as glycogen in the liver and muscle are the major source of energy, but the storing capacity is low. Fat intake, specifically with omega 3 fatty acids, avoids the immunosuppressive effect of the metabolization of omega 6 fatty acids, which produce prostaglandin E and thromboxane A_2. Carnitine is essential for a normal transport of fatty acids across the mitochondrial membrane and is necessary to maintain a normal oxidative process.

Minerals, vitamins, trace elements and electrolytes in adequate amounts are also necessary.

Cellular homeostasis has to allow a normal interplay between cell increase and growth, cell protection in case of imbalance due to any kind of injury, and final natural cell death. Macronutrients providing energy and multiple micronutrients, such as vitamins, trace elements and minerals, are essential as cofactors to maintain the balance. In all healthy individuals permanent oxidation-reduction processes take place for an optimal cellular functioning. As related in other sections, reactive species (ROS and RNS) are produced normally, in balance between the amount of these and the antioxidant response, which includes enzymatic and non-enzymatic antioxidants. Their action depends on cofactors like vitamins C and E, selenium, zinc, copper, chromium, cobalt, iron and many others.

Under- and overfeeding is associated with some similar risks and complications: immunosuppression, infections, slow wound healing and longer ICU stays. In the latter, there is also hyperglycemia, fatty liver, azotemia, CO_2 overproduction and hypercapnia. Weak respiratory muscles and decreased ventilator drive with a difficult weaning process from the mechanical ventilator are part of major practical consequences [12].

Clinical trials showed that otherwise healthy obese children may be under permanent oxidative stress exposing them to future cardiovascular diseases. This preexistence also enhances the risk of an augmented SMSR when exposed to prolonged starvation, trauma, surgery or any other stress situation [13].

The concept of immune-nutrition has been controversial. The specific target is a modulation of the inflammatory response and cellular immunity. Glutamine, arginine, omega3 fatty acids and nucleotides, among others, are involved in clinical trials and the elaboration of new industrial products. Results for each separated are still controversial.

3.2 Malnutrition

An imbalance between energy requirements and supply for the needs, in patients with an acute or chronic condition, gives way to this phenomenon. Disease-related malnutrition occurs quickly in any critically ill patient, more in infants and toddlers where reserves are less. Any of the macro- or micronutrients may be involved, or all of them.

Body composition, metabolic reserves, stress response and energetic requirements differ significantly from adults, making any comparison with children difficult. Children have significantly fewer fat and protein stores than adults and a higher water content, enhancing the overall physiologic and metabolic fragility [14]. Glucose and free fatty acids are the basic energy providers of the human organism. The most important metabolic cell fuel is glucose. Via glycolysis it is converted to pyruvate, than to acetyl coenzyme A in the mitochondria, and finally, by the tricarboxylic cycle, to energy, carbon dioxide and water. Fat and protein via other mechanisms also convert with this cycle and these final products, but with different efficiency in the liberation of calories per gram of substrate.

Insulin is the most important hormone interfering in glucose homeostasis. Its actions include the stimulation of glucose uptake by the muscle and adipose tissue, promotion of glycogen and protein synthesis, and inhibition of lipolysis and glycogenolysis. The counter-regulatory hormones, including growth hormone, cortisol, glucagon, and epinephrine directly oppose these effects and are therefore important in regulating glucose homeostasis as well.

Maintenance of normoglycemia is a complex process strictly regulated by neurohormonal and autoregulatory mechanisms [15].

The metabolic behavior will be different in previously healthy or malnourished patients, also in resting, fasting or stress response situations. The resting body needs less energy, slows down with oxygen consumption, but behaves as expected. Glucose is provided by normal mechanisms, such as glycogenolysis after an overnight fast. During starvation or longer fasting, the human organism tries to maintain an adequate energy provision: glucagon is released, insulin levels are reduced or suppressed, and the counter-regulatory hormones stimulate glycogenolysis and also gluconeogenesis. Catecholamines, cortisol and growth hormone are involved in this metabolic adaptation. Given that glycogen stores last no longer than 72 hours, the substrates for gluconeogenesis are then derived from lipolysis (glycerol) and the catabolism of skeletal muscle, and, later on, from visceral proteins. Glucose may also be synthesized from substrates like lactate, pyruvate, alanine, ketone bodies and glutamine. This last one also serves as intestinal energy source, and can be converted into alanine, transported via vena porta to the liver and then converted into glucose (glucose-alanine cycle).

The body storage of glucose is low; hepatic glycogen reserves are soon depleted. Protein muscle stores in children are reduced. As glucose supplies are further limited, the brain becomes dependent upon ketones as an alternative energy source [11].

Malnutrition has to be avoided, maintaining the energy provision and all the specific nutrients required for a balanced oxidative-reductive process and also avoiding the consumption of reduced body stores and the destruction of lean body mass.

3.3 The Systemic Metabolic Stress Response (SMSR)

It is a global unspecific systemic reaction to different triggers. It occurs in severe infections; trauma; renal, heart or respiratory failure and after surgery, among others. An activation of the sympathetic nervous system and the central hypothalamic-pituitary-adrenal axis is the starting point of an overall re-direction of energy providers, hormones, and counter-regulatory hormones, inducing a hypermetabolic and hyperdynamic state. Oxygen consumption increases. The hyper-inflammation can lead to an immunosuppressed state, enhancing the risk of in-hospital associated infections. In the context of surgery, trauma, and burns, this often results in sepsis, ARDS (Acute Respiratory Distress Syndrome) and MODS [16].

Clinical manifestations are drowsiness, irritability, tachycardia, tachypnea and changes in blood pressure. It is characterized by an increase in REE, which corresponds to up to 70-80% of the daily caloric need [17]. The SMSR is proportional to the degree of stress and causes an increase in the turnover of proteins, carbohydrates and fats. With an increased REE the whole body reorganizes to provide more energy by other means. Body protein degradation predominates over synthesis delivering free aminoacids for gluconeogenesis. SIRS, as a reaction to an imbalance between a pro- and anti-inflammatory process, activates a metabolic, immune, neuronal and hormonal response facilitating nutrients for the synthesis of acute phase proteins, energy production, tissue repair and immune defense. Oxidative stress, as a second imbalance between an oxidant and antioxidant response, enhances the damage. The control of hyperglycemia in safe ranges reduces oxidative stress. [18,19].

Presence of hyperglycemia, higher insulinemia, insulin resistance, and glucose intolerance is part of the expectable normal stress response in direct relationship to the intensity of the insult. Hypermetabolism with hypercatabolism, when present, is higher in the first 2-3 days after the initiation of the deleterious process. When properly managed, patients progressively return to a neutral state or even to anabolism after that.

The interference of this process with therapeutic measures other than the intent to recover stability and shorten the period of stress is not clear. Extremely strict glucose control has proven to be dangerous [20].

Malnourished and stressed patients handle errors in the supply of an excess of nutrients and water for their needs with difficulties. Respiratory dysfunction, reduced cardiac output, renal failure, and splanchnic functional disorders, among others, are expected to occur. Therefore, a correct comprehension of the pathophysiologic ongoing condition in each patient is vital for a correct nutritional support.

In ARDS the degree of SMSR is related to the underlying cause and if the respiratory syndrome is of primary (intra-thoracic) or secondary (extra-thoracic) origin. If the trigger is a systemic disease like burns, trauma or major surgery, the response is expected to be higher and a sum of that of the basic disease and the ARDS itself. The precocity of ventilator and hemodynamic support, and the prudency of oxygen-therapy, influence the systemic reaction of inflammation, SMSR, SIRS and the occurrence of OS [21,22].

In sepsis, the patient's previous nutritional status, age, degree of hypovolemia, hypoxemia, hypoxia and dysoxia, in a time-dependent magnitude of physiologic instability, also influence the degree of the metabolic response and the risk of further MODS (See chapter 6).

In case of a surgery, catabolism and muscle breakdown with negative nitrogen balance quickly occurs if nutrients are not supplied. SIRS, as part of the expectable physiologic postoperative reaction, activates the neuro-hormonal response, and substrates are facilitated to ensure energy provision for vital functions [23]. The preoperative nutritional status of the patient and, also, the type of surgery (length of intervention and anesthesia, severity of the disease), influence the outcome and magnitude of the metabolic response. SIRS has multisystem and multi-organic consequences with decreased vital functions, including respiratory, cardiovascular, splanchnic and renal failure. Infections and MODS are feared endpoints.

In trauma patients SMSR with the neuroendocrine response occurs soon after the accident, aimed at maintaining post-traumatic homeostasis. The sympathetic nervous system and the hypothalamic-pituitary-adrenal axis are involved. Meant to be a short adaptation process, if prolonged, it induces a systemic immune dissonance. The magnitude of the SMSR depends on the extension and severity of the acute injury and whether head trauma is included, increasing the deleterious response. As the brain is directly dependent upon glucose as an energy source, quick metabolic derangement takes place if it is not supplied. Primary traumatic tissue breakdown and loss, procedures, interventions, and fasting periods influence the metabolic response and high risk of OS.

The greatly burned is a "systemic" patient with a huge generalized hypermetabolic and inflammatory response, not only in the burned tissue zone. Liberation of inflammatory mediators (which act locally and also far from the burned zone), extension and deepness of the burned body surface, skin and protein/albumin loss, secondary immediate dehydration, hypoxemia and hypoxia influence the metabolic response and evolution. Initial tissue hypoperfusion and hypovolemic shock triggers the inflammatory reaction, SMSR and eventual imbalance of the oxidative-antioxidant response. The acute volume loss requires an immediate redistribution of fluids and may impair organ function, at least on a temporary basis. Tissue and red blood cells are destroyed and lost with the trauma. Enhanced permeability, hypovolemia, and cell dysfunction leads to hypoxia and dysoxia in a distributive shock context. Together with the hypermetabolism and catabolism, a hyperglycemic stress response is observed. Depending on the age of the patient and his nutritional reserves, this overall imbalance may give rise to OS.

3.4 Oxidative Stress (Details in Previous Chapters)

As a biological process, it is present in many acute and chronic severe diseases, contributing to clinical complications, MODS and worse outcomes. It is expectable in many critically ill patients. In catabolic conditions, as seen in these patients, physiologic disregulation takes place. An insulin receptor signaling pathway and signaling cascades of NF-kB and AP-1 induce, among other factors, inflammatory cytokines, leading to quick muscle wasting. The insulin receptor signal, not adequately down-regulated, compromises glucose homeostasis. If hypoglycemia occurs and exogenous glucose is not provided, a stress response with glucagon, cortisol, growth hormone and adrenaline release is activated, enhancing catabolism intended to provide energy to this stressed organism [24].

The production of oxidative and nitrosative species is permanent, but they are normally detoxified efficiently. Only when this protective capacity is overwhelmed is the concept of oxidative stress applicable. Oxidative stress is not only a consequence of the primary insult but also of some of the ICU-therapies, due to mechanical injury or contact of biological fluids with non-biological elements [17].

ARDS (see chapter 9), or at least ALI (Acute Lung Injury), is in the mind of every intensivist when a critically ill patient is admitted to the ICU. The planning includes the intent to avoid the occurrence. The intensity of OS will be related not only to the primary factor conditioning ALI or ARDS, but also to some elements of the therapy in ICU, including oxygen-therapy and mechanical ventilation. Exposure to high concentrated oxygen induces a lung inflammatory response with airway deposition of neutrophils and macrophages, after an endothelial and epithelial damage occurs, causing fibrosis [25]. Volutrauma, barotrauma and biotrauma due to mechanical ventilation add possible damage and the risk of OS. A lung protective strategy has been the goal over the past years, beyond the scope of this chapter.

Sepsis (see chapter 2) and septic shock are major causes of morbi-mortality in ICU. As a primary disease conditioning the admission to ICU, or secondary to any other condition in just critically ill patients, it has been a model to study the inflammatory response and OS. In the absence of new antibiotics over recent years and an increasing bacterial resistance to them, more in developed countries due to over-use, the emphasis has changed from avoiding the circumstance of severe infections to prevention. Controlling OS and enhancing the antioxidant response capacity has been in the center of the discussion and research, still lacking objective results for clinical practice.

Surgery is a major trauma or insult to the whole body independent of the cause. The procedure of surgery is an initiator of a SMSR, on a multifactorial way, and oxidative stress again can follow each intervention. Involved factors are preoperative stress as a consequence of major trauma, accidental burning, an infectious focus not immediately diagnosed (wound infection, appendicitis followed by peritonitis, abscesses, phlegmons), intraoperative hemorrhage or hypovolemic shock, prolonged operative time with hypothermia, and different complications in the postoperative period.

Discussion persists as to whether open or closed surgery causes a greater degree of OS.

Trauma is a frequent admission cause in tertiary care ICUs. Characteristics vary over the world dependent on local epidemiology. High-energy accidents impact profoundly on the whole organism with tissue destruction and loss, vital organ failure, OS and further MODS.

Bone fractures need calcium and antioxidants for reconstruction. FR produced after a fracture may help to modulate osteoclast activity when in controlled amounts. If not, an osteoporotic process takes, place delaying fracture healing [26].

Traumatic brain injury is the result of a primary (energy of the trauma itself) and, in general, a secondary organic and functional insult due to the consequences of the former. OS when present results in DNA-damage and further neuronal loss. In spinal cord injury with a known huge OS, further damage must be avoided. Acrolein, a reactive aldehyde, product of lipid peroxidation with longer half-life than other FR, is in the mirror. Its control may be a target in future therapeutic interventions to attenuate OS [27]. Micronutrient loss, together with the trauma itself, in the context of elevated requirements for the physiologic stabilization, tissue repair and OS detention, need a quick medical response. Different trace elements like copper, selenium, zinc and vitamins are lost in major trauma [28].

Burning is a major thermal injury triggering a local and systemic inflammatory response and OS. After the injury, tissue loss, dehydration, loss of nutrients and albumin reduces the defense system. Liberation of inflammatory mediators activates inflammatory cells and endothelial dysfunction. Oxidative species are produced in excess for the normal capacity to counterbalance. Elevated end products of lipid peroxidation and reduced antioxidants, vitamins and trace elements have been found in different studies in patients with at least 30% burned body surface. Free radicals with antimicrobial action and wound healing effects when in physiologic amounts, lose their beneficial effect. Oxidative stress recovered around the fifth day after the thermal trauma, in a group with few added complications [29]. The loss of vitamins and trace elements, as in every trauma, influences the outcome. The rebuilding of tissue, collagen and the functional performance of vital systems in this scenario, requires the presence and support of higher amounts than normal of these elements [30].

If we remember the known, frequent fact of malnourishment in hospitalized patients or with fasting periods of variable time waiting for surgery, the imbalance of the oxidant and antioxidant response is almost part of the clinical process in many patients. In spite of this documented knowledge and huge amount of related research, little has changed until now in clinical settings regarding the avoidance and taking into account of oxidative stress and its deleterious effects.

In summary, the inflammatory response, cell and tissue destruction, and the occurrence of oxidative stress influences tissue repair and the healing process. This, together with insufficient nutrition and specific antioxidants necessary to counterbalance oxidative response, enhance the risk of a negative outcome.

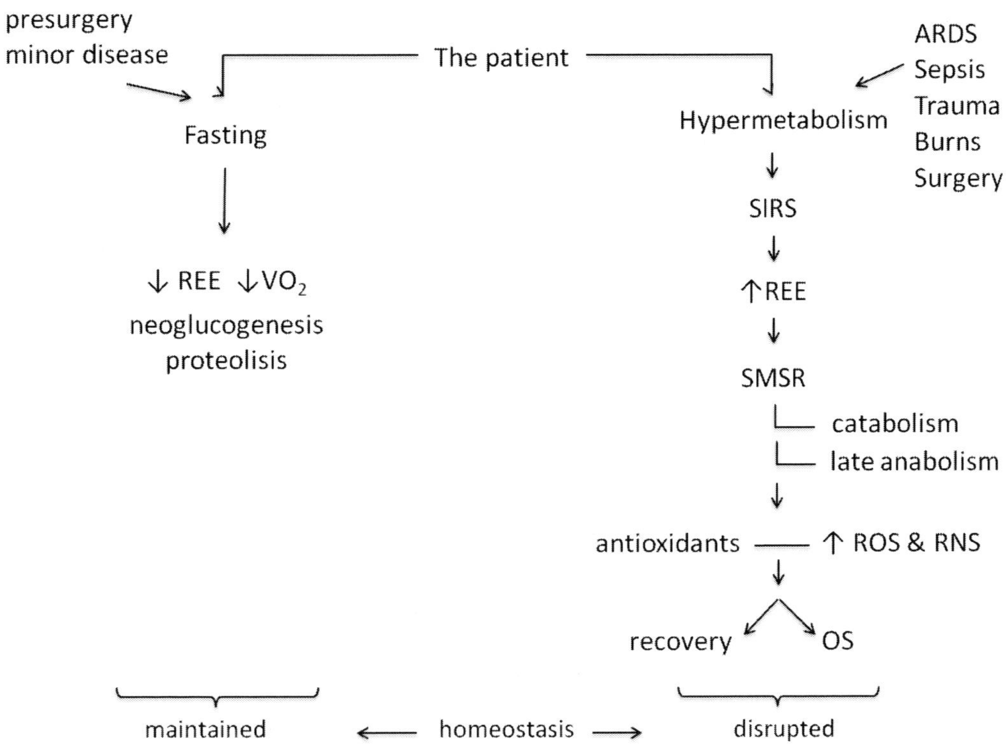

Diagram. Metabolic response during fasting and in stress situations.

4. Clinical Aspects and Studies

In the discussion about nutritional needs in critically ill patients, with the aim of preventing a further deterioration and finally MODS, many facts have to be taken into account. The total amount of calories and quality and quantity of nutrients have to be adapted to each patient, depending on the diagnosis, degree of vital functional derangement, metabolic stress response, presence of oxidative stress, programmed medical support and vital function support (available feeding formulas, vasoactive drugs, ventilator care, renal replacement and general care, temperature control, among others). Formerly used validated formulas to calculate energy requirements (Benedict, Schoffield, FAO/WHO) have demonstrated in clinical studies with indirect-calorimetry to overestimate needs for the actual critical care management in most ICUs [31].

The most important factor to be changed is the professional behavior: consciousness about the value of an early, tailor-made individual planned nutrition or at least, to keep in mind that starving and fasting can be minimized or avoided with an adequate therapeutic planning in clinical settings, as with every other component of the therapeutic program.

Better clinical outcomes based on early diagnosis and initiation of treatment maintaining the nutritional status and avoiding secondary complications, help to induce a quickder recovery of physiologic derangements, shorter hospital/ICU stays and are of known cost/effectiveness.

Huge gaps existed until now in the nutrition support between ICUs, in spite of published guidelines and recommendations. Enteral nutrition is still later initiated than in the recommended first 24-48 hours after ICU admission, often in an insufficient amount or without a reasonable argument for the delay. Parenteral nutrition is overused in cases when the enteral route is possible. Fasting and starvation in patients able to be fed is not an exception. About one-third of the time in the ICU the patients of a worldwide multicenter study never received nutrition [32]. Discrepancy around strict glucose control persists.

Critically ill patients experience a severe inflammatory response, cellular immune dysfunction, oxidative stress and mitochondrial dysfunction. Supplementation with key nutrients, such as glutamine and antioxidants, is most likely to have a favorable effect on these physiological derangements, leading to an improvement in clinical outcomes [33].

Oxidative injury from pathologic conditions, such as sepsis, may have more serious consequences in pediatric patients than in elderly people because of the lower functional reserve and the need for subsequent tissue growth to match somatic and normal development.

Early enteral feeding and directed nutritional support with carbohydrates, proteins, fat, vitamins and trace elements, including different antioxidants, reduces the risk of severe oxidative stress in burned patients [34]. Controversial results have been observed in patients with low-volume enteral supplement containing mostly key nutrients.

A first step to improve the clinical approach would be to precisely determine the optimal dose that could have a maximal positive effect on the underlying inflammatory, immunologic, and metabolic processes and minimum eventual deleterious effects due to overdose.

In surgical patients, glutamine supplementation may be associated with a reduction in infectious complication rates and shorter hospital stay. In critically ill patients, glutamine supplementation may be associated with a reduction in complications and mortality rates. The greatest benefit has been observed in patients receiving high-dose, parenteral glutamine [35]. There is growing evidence that antioxidant supplements, particularly high-dose selenium, may reduce mortality, infectious complications, and improve wound healing. Deleterious effects may result from prolonged high doses, whereas short-term high dose supplements are probably safe in most critically ill patients.

5. Management

5.1 Monitoring

As mentioned before, different standard equations are available to calculate REE but they are only approximations when compared with indirect calorimetry. The inconvenience is that they were formulated for healthy persons and may overestimate nutritional needs in critically ill mechanically supported patients. Calorimetry is more precise to measure REE, but it is instant and technology dependent so not always available. It measures O_2 consumption and CO_2 production. Intermittent measurement requires the absence of air-leak in invasive ventilated patients and only moderate oxygen supply, up to 40% IFO_2 (Inspired Fraction of O_2). This diagnostic procedure would be of greatest interest for a goal directed therapy in younger malnourished children, patients of any age staying more than 5 days in the PICU, and also in stabilized chronic patients whose functional performance depends on an optimal nutritional status [36].

Respiratory quotient (RQ) is a formula establishing a relationship between the oxygen extraction and CO_2 production. It reflects the energy produced by the metabolism of carbohydrates, fat and proteins. It ranges between 1 and 0.7, lower values indicating more oxidation of fat and higher more of carbohydrates.

Albumin, with a long half-life, is an important predictor of outcome in any critical patient with SIRS, including postsurgery, as a difference to the short half-life of prealbumin. It is not meant to be an indicator of nutritional status [37]. No single biomarker is available for the determination of oxidative stress in normal clinical settings. Laboratory sample recollection requires standards and stabilization by quick freezing. Reference values are not always available [17].

In burned patients, liver function integrity, expressed as the ability to produce acute phase proteins like C Reactive Protein, prealbumin, retinol-binding-protein and others, is related to outcome.

Measurement of the antioxidant response system is in the mirror of clinicians, but still mostly as part of research (See chapter 11).

5.2 Treatment

Early enteral nutrition (EN) reduces the hypercatabolic phase, prevents intestinal permeability and atrophy, bacterial translocation, inflammation and modulates the stress response [38].

Prudent control of stress hyperglycemia is important. It tends to normalize in the first 24 hours together with the overall stabilization of the patient. The strict glucose control of the past decade has been abandoned after the evidence of an increasing rate of harmful hypoglycemia [39].

Supplements with omega 3 fatty acids, aminoacids, electrolytes, vitamins, minerals and trace elements depend on a lot of particular, not completely cleared, variables and require future research. Plasma micronutrient concentrations are low during critical illness as a result of losses, low intake, dilution and redistribution from plasma to tissues. An assessment of the real reserve and disponibility is difficult. Micronutrient supplements appear beneficial in conditions such as major burns, trauma and sepsis and stroke, and are most likely to benefit patients with previous or acute depletion. Selenium is necessary in any critically ill patient, aespecially when myocardial compromise is expected. Glutamine supplement is recommended in burn and trauma patients, fish oil in ALI and ARDS, and zinc and vitamin C when tissue repair is a primary goal. Nucleotides, copper, N-acetyl-cysteine and others have been studied for their particular action [16,40].

The intravenous route seems to be more efficient and secure than the enteral one for this micronutrient supply in critically ill patients with expectable systemic perfusion disorders and possible altered intestinal absorption. Although chronic high intakes may be harmful, short-term interventions appear to be free of deleterious effects. Further research is required to determine the optimal micronutrient combinations and the doses required according to the timing of intervention and severity of disease [41].

Vitamin C supplement, an important antioxidant, is also a cofactor of enzymatic pathways. Ascorbate plasma levels are reduced after trauma or shock. Requirements are much higher than the traditional 100 mg/day in trauma, burn, perioperative and septic patients. Definitive amounts are not yet clear [42].

In respiratory failure, with ARDS on the top, maintenance of lean body mass and respiratory muscle strength is important. Energy, micronutrients and electrolytes are necessary for the REE, enhanced requirements due to hypermetabolism, enhanced ATP production and antioxidant response. Ventilator weaning and functional recovering depend on the nutritional status, critical care management (sedation, vasoactive drugs, procedures, surgery) and the underlying cause of ARDS, including trauma, burns, surgery and severe primary or secondary respiratory infections and disorders. Exact needs, again, are difficult to determine for rapidly changing conditions and in the absence of an available monitoring tool. Indirect calorimetry in severe respiratory failure is technically still not applicable.

Free radicals are constantly delivered resulting in inflammation, edema and cell damage and death. Arachidonic acid mediators are included [12]. Avoidance of hyperoxia, barotrauma, volutrauma, and biotrauma are essential to reducing inflammation.

Omega 3 fatty acid enriched diets, specifically EPA (eicosapentaenoic acid) and GLA (γ-linoleic), modify arachidonic acid availability and shift the production of high pro-inflammatory cytokines to less inflammatory series. GLA metabolized to prostaglandin E1 reduces inflammatory lung injury and induces vasodilation, better perfusion and oxygenation. This, together with the supply of antioxidants, showed reduction of the metabolic response and modulation of inflammation. From the clinical point of view it was associated with improved outcome and lower costs due to less complications and ICU [43].

Later studies (ARDSNet EDEN-Omega study 2011) didn´t confirm the results, so the controversy is still open.

The amount of variables influencing the outcome makes it difficult to individualize if a particular nutritional immune-modulating strategy is break-pointing. It seems that up to now the opportunity of re-initiation (early nutritional support) is more important than the type and the route of the nutritional supply, should stop in part the cascade of negative physiologic events, and is fundamental for a better evolution of ARDS. The previous nutritional status is an additional factor to analyze, given that this influences the antioxidant endogenous reserve.

In sepsis early EN after resuscitation has a demonstrated positive outcome modulating effect. The presence of SIRS, a generalized endothelial dysfunction with increased permeability, hypercatabolism with muscle breakdown, and oxidative stress with reduced antioxidant response to maintain the balance are cornerstones to keep in mind in the planning of the nutritional support. Macronutrients, but also micronutrients, specifically antioxidants, are involved in the control of the pathophysiologic events. Vitamin C, vitamin E, selenium, and N-actetil-cysteine, among others, have been expected to benefit septic patients. Propranolol, a beta-adrenoceptor blocker, has been studied for an eventual beneficial effect attenuating an exaggerated catecholamine sympathetic response [44].

Any medical procedure is a stress per se. As previously related, many factors influence the needs in quantity and quality of nutrition in this scenario. The goal today is not only a provision of energy and macronutrients, but avoiding acute malnutrition due to failure in the support. More decisive is an early goal directed therapy pretending to stop the SMSR, OS and avoid MODS [45].

Correcting albumin was reported to influence a better outcome in major abdominal surgery. The long half-life of 21 days, more than of nutritional value is an indicator of permeability and interstitial leak, loss (burns) and severity of inflammation, SMSR and general stability of the patient. Prealbumin with a short half-life (2 days) is a better indicator of the re-building of proteins when inflammation and catabolism is being controlled.

The enteral route is preferred a soon as possible, enhancing the patient-tolerance based support. Few exceptions to use the bowel remain up to today, when consciousness of the importance exists, nursery care is optimized and subjective fear to use the intestines is excluded. An enriched immune-modulating preoperative diet with arginine, omega 3 fatty acids and nucleic acids showed an improvement of postoperative evolution of overall ICU stay quality assessment parameters and infections [46].

Controversy about preoperative fasting exists. In small children physiologic reserves are small and benefits of this custom are not clear. Parenteral support should be used to replace enteral feeding when needed. Postoperative fasting has been shortened in recent years, trying to recover splanchnic perfusion and function as soon as possible.

A vitamin C supplement of 500 mg/day in surgical patients reduced OS and improved outcome, but the optimal safe dosage is still not known [47]. The generally proposed recommendation for elective surgical patients is a tailor-made supplemented nutrition 10 days prior to and 7 days post-surgery in malnourished patients, favoring the enteral route whenever possible, at least in part [40]. Considerations are similar for trauma patients.

In the greatly burned patients early enteral nutrition with enhanced special micronutrient support, but mostly early recovery of volemia, burn-wound excision, coverage of the burned clean surface and avoidance of secondary infections are primary goals. Growth hormone increases the speed of tissue repair. The global aim is to control the inflammatory response as soon as possible, shortening the period of exposed burned tissue. Melatonin, a powerful antioxidant, has been proposed as a complement therapy, enhancing the inflammatory and oxidative response system with activation of the immune system and its detoxifying effect [48].

In summary every patient can be fed when knowledge and consciousness about the transcendental role of nutrition in critically ill patients is taken into account. A tailor made feeding plan, individualized design based on nutrigenomics and nutrigenetics may be the future, trying to achieve the goal of specific needs for each circumstance and individual case. Not only macronutrients, but also micronutrients, including vitamins, minerals and trace-elements, are important. Control of inflammation, reduction of oxidation-reduction phenomena and avoidance of MODS are part of the goal. An early use of the enteral route has been demonstrated to modulate and reduce the metabolic stress response, shortening the catabolic phase. Early enteral feeding of the critically ill doesn´t mean feeding the total amount of calculated needs immediately, but at a constant increase according to the capacity of the patient in the recovering period. Avoidance of catabolism and auto-consumption may be enough in the first phase. The concept of "physiologic underfeeding" is mentioned in the literature [49].

This is congruent in the context of actual ICU management, with lower needs measured by indirect calorimetry compared with former equations. In adults a cut off of daily energy supply is around 25 kcal /kg/day, avoiding liver dysfunction. In adolescents it is 20-30 kcal/kg/day, , up to 60-80 kcal/kg/day, in infants are is normally prudent. Not only the amount, but also the distribution of the quality and quantity of the different macro-and micronutrients, is important for a correct metabolic utilization [50].

Conclusions and Future Goals

Research is still lacking as to precise, real individual needs in most patients, more in the critically ill. Monitoring tools allowing an identification and follow-up of fast changing needs have to be individualized. End-points have to be established for a goal-directed nutritional therapy.

For the moment, more consciousness about the role of nutrition in every hospitalized patient, considering it a prima facie right of anyone from the bioethical perspective, and an obligation from the clinical point of view to prevent complications, reduce morbimortality and higher costs by reducing hospital stay may be the starting point. Metabolic stress response and oxidative stress may not be avoidable in all cases but they are partially preventable, detectable early when present and able to be reduced and modulated with different strategies.

Studies concluded that nutritional support was better and earlier where guidelines existed. The enteral route as early as possible has to be preferred. This basic approach is more efficient and beneficial to the patient than more sophisticated strategies.

References

[1] Briassoulis G, Zavras N, Hatzis T. Malnutrition, nutritional indices, and early enteral feeding in critically ill children. *Nutrition* 2001;17:548-557.

[2] Mehta N, Duggan C. Nutritional deficiencies during critical illness. *Pediatr Clin N Am* 2009;56:1143-1160.

[3] Flaring U, Finkel Y. Nutritional support to patients within the pediatric intensive setting. *Pediatric Anesthesia* 2009;19:300-312.

[4] Heyland D, Dhaliwal R, Day A, Jain M, Drover J. Validation of the Canadian clinical practice guidelines for nutrition support in mechanically ventilated, critically ill adult patients: Results of a prospective observational study. *Crit Care Med* 2004;32:2260-2266.

[5] Berger M, Mechanik J. Optimizing nutrition therapy in the ICU. *Curr Opin Clin Nutr Metab Care* 2009;12:159-160.

[6] Mc Clave SA, Martindale PG, Vanek VW et al. A.S.P.E.N Board of directors. Guidelines for the provision and assessment of nutrition support therapy in the adult critically ill patient: Society of Critical Care Medicine and American Society for Parenteral and Enteral Nutrtion. *JPEN J Parenter Enteral Nutr* 2009;33:277-316.

[7] Taylor R, Cheeseman P, Preedy V, Baker A, Grimble G. Can energy expenditure be predicted in critically ill children? *Ped Crit Care Med* 2003;4:176-180.

[8] Heyland DK, Schtoter-Noppe D, Drover JW. Nutrition support in the critical care setting: Current practice in Canadian ICUs - Opportunities for improvement. *JPEN J Parenter Enteral Nutr* 2003;27:74-83.

[9] Mishra V. Oxidative stress and role of antioxidant supplementation in critical illness. *Clin Lab* 2007;53:199-209.
[10] Kreymann KG, Berger MM, Deutz NEP. E.S.P.E.N Guidelines on Enteral Nutrition: Intensive Care. *Clin Nutr* 2006;25:210-223.
[11] Khan LUR, Ahmed J, Mac Fie J. Refeeding syndrome: a literature review. *Gastroenterology Research and Practice* 2011;doi 1155/2011/41097.
[12] Krzak A, Pleva M, Napolitano L. Nutrition therapy for ALI and ARDS. *Crit Care Clin* 2011;27:647-659.
[13] Oliver SR, Rosa JS, Milne GL, Pontello AM, Borntrager HL, Heydari S, Galassetti PR. Increased oxidative stress and altered substrate metabolism in obese children. *Int J Pediatr Obes* 2010;5:436-444.
[14] Agus M, Jaksic T. Nutritional support of the critically ill child. *Current Opinion in Pediatrics* 2002;14:470-481.
[15] Mizock BA, Alterations in fuel metabolism in critical illness: Hyperglycemia. *Best Pract Res Clin Endocrinol Metab* 2001;15:533-551.
[16] Calder PC. Immunonutrition in surgical and critically ill patients. *Br J Nutr* 2007;98:33-39.
[17] Grune T, Berger M. Markers of oxidative stress in ICU settings: present and future. *Curr Opin Clin Nutr Metab Care* 2007;10:712-717.
[18] Von Dessauer B, Bongain J, Molina V, Quilodrán J, Castillo R, Rodrigo R. Oxidative stress as a novel target in pediatric sepsis management. *J Crit Care* 2011; 26:103-107.
[19] Zimmerman J.Defining the role of oxyradicals in the pathogenesis in sepsis. *Crit Care Med* 1995;23:616-617.
[20] Kavanagh B, McCowen K. Glycemic control in the ICU. *N Engl J Med* 2010;363:2540-2546.
[21] Dahlem P, van Aalderen WM, Bos AP. Pediatric acute lung injury. *Paed Resp Review* 2007;8:348-362.
[22] Suter PM. Lung inflammation in ARDS-friend or foe? *N Engl J Med* 2006;354:1671-1684.
[23] Anand K. The stress response to surgical trauma: From physiological basis to therapeutic implications. *Progr Food Nutr Sci* 1986;10:67-132.
[24] Dröge W. Redox regulation in anabolic and catabolic processes. *Curr Opin Clin Nutr Metab Care* 2006;9:190-196.
[25] Ward PA. Oxidative stress; acute and progressive lung injury. *Ann N Y Acad Sci* 2010;1203:53-59.
[26] Sheweita SA, Khoshhal KI. Calcium metabolism and oxidative stress in bone fractures: role of antioxidants. *Curr Drug Metab* 2007;8:19-25.
[27] Hamann K, Shi R. Acrolein scavenging: a potential novel mechanism of attenuating oxidative stress following spinal cord injury. *J Neurochem* 2009;111:1348-1356.
[28] Berger M, Chiolero C, Dirren H. Copper, selenium, and zinc status and balances after major trauma. *J Trauma* 1996;40:103-109.
[29] Bertin-Maghit, Goudable J, Dalmas E, Steghens JP; Bouchard C, Gueugniand PY, Petit P, Delafosse B. Time course of oxidative stress after major burns. *Int Care Med* 2000;26:800-803.
[30] Parihar A, Parihar MS, Milner A, Bhat S. Oxidative stress and antioxidative mobilization in burn patients. *Burns* 2008;34:6-17.

[31] Alexander E, Susla G, Burstein AH et al. Retrospective evaluation of commonly used equations to predict energy expenditure in mechanically ventilated, critically ill patients. *Pharmacotherapy* 2004;24:1659-1667.

[32] Cahill N, Dhaliwal R, day A, Jinag X, Heyland D. Nutrition therapy in the critical care setting: What is "best achievable" practice"? An international multicenter observational study. *Crit Care Med* 2010;38:395-401.

[33] Heyland DK, Dhaliwal R, Day AG, Muscedere J, Drover J, Suchner U, Cook D; Canadian Critical Care Trials Group. Reducing Deaths due to Oxidative Stress (The REDOXS Study): Rationale and study design for a randomized trial of glutamine and antioxidant supplementation in critically ill patients. *Proc Nutr Soc* 2006;65:250-263.

[34] Venter M,Rode H, Sive M. Enteral resuscitation and early enteral feeding in children with major burns –Effect on McFarlane response to stress. *Burns* 2007;33:464-471.

[35] Novak F, Heyland DK, Avenell A, Drover JW, Su X. Glutamine supplementation in serious illness: a systematic review of the evidence. *Crit Care Med* 2002;30:2022-2029.

[36] Kyle U, Arriaza A, Esposito M, Coss-Bu J. Is indirect calorimetry a necessity or a luxury in the Pediatric Intensive Care Unit. *JPEN J Parenter and Enteral Nutr* 2011;e-pub 8 august 2011.

[37] Kudsk KA, Tolley EA, DeWitt RC. Preoperative albumin and surgical site identify surgical risk for major postoperative complications. JPEN *J Parent and Enteral Nutr* 2003;27:1-9.

[38] Marik PE, Zaloaga GP. Early enteral nutrition in acutely ill patients: a systematic review. *Crit Care Med* 2001;29:2264-2270.

[39] Griesdale D, de Souza R, van Dam R. Intensive insulin therapy and mortality among critically ill patients: a metanalysis including NICE-SUGAR study data. *CMAJ* 2009;180:821-827.

[40] Xu J, Yunshi Z, Li R. Immunonutrition in surgical patients. *Curr Drug Targets* 2009;10:771-777.

[41] Berger MM, Shenkin A. Update on clinical micronutrient supplementation studies in the critically ill. *Curr Opin Clin Nutr Metab Care* 2006;9:711-716.

[42] Berger M.Vitamin C requirements in parenteral nutrition. *Gastroenterology* 2009;137:70-78.

[43] Mizock SA, DeMichele SJ. The acute respiratory distress syndrome: role of nutritional modulation through dietary lipids. *Nutr Clin Pract* 2004;19:563-574.

[44] Norbury WB, Jeschke MG, Herndon DN. Metabolism modulators in sepsis: propranolol. *Crit Care Med* 2007;35:616-620.

[45] Martindale R, Maerz L Management of perioperative nutrition support. *Curr Opin Crit Care* 2006;12:290-294.

[46] Braga M, Gianotti L, Nespoli L et al. Hospital resources consumed for surgical morbidity: effects of preoperative arginine and omega 3 fatty acid supplementation on costs. *Nutrition* 2005;21:1078-1086.

[47] Fukushima R, Yamazaki E. Vitamin C requirement in surgical patients. *Curr Opin Clin Nutr Metab Care* 2010;13:669-676.

[48] Maldonado MD, Murillo-Cabezas F, Calvo JR, Lardone PJ, Tan DX, Guerrero JM, Reiter RJ. Melatonin as pharmacologic support in burn patients: a proposed solution to thermal injury-related lymphocytopenia and oxidative damage. *Crit Care Med* 2007;35:1177-1185.

[49] Krishnan et al. JA, Parce PB, Martinez A. Caloric intake in medical ICU patients: consistency of care with guidelines and relationships of clinical outcome. *Chest* 2003;124:297-305.

[50] Mechanik JI, Chiolero R. Special commentary: a call for intensive metabolic support. *Curr Opin Clin Metab Care* 2008;11:666-670.

In: Oxidative Stress and the Critically Ill Patient
Editors: Ramón Rodrigo and Bettina von Dessauer
ISBN: 978-1-62081-576-2

Chapter VIII

Contribution of Oxidative Stress in Pneumonia

Rodrigo Carrasco Loza
PhD student, Faculty of Medicine, University of Chile

1. Abstract

The pathophysiology of pneumonia includes various mechanisms such as microorganism invasion, airway damage and activation of defense mechanisms, characterized by a massive influx of activated phagocytes. Polymorphonuclear neutrophils and macrophages kill microorganisms by using ROS, increasing oxidative stress in the lung, which may cause a direct injury in the tissue and activate transcription factors. This leads to a local inflammatory response, which could progress to a systemic inflammatory response.

Although the generation of reactive species is nonspecific for any site affected by an infectious agent, modulation of redox balance could be most affected in the lungs due to functional characteristics such as their permanent exposition at high concentrations of oxygen and pro-oxidant agents from environmental contaminants. This permanent oxidative stimulus, has allowed the development of the lung's antioxidant defense system very suitable in basal conditions, but it may be surpassed by lung infections such as community-acquired pneumonia, which can have a great generation of reactive species.

Thus, as the imbalance of redox state and oxidative injury are part of direct mechanisms of damage and mediate the immune response is that we can argue that some of the biomarkers could be related to the severity of pneumonia, as well it allow us to propose a potential therapeutic target that could intervene.

Abbreviations

AP-1	activator protein 1
CAP:	community-acquired pneumonia
CAT:	catalase
COPD:	chronic obstructive pulmonary disease
FRAP:	ferric reducing ability of plasma
Gamma-GCS	gamma-glutamylcysteine synthetase
GSH:	reduced glutathione
GSH-Px:	glutathione peroxidase
GSSG:	glutathione disulfide
ICU:	intensive care unit
MDA:	malondialdehyde
MPO	myeloperoxidase
NAC:	N-acetylcysteine
NADPH:	nicotinamide adenine dinucleotide phosphate
(Nrf2)	nuclear factor erythroid 2-related factor 2
(NF)-kappaB kappa B	nuclear factor
PCR:	polymerase chain reaction
PMNs	poly-morphonuclear cells
REDOX	reduction-oxidation
ROS:	reactive oxygen species
RNS:	reactive nitrogen species
SOD:	superoxide dismutase
XOR:	xanthine oxidoreductase

2. Introduction

Community-acquired pneumonia (CAP) is a frequent cause for hospital admission that results in significant costs for health care systems [1] and represents the most frequent cause of death of infectious origin. About 10% of patients hospitalized for CAP require admission to intensive care units (ICU), and the lethality varies from 20% to 50% [2].

Although multiple pathophysiologic mechanisms are involved in the development of community-acquired pneumonia, this chapter focuses on a less common approach related to the role of redox status in patients with pneumonia.

Classically, the most relevant pathophysiological events are the invasion of microorganisms, airway damage and the activation of defense mechanisms. During CAP, a massive influx of activated phagocytes into the lower airways is observed, which represents the first line of defense against invading microorganisms. Polymorphonuclear neutrophils (PMNs) and macrophages kill these microorganisms using reactive oxygen species (ROS) and lysosomal enzymes, including proteinases [3]. This increase in pulmonary ROS concentration and proteolytic enzymes could be reflect at the systemic level as an increase in the biomarkers of oxidative stress and airway remodeling in these patients [4,5].

The local response primarily involves the lower airways that represent distal airways. The distal airways, lined by alveolar epithelial cells (Types I and II), contain capillaries, the interstitial compartment and the alveolar compartment. When oxidant injury overwhelms the repair capacity of the distal airway compartment, alveolar collapse may result together with extensive fibrotic scars, which effectively destroy the exchange of air between affected airways and the capillary system [6].

Therefore, considering that in an infection of any origin, the innate immune response of PMN activation causes an increase in the generation of ROS, the redox (reduction-oxidation) state could be affected in any infectious process.

However, does a lung infection exhibit a different redox response compared with other parenchymal areas affected by infectious agents? Would there be any difference in relation to effects on the redox state? To answer these questions, we must understand the nature of the pulmonary redox balance, so we must first understand the sources of reactive species and antioxidant defense systems.

3. Special Features of the Lung Parenchyma in Relation to Redox Balance

The lung, because of its structural and functional features, is a unique organ in terms of its permanent direct exposure to high levels of oxygen and reactive compounds. This permanent direct exposure results in particular characteristics in terms of the redox balance with respect to other tissues. This organ is exposed continuously to reactive species as a result of the permanent exposure of the alveolar compartment to endogenous sources, such as reactive oxygen (ROS) and nitrogen species (RNS), as well as external sources of reactive species that come from pollutants and inhaled particles present in ambient air.

For this reason, the lung tissue has developed an optimal antioxidant defense system designed to maintain an adequate balance in the redox state and thus prevent damage by reactive species. The antioxidant defense system of the epithelial lining fluid consists of several low molecular weight compounds, such as reduced glutathione (GSH), ascorbic acid (vitamin C) and uric acid; lipophilic antioxidants, such as α-tocopherol (vitamin E), retinol (vitamin A) and plasmalogens (1-alkenyl-phospholipids); and antioxidant enzymes, such as superoxide dismutase, catalase and glutathione peroxidase. Thus, under normal conditions in the lung, complex and coordinated interactions occur among all these antioxidant compounds to maintain an adequate balance in the redox state and thus prevent damage from reactive species [7].

Some conditions can disrupt the balance between ROS production and the defensive capacity of the antioxidant system, leading to pathological reactions that can result in injury or disease. One example is the action of some external agent that disrupts the redox balance and that can generate a greater oxidative insult than that produced in other systems with similar insults. In this sense, an infectious agent can cause an immune response initiated by poly-morphonuclear cells (PMNs), which will generate an inflammatory response that is associated with the generation of reactive oxygen species to act on the infectious agent involved.

Although this situation may occur in any organ affected by an infection, the oxidative injury may be greater in the lung if the generation of reactive species is of a magnitude that causes an imbalance in the redox state, as this system has a permanently high production of reactive species.

Considering the background discussed thus far, community-associated pneumonia is a pathology that disrupts the redox balance in the lung and that is associated with a subsequent inflammatory process.

3.1 Sources of Reactive Species in the Lung

Reactive oxygen species (ROS) and reactive nitrogen species (RNS) are free radicals that are generated physiologically during oxidative phosphorylation, but reactive species in the lung may also arise from other sources. For example, the different cell types prevalent in the lung, particularly the PMNs, may generate significant amounts of reactive species, as they are part of the innate immune response [8].

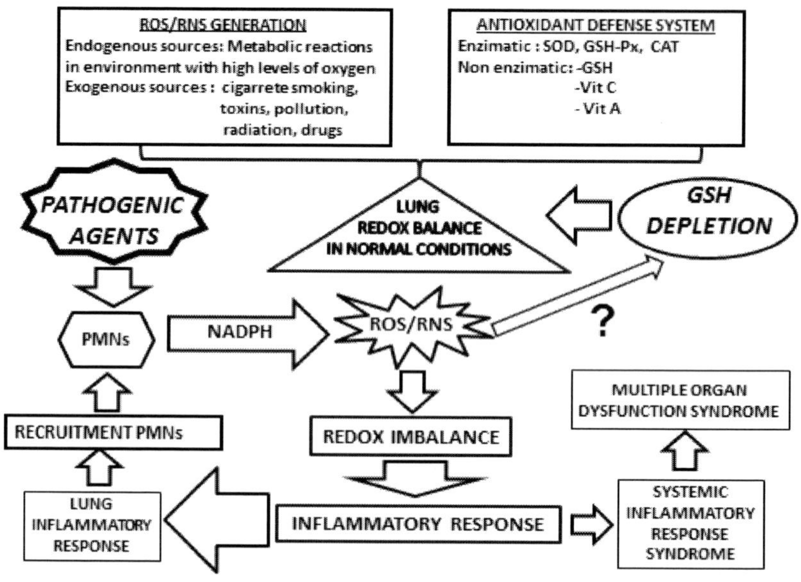

Figure 1. Pathophysiology of Community-acquired pneumonia and alteration of redox state. Under normal conditions the lung is in a balance between the generation of reactive species (ROS/ RNS) and the antioxidant defense system. The action of a pathogenic agent causes an innate immune response, characterized mainly by the action of PMNs. PMNs produce large amounts of ROS generated by NADPH oxidase cytoplasmic as part of their bactericidal activity, a phenomenon known as "respiratory burst". Under certain circumstances this increased generation of ROS / RNS in an environment with decreased antioxidant defense system, occasioned for example by a GSH depletion, which decreases mechanism is not well known, causes an imbalance in the redox state. The redox imbalance causes a direct injury on the pulmonary parenchyma and mediates initially the activation of a local inflammatory response which may at the same time promote further recruitment of PMNs. When the inflammatory response progresses in magnitude can produce systemic effects, which in the highest degree of severity may lead to MODS. ROS, reactive oxygen species; RNS, reactive nitrogen species; SOD, superoxide dismutase; GSH, reduced glutathione; GSH-Px, glutathione peroxidase; CAT, catalase; Vit C, vitamin C; Vit A, vitamin A; PMNs, poly-morphonuclear cells; NADPH, nicotinamide adenine dinucleotide phosphate.

ROS and RNS have various physiological roles and are quickly removed from the body because their persistence can cause cellular dysfunction and cell death. For this reason, biological systems have developed several defense mechanisms against oxidants, including enzymatic and non-enzymatic antioxidant systems. An imbalance between the generation of ROS/RNS and antioxidant defenses leads to a harmful condition known as oxidative/nitrosative stress, in which antioxidant mechanisms are insufficient to keep ROS/RNS below a toxic threshold as a result of the excessive production of ROS/RNS and/or the loss of antioxidant defenses. Oxidative/nitrosative stress can affect proteins, lipids, carbohydrates and nucleic acids, i.e., all the main cellular components [9].

Oxidizing agents can be produced endogenously by metabolic reactions (including by the activation of phagocytes or mitochondrial electron transport during respiration) or exogenously by cigarette smoking, toxins, pollution, radiation, drugs and other causes [10].

3.2 Cellular Sources of ROS in the Lungs

Neutrophils have been known to produce ROS as part of their bactericidal activity. The cytoplasmic membranes of neutrophils contain NADPH oxidase, which generates large amounts of O_2^-. This phenomenon is known "respiratory burst". Another enzyme contributing to the complex defense mechanism is myeloperoxidase (MPO), which catalyzes the reaction of H_2O_2 with halide anions upon neutrophil stimulation. This reaction occurs by far the most frequently with the chloride anion, so MPO produces mostly hypochlorous acid $HOCl^-$, which is highly reactive. Xanthine oxidoreductase (XOR) has also been detected in neutrophils, and it would also be another source of reactive species [11].

However, neutrophils constitute only a minor portion of the cellular population in the lungs under physiologic conditions, they migrate into the pulmonary circulation in large amounts only after stimulation during inflammation [11]. Therefore, the source of reactive species is of interest when evaluating oxidative injury during the development of community-acquired pneumonia.

Eosinophils are also a potent cellular source of ROS, especially in some allergic or infectious diseases. Similarly to neutrophils, their membranes contain NADPH oxidase, which generates superoxide. Cytoplasmic peroxidase (eosinophilic peroxidase, an analogue of myeloperoxidase in neutrophils) contributes significantly to the bactericidal activity or damaging effects of eosinophils, producing mostly hypochlorous acid (HOCl) [12].

Alveolar macrophages are phagocytic cells that are present in large numbers in the lungs and therefore form the first line of lung defense against infection. Similarly to neutrophils, their main source of ROS is the membrane NADPH oxidase, generating O_2^-. Alveolar macrophages have been suggested to be the major source of ROS under physiologic conditions [13].

Peripheral monocytes-macrophages attracted by inflammatory cytokines contribute substantially to the damage in pulmonary diseases after stimulation and differentiation into macrophages, these cells have recently shown the ability to produce superoxide by XOR, which plays a significant role in acute lung injury (as opposed to invading neutrophils, where XOR is silent) [14].

Mast cells are also present in the lungs, but so far, reports on their ROS production are rather confusing. However, some data suggest that they might be able to generate ROS [10].

Type II pneumocytes form part of the alveolar epithelium. These cuboidal cells with a highly active metabolism produce surfactant and are thought to function as precursor cells for type I pneumocytes in the case of increased destruction of the alveolar epithelium. Recent studies show that even type II epithelial cells exhibit enzymatic production of some ROS [15].

Endothelial cells represent another substantial cellular mass because of rich lung vascularization. In recent years, increasing evidence has shown that even these cells can represent a source of ROS and participate in oxidative stress and lung injury under pathological conditions. These cells contain xanthine oxidoreductase complex, which seems to become stimulated mostly after hypoxia [16].

Endothelial cells are capable of releasing substantial amounts of O_2^- into the extracellular space, possibly via membrane anion channels. The formation of another ROS, highly reactive OH, can be catalyzed by iron ions present in the proximity of the endothelial surface [17].

Cells of practically every type present in the lungs are capable of producing some ROS. The roles of the different cell types in the pathogenesis of specific diseases are far from clear. While phagocytes are believed to be the main source of the oxidative stress during inflammation, the roles of the different cell types in a variety of other conditions remain unknown. This deficit in our knowledge is partly due to the lack of appropriate methods of localization of the ROS formation in the lung tissue in situ. However, the role of ROS in various physiological processes such as signaling or apoptosis seems to be even more important.

3.3 Antioxidant Defense in the Lung

Practically every cell is endowed with mechanisms protecting it against the damaging effects of ROS. Antioxidants can be divided into intra- and extracellular antioxidants as well as enzymatic and non-enzymatic categories.

Gutteridge and Halliwell classified antioxidants as primary (preventing oxidant formation), secondary (scavenging ROS) and tertiary (removing or repairing oxidatively modified molecules), which may be constitutive, inducible or dietary according to their origin [18].

The lung is directly exposed to the environment and to oxygen at higher partial pressure than other organs, making its antioxidant defense particularly important. First in the line of enzymatic ROS degradation is superoxide dismutase (SOD). This enzyme exists in 3 forms: a) Cu/Zn SOD, which is present mainly in the cytosolic matrix; b) MnSOD, which is localized preferentially in mitochondria; and c) extracellular SOD. All SODs efficiently catalyze the transformation of O_2^- into H_2O_2, yet the role of SOD in the antioxidant defense is not clear. Adding SOD was reported to enhance and in other cases to limit lipid peroxidation and membrane damage, with these contradictory effects potentially resulting from differences in the local concentrations of Fe^+ and/or differences in the enzyme concentrations protecting the cells against hydrogen peroxide. Moreover, cells contain another enzyme protecting them against hydrogen peroxide [19].

This function is fulfilled by the catalase and glutathione system. Catalase is localized intracellularly, especially in peroxisomes, and works efficiently under high concentrations of H_2O_2. At low concentrations, the reduced form of glutathione (GSH) mainly transforms hydrogen peroxide. The ability of the glutathione system to reduce H_2O_2 depends on the ratio between GSH and the oxidized form (GSSG), which in turn depends on two processes: transport of GSSG out of the cell and the capacity of GSH reductase, an enzyme that converts GSSG to GSH. The GSH concentration in the alveolar lavage fluid exceeds its plasmatic concentration by more than 100-fold, demonstrating the high capacity of this system in the lung. The regeneration of GSH requires reduced nicotinamide adenine dinucleotide phosphate (NADPH), which is supplied through glucoso-6-phosphate dehydrogenase (G6PD) activity in the hexoso monophosphate shunt. Moreover, other enzymatic systems may contribute directly or indirectly to the defense against oxidative stress, including thioredoxins, which exert a protective effect through the reduction of disulfide bonds.

The non-enzymatic antioxidants are mostly "scavengers" of free radicals and will be discussed later when presenting the therapeutic interventions that aim to prevent damage by oxidative stress.

4. Pathophysiology of Community-Acquired Pneumonia

4.1 Sources of Reactive Species and Antioxidant Defenses in CAP

As mentioned above, in normal conditions, organisms living in an aerobic environment are continuously and obligatorily exposed to ROS. These species includes a variety of partially reduced oxygen metabolites (e.g., superoxide anions, hydrogen peroxide and hydroxyl radicals) that display higher reactivities than molecular oxygen [20]. Reactive oxygen species are generated intracellularly through a variety of pathways, i.e., as products of normal aerobic metabolism or as second messengers in various signal transduction pathways. However, ROS may also be derived from exogenous sources and may be taken up directly by cells from the extracellular surroundings or produced by exposure of the cells to some environmental insult [21]. At high and/or sustained levels, ROS can cause severe damage to DNA, proteins, and lipids; in contrast, low to moderate levels of ROS can trigger survival mechanisms. A number of defense systems are involved in protection against ROS injury. These systems include various non-enzymatic scavenger molecules (e.g.., glutathione, vitamins A, vitamin E, and flavonoids) as well as antioxidant enzymes [e.g., superoxide dismutase (SOD), catalase (CAT), and glutathione peroxidase (GSH-Px)]. In some cases, these defense mechanisms are not sufficiently effective to counteract the production of ROS, resulting in a state called "oxidative stress". Oxidative injury has been implicated in a wide variety of diseases including atherosclerosis, diabetes, pulmonary fibrosis, neurodegenerative disorders, and arthritis [22].

In CAP, increased concentrations of ROS in the lungs of such patients are reflected by elevated concentrations of oxidative stress markers in the breath, airways, lung tissue and blood. Traditionally, the measurement of these biomarkers has involved invasive procedures to procure the samples or to examine the affected compartments, causing the discomfort for the patient. As a consequence, there is a need for less or non-invasive approaches to measure oxidative stress [23] to enable use as biomarkers in clinical practice.

4.2 Prognostic Factors and Biomarkers

After the CAP diagnosis, a key element is the ability to assess the severity of the symptoms and the possible further evolution of this pathologic process, as this ability determines when and how each patient should be treated. Knowing when to treat a patient is considered very useful, with prognostic scales that estimate the probability of the death of a patient from CAP leading to the decision of hospital admission. This information is especially valuable if complemented by individual clinical trials for each case [24]. Indeed, interest has existed for many years in identifying early prognostic factors for CAP complications and developing tools able to predict prognostic factors and mortality [25].

Some of the prognostic scales that provide better results in their application at admission of CAP patients are the PSI (Pneumonia Severity Index), Fine scale, [25, 26] and the CURB-65. [27]. However, these tools utilize only clinical aspects and routine laboratory tests, so interest exists in finding new prognostic biomarkers that could be useful in enhancing the sensitivity of these prognostic tests. These scales have been widely validated in clinical trials [28]; however, they only show the probability of death at diagnosis. These scales do not determine the inflammatory response of the host, which is currently considered a key aspect in the prognosis of the patient [29]. To obtain this information, a new approach is required including the evaluation of biological biomarkers as an expression of the host's inflammatory response against the microorganism to identify the defense capacity of the patient and to individualize the prognosis. In this response, the host produces pro-inflammatory and anti-inflammatory mediators that depend on genetic polymorphisms, the microorganism and the initial severity of the disease [29].

Biomarkers of infection and inflammation have generated considerable interest because of their ability to rapidly and feasibly reflect the inflammatory response of the host. Previous studies with C-reactive protein (CRP), procalcitonin (PCT) and, more recently, proadrenomedullin have demonstrated a correlation with initial severity and poor clinical outcomes [30, 31].

Although these compounds have a beneficial effect, an excessive release of mediators has been associated with deleterious effects. For example, excessive releases of cytokines induce hypotension, myocardial dysfunction, hypoperfusion of vital organs and lactic acidosis and are associated with higher mortality [29, 32, 33]. Other mediators are involved in the immune response and the generation of ROS, which in the case of an induction of oxidative stress could be associated with major morbi-mortality in CAP patients.

4.3 Oxidative Stress in CAP

ROS unquestionably have an important role in the pathogenesis of pulmonary diseases and many regulatory physiologic functions. Their importance depends on the subtle balance between ROS production and the defensive capacity of antioxidant systems. In addition, the location of their production also plays an important role in the pathogenesis of pulmonary diseases. Many cells of the pulmonary tissue have the capacity to form ROS; however, the real sources of ROS specified in each different pathological process in the lung remain unclear.

The studies conducted thus far have demonstrated that independent of the etiology of pneumonia, the clinical event is associated with a pro-oxidant state, represented by a lower antioxidant capacity and increased systemic lipid peroxidation.

In CAP, similarly to other causes of infectious disease, is highly relevant as an early indication of patients with higher risk. A reliable method of assessing the severity of pneumonia may potentially improve the triage or initial management of patients by helping clinicians to determine whether close monitoring and aggressive treatment is more appropriate than conservative management. However, because accurately assessing the severity of pneumonia can be challenging, a number of scales based on prognostic factors have been designed to identify patients at high risk of death and those at low risk who may require less vigilance [31]. The sensitivity and prognostic value of these scales could be enhanced by an association with current biomarkers, in this case to oxidative stress-related parameters, which would be added to the risk factor given by the redox imbalance, with the highest score associated with the highest severity.

An impairment of the antioxidant defense system in CAP patients is demonstrated by a decrease in antioxidant capacity associated with higher values of lipid peroxidation plasma and erythrocytes [34, 35]. In addition, an enhancement in superoxide production and a lower total antioxidant capacity has also been reported in this setting, explained partly through a decrease in extracellular superoxide dismutase activity (ECSOD). Other trials have also demonstrated the elevation of lipid peroxidation products in the whole blood of these patients. Accordingly, serum MDA levels have been reported to be elevated in acute pneumonia in both children [36] and adult patients [37,38].

Phagocyte response, an essential component of the defense system, results in increased ROS production. The effects of these substances in the airway as well as in other organs depend on ROS concentration and the time of exposure. In general, higher levels of ROS induce damage in biomolecules (e.g., lipid peroxidation) and induce intracellular signaling pathways, leading to cell death, mainly through apoptosis [39]. Together with this effect, an impairment of the antioxidant power could also contribute to the enhancement of cell damage. Thus, glutathione depletion in lung epithelial cells is reported to be associated with the initiation of apoptosis, as assessed by ceramide accumulation [40]. In contrast, the defense mechanism could be activated by moderately increased ROS through survival pathways, as demonstrated *in vitro* [41, 42] and in an *in vivo* model of lung injury (e.g., anti-inflammatory effects) [43, 44]. Cytoprotection is partly mediated by the nuclear factor erythroid 2-related factor 2 (Nrf2) that controls the antioxidant response element (ARE)-dependent gene regulation in response to oxidative stress. Upon activation, Nrf2 mediates the induction of a spectrum of cytoprotective proteins including antioxidant enzymes that protect against epithelial damage in oxidative stress settings, such as asthma, chronic obstructive pulmonary disease and CAP. The temporal analysis of pulmonary global gene expression after LPS challenge revealed an increase in the expression of large numbers of proinflammatory genes associated with the innate immune response at as early as 30 minutes in the lungs of Nrf2-deficient mice, indicating severe immune dysregulation [45]. Nrf2 was consistently required for LPS-mediated ARE induction as revealed by chromatin immunoprecipitation using antibodies specific for c-Jun and c-Fos and the observation of low ARE induction in Nrf2-null bone epithelial lung-derived macrophages. Moreover, chemical antioxidants such as N-acetylcysteine and butylated hydroxyanisole and the NADPH oxidase inhibitor diphenyleneiodonium inhibited ARE induction as well as the generation of reactive oxygen species, both of which were also suppressed in Nox2 (NADPH oxidase 2)-deficient lung-derived macrophages [46]. In CAP, the magnitude of infectious and inflammatory processes (ROS burst) in the airway as a consequence of the acute microbial invasion is not adequately counteracted by the response of the antioxidant defense system. However, no association has been observed between this pro-oxidant status and the clinical severity of CAP. For this reason, it is very important to determine the antioxidant status in CAP patients to estimate the magnitude of the organismal response to the infection at admission.

Regarding oxidative stress biomarkers, 8-isoprostane has been validated as a measure of oxidative stress in various lung diseases, such as sarcoidosis, streptococcal pneumonia, chronic obstructive pulmonary disease and asthma [47]. Some studies suggest that this depletion of antioxidants would occur prior to the establishment of systemic inflammation [48]. Recently, an elevated lipid peroxidation in the erythrocytes in the acute phase of CAP has been reported, as well as a decrease in both the content of reduced glutathione and the activities of superoxide dismutase and catalase [46, 49]. However, these studies have mainly been performed on bronchoalveolar lavage fluid, which requires an invasive procedure.

The glutathione system has an important role in the control of pro-inflammatory processes in the lungs, being involved in immune modulation, extracellular matrix remodeling, apoptosis and mitochondrial respiration [48, 50]. In CAP, the role of glutathione in the pathogenesis of microorganism invasion or the antioxidant non-enzymatic response has not been characterized. Cemek et al. [36] studied antioxidant status in children with acute pneumonia, finding that all antioxidant compounds were decreased compared with the control group, i.e., vitamin C, vitamin E and GSH levels. Recently, macrolide antibiotics demonstrated anti-inflammatory effects, suggesting that they could be advantageous in patients with CAP and chronic obstructive pulmonary disease based on the suppression of oxidant-induced glutathione synthesis by erythromycin in human bronchial epithelial cells [51, 52]. The molecular mechanisms of this anti-inflammatory effect are associated with the inhibition of activator protein 1 (AP-1) and nuclear factor (NF)-kappaB. These transcriptional factors are involved in the expression of gamma-glutamylcysteine synthetase (gamma-GCS), suggesting that these drugs influence the oxidant-antioxidant balance in human bronchial epithelial cells. However, few clinical trials support the relationship between GSH levels and CAP severity [37, 53]. The protective mechanism is based on the redox environment of pulmonary fluid, one of the important factors in determining the contribution of the innate and adaptive immune systems against infection, independent of etiology. In the normal lung, an extremely high level of extracellular antioxidants is able to maintain this compartment in a highly reduced state to facilitate the maintenance of an efficient immune response [54].

Conclusions and Perspectives

Current data suggests that because of the importance of oxidative stress in the development of community-acquired pneumonia, the potential development of antioxidant treatments should be considered a supplementary therapy in patients with CAP. Therefore, measurement of oxidative stress biomarkers may be useful as an additional criterion indicating the severity of pneumonia, although its clinical significance needs to be further explored.

Regarding antioxidant strategies that have already been tested, non-enzymatic antioxidants are mostly "scavengers" of free radicals such as vitamin C, vitamin E (inhibits oxidation of membrane lipids), uric acid (an efficient scavenger of peroxynitrite, present in plasma and airway lining fluid), albumin, bilirubin, glutathione or N-acetylcysteine (NAC). NAC is a potent drug that acts directly by reacting with ROS (forming NAC disulfides) and indirectly, serving as a GSH precursor. NAC does not prevent neutrophil influx to the lungs, but it does prevent their oxidative burst. However, as with many antioxidant substances, NAC in high doses can exhibit pro-oxidative effects [55].

Another non-enzymatic antioxidant that may also prevent ROS formation is allopurinol, a potent inhibitor of xanthine oxidoreductase. As the knowledge about ROS and their role in many pathologic processes increases, many natural and synthetic substances (some mentioned above) are being tested in search of new therapeutic approaches utilizing their antioxidant properties. Among the most frequently investigated experimentally are glutathione, vitamins C and E, [56] N-acetylcysteine melatonin or allopurinol in a model of acute lung injury [57]. Another line of research has focused on enhancing the enzymatic defense system by administering SOD or catalase either intravenously or intratracheally. Some of the agents tested were already used in small clinical trials on human patients with promising results: glutathione [58, 59, 60], vitamin C [61], SOD [62], and NAC [63]. However, so far, none of these compounds has become routinely used in clinical practice, as there are still some confusing points to be resolved regarding their activity.

REFERENCES

[1] Butt S, Swiatlo E. Treatment of community-acquired pneumonia in an ambulatory setting. *Am J Med.* 2011; 124: 297-300.

[2] Ewig S, Ruiz M, Mensa J, et al. Severe community-acquired pneumonia. Assessment of severity criteria. *Am J Respir Crit Care Med.* 1998; 158: 1102–8.

[3] Jones MR, Simms BT, Lupa MM, et al. Lung NF-kappaB activation and neutrophil recruitment require IL-1 and TNF receptor signaling during pneumococcal pneumonia. *J Immunol.* 2005; 175: 7530–5.

[4] Katsoulis K, Kontakiotis T, Baltopoulos G, et al. Total antioxidant status and severity of community-acquired pneumonia: are they correlated? *Respiration* 2005; 72: 381–7

[5] Laskaj R, Dodig S, Cepelak I, et al. Gamma-glutamyltransferase activity and total antioxidant status in serum and platelets of patients with community-acquired pneumonia. *Arch Med Res.* 2007; 38: 424–31.

[6] Ward PA. Oxidative stress: acute and progressive lung injury. *Ann N Y Acad Sci.* 2010; 1203:53-9.

[7] Schmidt R, Luboeinski T, Markart P, Ruppert C, Daum C, Grimminger F, Seeger W, Günther A. Alveolar antioxidant status in patients with acute respiratory distress syndrome. *Eur Respir J* 2004; 24:994-9.

[8] Ivanov I, Saam J, Kuhn H, Holzhütter HG. Dual role of oxygen during lipoxygenase reactions. *FEBS J* 2005; 272: 2523–2535.

[9] Nagata M. Inflammatory cells and oxygen radicals. *Curr. Drug Targets Inflamm Allergy* 2005; 4: 503–504.

[10] Kim JY, Lee KH, Lee BK, Ro JY. Peroxynitrite modulates release of inflammatory mediators from Guinea pig lung mast cells activated by antigen-antibody reaction. *Int. Arch. Allergy Immunol* 2005; 137: 104–114.

[11] Hammerschmidt S, Büchler N, Wahn H. Tissue lipid peroxidation and reduced glutathione depletion in hypochlorite-induced lung injury. *Chest* 2002; 121: 573–581.

[12] Nagata M. Inflammatory cells and oxygen radicals. *Curr Drug Targets Inflamm Allergy* 2005; 4: 503–504.

[13] Forman HJ, Torres M. Reactive oxygen species and cell signaling. *Am J Resp Crit Care Med* 2002; 166: S4–S8.

[14] Wright RM, Ginger LA, Kosila N, Elkins ND, Essary B, Mcmanaman JL, Repine JE. Mononuclear phagocyte xanthine oxidoreductase contributes to cytokine-induced acute lung injury. *Am J Respir Cell Mol Biol* 2004; 30: 479–490.

[15] Van Klaveren RJ, Roelant C, Boogaerts M, Demedts M, Nemery B. Involvement of an NAD(P)H oxidase-like enzyme in superoxide anion and hydrogen peroxide generation by rat type II cells. *Thorax* 1997; 52: 465–471.

[16] Kelley EE, Hock T, Khoo NK, Richardson GR, Johnson KK, Powell PC, Giles GI, Agarwal A, Lancaster JR, Tarpey MM. Moderate hypoxia induces xanthine oxidoreductase activity in arterial endothelial cells. *Free Radic Biol Med* 2006; 40: 952–959.

[17] Terada LS. Hypoxia-reoxygenation increases O2-× efflux which injures endothelial cells by an extracellular mechanism. *Am J Physiol* 1996; 270: H945–950.

[18] Gutteridge JMC, Halliwell B. Free radicals and antioxidants in the year 2000. A historical look to the future. *Ann. N Y Acad Sci* 2000; 899: 136–147.

[19] Comhair SA., Erzurum SC. Antioxidant responses to oxidant-mediated lung diseases. *Am J Physiol Lung Cell Mol Physiol.* 2002; 283: L246–255.

[20] Thannickal VJ, Fanburg BL. Reactive oxygen species in cell signaling. *Am J Physiol. Lung Cell Mol Physiol.* 2000; 279: L1005–28.

[21] Valko M, Leibfritz D, Moncol J, et al. Free radicals and antioxidants in normal physiological functions and human disease. *Int J Biochem Cell Biol.* 2007; 39: 44–84.

[22] Libby P. Inflammatory mechanisms: the molecular basis of inflammation and disease. *Nutr Rev.* 2007; 65: S140–6.

[23] Rahman I, Biswas SK. Non-invasive biomarkers of oxidative stress: reproducibility and methodological issues. *Redox Rep.* 2004; 9: 125-43.

[24] Loke YK, Kwok CS, Niruban A, et al. Value of severity scales in predicting mortality from community-acquired pneumonia: systematic review and meta-analysis. *Thorax* 2010; 65: 884-90.

[25] Fine MJ, Auble TE, Yealy DM, et al. A prediction rule to identify low-risk patients with community-acquired pneumonia. *N Engl. J Med.* 1997;336: 243-50.

[26] Lim WS, van der Eerden MM, Laing R, et al. Defining community acquired pneumonia severity on presentation to hospital: an international derivation and validation study. *Thorax* 2003; 58: 377-382.

[27] Capelastegui A, Espana PP, Quintana JM, et al. Validation of a predictive rule for the management of community-acquired pneumonia. *Eur. Respir. J.* 2006; 27:151–7.

[28] Deng JC, Standiford TJ. The systemic response to lung infection. *Clin. Chest Med.* 2005; 26: 1–9.

[29] Christ-Crain M, Morgenthaler NG, Stolz D, et al. Pro-adrenomedullin to predict severity and outcome in community-acquired pneumonia. *Crit. Care* 2006; 10: R96.

[30] Menéndez R, Martínez R, Reyes S, et al. Biomarkers improve mortality prediction by prognostic scales in community-acquired pneumonia. *Thorax* 2009 ; 64: 587-91.

[31] Nelson S. Novel nonantibiotic therapies for pneumonia: cytokines and host defense. *Chest* 2001; 119:419S–25S.

[32] Skerrett SJ, Park DR. Anti-inflammatory treatment of acute and chronic pneumonia. *Semin. Respir. Infect.* 2001;16: 76–84.

[33] Fine MJ, Smith MA, Carson CA, et al. Prognosis and outcomes of patients with community-acquired pneumonia. *A meta-analysis. JAMA* 1996; 275: 134–41.

[34] Pierrou S, Broberg P, O'Donnell RA, et al. Expression of genes involved in oxidative stress responses in airway epithelial cells of smokers with chronic obstructive pulmonary disease. *Am. J. Respir. Crit. Care Med.* 2007; 175: 577–86.

[35] Kinnula VL, Myllärniemi M. Oxidant-antioxidant imbalance as a potential contributor to the progression of human pulmonary fibrosis. *Antioxid. Redox Signal* 2008; 10: 727–38.

[36] Cemek M, Caksen H, Bayiroğlu F, et al. Oxidative stress and enzymic-non-enzymic antioxidant responses in children with acute pneumonia. *Cell Biochem. Funct.* 2006; 24: 269–273.

[37] Duflo F, Debon R, Goudable J, et al. Alveolar and serum oxidative stress in ventilator-associated pneumonia. *Br. J. Anaesth.* 2002; 89: 231–6.

[38] Li GF, He YF, Huang MR, et al. Determination of serum superoxide dismutase, glutathione peroxidase, total antioxidative capacity, malondialdehyde in patients with pneumonia. *Di Yi Jun Yi Da Xue Xue Bao*. 2003; 23: 961–2.

[39] Tasaka S, Amaya F, Hashimoto S, et al. Roles of oxidants and redox signaling in the pathogenesis of acute respiratory distress syndrome. *Antioxid. Redox Signal* 2008; 10: 739–53.

[40] Goldkorn T, Ravid T, Khan EM. Life and death decisions: ceramide generation and EGF receptor trafficking are modulated by oxidative stress. *Antioxid. Redox Signal* 2005; 7: 119–28.

[41] Slebos DJ, Ryter SW, Choi AM. Heme oxygenase-1 and carbon monoxide in pulmonary medicine. *Respir. Res.* 2003; 4: 7.

[42] Jia L, Xu M, Zhen W, et al. Novel anti-oxidative role of calreticulin in protecting A549 human type II alveolar epithelial cells against hypoxic injury *Am. J. Physiol. Cell Physiol.* 2008; 294: C47-C55.

[43] Dandona P, Kumar V, Aljada A, et al. Angiotensin II receptor blocker valsartan suppresses reactive oxygen species generation in leukocytes, nuclear factor-kappa B, in mononuclear cells of normal subjects: evidence of an antiinflammatory action. *J. Clin. Endocrinol. Metab.* 2003; 88: 4496–4501.

[44] Geraets L, Moonen HJ, Brauers K, et al. Dietary flavones and flavonoles are inhibitors of poly(ADP-ribose)polymerase-1 in pulmonary epithelial cells. *J. Nutr.* 2007; 137: 2190–95.

[45] Thimmulappa RK, Lee H, Rangasamy T, et al. Nrf2 is a critical regulator of the innate immune response and survival during experimental sepsis. *J. Clin. Invest.* 2006; 116: 984–995.

[46] Kim H, Jung Y, Shin BS, et al. Redox regulation of lipopolysaccharide-mediated sulfiredoxin induction, which depends on both AP-1 and Nrf2. *J. Biol. Chem.* 2010; 285: 34419–28.

[47] Psathakis K, Papatheodorou G, Plataki M. 8-Isoprostane, a marker of oxidative stress, is increased in the expired breath condensate of patients with pulmonary sarcoidosis. *Chest* 2004; 125: 1005–11.

[48] Von Dessauer B, Bongain J, Molina V, et al. Oxidative stress as a novel target in pediatric sepsis management. *J. Crit. Care*. 2011; 26: 103.e1-7.

[49] Ageeva TS, Zhavoronok TV, Teteneva FF, et al. Extrahospital pneumonias: the clinico-scintigraphic characterization and oxidative balance of cells. *Klin. Med.* 2007; 85: 43–8.

[50] He Z, Li B, Yu L, Liu Q, et al. Suppression of oxidant-induced glutathione synthesis by erythromycin in human bronchial epithelial cells. *Respiration* 2008; 75: 202–9.

[51] Rahman I, MacNee W. Oxidative stress and regulation of glutathione in lung inflammation. *Eur. Respir. J.* 2000; 16: 534–54.

[52] Berger MM, Eggimann P, Heyland DK, et al. Reduction of nosocomial pneumonia after major burns by trace element supplementation: aggregation of two randomised trials. *Crit. Care* 2006; 10: R153.

[53] Crapo JD. Oxidative stress as an initiator of cytokine release and cell damage. Eur. Respir. *J. Suppl.* 2003; 44: 4s-6s.

[54] Berger MM, Eggimann P, Heyland DK, et al. Reduction of nosocomial pneumonia after major burns by trace element supplementation: aggregation of two randomised trials. *Crit. Care* 2006; 10: R153.

[55] Dekhuijzen PNR. Antioxidant properties of N-acetylcysteine: their relevance in relation to chronic obstructive pulmonary disease. *Eur. Respir J* 2004; 23: 629–636.

[56] Panda K., Chattopadhyay R, Chattopadhyay DJ, Chatterjee IB. Vitamin C prevents cigarette smoke-induced oxidative damage in vivo. *Free Radic Biol Med* 2000. 29: 115–124.

[57] Wright RM, Ginger LA, Kosila N, Elkins ND, Essary B, Mcmanaman JL, Repine JE. Mononuclear phagocyte xanthine oxidoreductase contributes to cytokine-induced acute lung injury. *Am J Respir Cell Mol Biol* 2004, 30: 479–490.

[58] Griese M, Ramakers J, Krasselt A, Starosta V, Van Koningsbruggen S, Fischer R , Ratjen F, Mullinger B, Huber RM, Maier K, Rietschel E, Scheuch G. Improvement of alveolar glutathione and lung function but not oxidative state in cystic fibrosis. *Am J Respir Crit Care. Med.* 2004: 169: 822–828

[59] Roum JH, Borok Z, Mcelvaney NG, Grimes GJ, Bokser AD, Buhl R, Crystal RG. Glutathione aerosol suppresses lung epithelial surface inflammatory cell-derived oxidants in cystic fibrosis. *J Appl Physiol*. 1999; 87: 438–443.

[60] Cooke RW, Drury JA. Reduction of oxidative stress marker in lung fluid of preterm infants after administration of intra-tracheal liposomal glutathione. *Biol. Neonate*. 87: 178–180, 2005.

[61] Nathens AB, Neff MJ, Jurkovich GJ, Klotz P, Farver K., Ruzinski JT, Radella F, Garcia I, Maier RV. Randomized, prospective trial of antioxidant supplementation in critically ill surgical patients. *Ann. Surg*. 236: 814–822, 2002.

[62] Davis JM, Parad RB, Michele T, Allred E, Price A, Rosenfeld W. Pulmonary outcome at 1 year corrected age in premature infants treated at birth with recombinant human CuZn superoxide dismutase. *Pediatrics*. 111: 469–476, 2003.

[63] Bernard GR, Wheeler AP, Arons MA, Morris PE, Paz HL, Russell JA, Wright PE. A trial of antioxidants N-acetylcysteine and procysteine in ARDS. *Chest* 112: 164–172, 1997.

In: Oxidative Stress and the Critically Ill Patient
Editors: Ramón Rodrigo and Bettina von Dessauer
ISBN: 978-1-62081-576-2

Chapter IX

Oxidative Stress and Acute Respiratory Distress Syndrome

Rodrigo Carrasco[1], and Cristian Carvajal[2]
PhD student, Faculty of Medicine, University of Chile[1]
Pediatric Intensivist, Hospital Roberto del Río, Chile[2]

1. Abstract

Acute Respiratory Distress Syndrome (ARDS) is a clinical condition secondary to a variety of insults that is characterized by diffuse inflammation of the lung tissue, protein exudate and non-orthostatic alveolar edema, leading to a severe impairment in gas exchange and high morbi-mortality in critically ill patients. The inflammatory response, via the activation of neutrophils and macrophages, enhances the production of reactive oxygen and nitrogen species, which leads to oxidative phenomena and tissue injury. Another factor that may increase lung injury in this clinical condition is the effect of mechanical ventilation, which can cause ventilator-induced lung injury secondary to oxidative stress.

Abbreviations

ALI	acute lung injury
ARDS	acute respiratory distress syndrome
ARF	acute Respiratory Failure
ELF	epithelial lining fluid
BALF	bronchoalveolar lavage fluid
DAD	diffuse alveolar damage
GSH	glutathione
H_2O_2	oxygen peroxide
IgG IC	IgG immune complexes

LPS	lipopolysaccharide
MV	mechanical ventilation
MODS	multiple organ dysfunction syndrome
NADH	reduced nicotinamide adenine dinucleotide
NO•	nitric oxide
NOS	nitric oxide synthase
O_2	molecular oxygen
O_2•−	superoxide
ONOO−	peroxynitrite
$PaFiO_2$	PaO_2/FiO_2 ratio
PCWP	pulmonary Capillary Wedge Pressure
PEEP	positive end expiratory pressure
RNS	reactive nitrogen species
ROS	reactive oxygen species
SOD	superoxide dismutase
TNF	tumor necrosis factor
VILI	ventilator-induced lung injury

2. Introduction

The most severe form of acute lung injury (ALI), acute respiratory distress syndrome (ARDS), is a relatively frequent complication in critically ill patients that is responsible for significant co-morbidity and mortality [1, 2].

Multiple studies currently aim to determine the mechanisms of generation and progression of ARDS. The research areas of investigation for these studies include the recognition of subtypes of ALI/ARDS and the identification of risk factors and prognostic factors to aid in the development of new therapeutic strategies through specific interventions that allows the stabilization of, prevent the progression of and/or reverse damage already caused by the primary injury. However, despite multiple studies evaluating different types of interventions, only a few studies have shown significant effectiveness for these interventions. In particular, only the early treatment of the underlying triggering disease and supportive care using "lung-protective" strategies of mechanical ventilation have contributed to better clinical outcomes.

In essence, these syndromes reflect a pulmonary injury that leads to dysfunction and the compromise of the barrier properties of the pulmonary endothelium and epithelium as a consequence of an unregulated acute inflammatory response. In this hypothetical construct, an initiating event (e.g., sepsis, shock, trauma, multiple transfusions, or pancreatitis) leads to the activation of a systemic acute inflammatory response. One of the earliest manifestations of ALI/ARDS is the activation of the pulmonary endothelium and macrophages (alveolar and interstitial ones), up-regulation of adhesion molecules and production of cytokines and chemokines, contributing to massive sequestration of neutrophils within the pulmonary microvasculature. These cells migrate across the endothelium and epithelium into the alveolar space and release a variety of cytotoxic and pro-inflammatory compounds, including proteolytic enzymes, reactive oxygen (ROS) and nitrogen species (RNS), cationic proteins, lipid mediators, and additional proinflammatory cytokines. This release perpetuates a vicious cycle by recruiting additional inflammatory cells that in turn produce more cytotoxic mediators, ultimately leading to a profound injury to the alveolar-capillary membrane and respiratory failure. Note that although the most obvious initial manifestations may be respiratory in nature, ALI and ARDS are part of a systemic process involving microvascular dysfunction of diverse organs, including the heart, kidneys, intestines, liver, muscle, and brain. This phenomenon may finally converge and manifest as a multi-organ dysfunction syndrome (MODS).

To contextualize the problem, we first present some general aspects of ALI/ARDS and then describe some of the pathophysiological events that occur during its development. Finally, we focus on the mechanisms of damage related to REDOX imbalance.

The purpose of this chapter is to present an approach to the pathophysiology of lung injury related to the redox imbalance and the subsequent oxidative stress injury. A more complete understanding of these mechanisms may allow for the development of new therapeutic strategies to reduce the damage resulting from oxidative stress in patients with ALI/ARDS and may prevent ventilator-induced lung injury.

3. General Aspects

Definition and Diagnostic Criteria of ARDS

ARDS is caused by several conditions that induce pulmonary tissue inflammation and damage of the cells that form the alveolar-capillary membrane, progressively leading to diverse degrees of hypoxemia and multi-organ failure. The degree of failure varies along a continuum between the severity of pulmonary involvement and the level of hypoxemia, with the initial step known as ALI and the later stages as ARDS. This syndrome was previously referred to as "adult" respiratory distress syndrome but has now been renamed "acute respiratory distress syndrome" because it also occurs in the pediatric population.

The diagnosis of ALI/ARDS includes histological evidence of increased alveolar-capillary permeability and diffuse alveolar damage, which is unlikely to be obtained in a clinical setting considering the instability of these patients. Thus, in practical terms, there is no "gold standard" with which to compare the results of studies using different diagnostic criteria as discussed below.

Since the initial description by Ashbaugh and colleagues in 1967 of a syndrome characterized by severe dyspnea, tachycardia, cyanosis refractory to oxygen therapy, decreased lung compliance and diffuse alveolar infiltrate in the chest X-ray, the optimal definition of ARDS remains a controversial subject [2].

In 1994, the American-European Consensus Conference (A-ECC) on ARDS defined ALI/ARDS as the acute onset of respiratory failure (expressed as an alteration in $PaFiO_2$, the PaO_2/FiO_2 ratio, with ALI defined as $PaFiO_2 \leq 300$ and ARDS as $PaFiO_2 \leq 200$), bilateral pulmonary infiltrates on chest x-ray excluding cardiogenic pulmonary edema (expressed as pulmonary capillary wedge pressure, PCWP, of 18 mmHg or less, or no evidence of left atrial hypertension) [3] (Table 1).

Although the establishment of this classification system was a significant advance for clinical purposes, it had also several disadvantages. First, in clinical settings, the boundary between ALI and ARDS is less clear when it is only defined by the $PaFiO_2$ ratio, since it does not take into account the influence of therapy and ventilator support in relation to these criteria (e.g., the effect of the PEEP or FiO_2 on blood sampling). In addition, not all clinicians accept the concomitant diagnosis of ARDS for conditions that meet the diagnostic criteria of ALI/ARDS when there are no significant differences in management (e.g., severe pneumonia).

Table 1. A-ECC ARDS Criteria

A-ECC ARDS Criteria
Oxygenation ALI $PaO_2/FiO_2 < 300$ (regardless of positive end expiratory pressure level) ARDS $PaO_2/FiO_2 < 200$ (regardless of positive end expiratory pressure level)
Chest radiograph bilateral infiltration seen on frontal chest radiograph
Pulmonary artery occlusion pressure <18 mm Hg when measured or no clinical evidence of left atrial hypertension

Second, given the less frequent use of the Swan-Ganz catheter in modern ICU settings, PCWP is determined less often for diagnostic purposes, and frequently, the diagnosis is obtained by indirect tools, such as echocardiography. Other diagnostic criteria involve radiological interpretation, introducing significant interobserver variability. Nevertheless, the AECC definition has been used in several clinical trials, including by the entire ARDS Network group.

Third, and important for studying the pathophysiological mechanisms involved in the development of ARDS, although the AECC definition of ALI/ARDS is simple to apply and is the most commonly used definition in clinical practice, the definition has serious deficiencies in its ability to discriminate diffuse alveolar damage (DAD), which is widely considered to be a major characteristic histologic feature of ALI/ARDS. In that sense, a comparison of the AECC definition with autopsy findings of DAD in a series of 382 patients found the sensitivity (75%) and specificity (84%) to be only moderate.

Another ALI/ARDS classification scheme was proposed in 1988 by Murray *et al.* [4] called the Lung Injury Score (Table 2), which determines the presence of ARDS by two to four criteria, each based on a four point scale, including a "scoring" of hypoxemia, a "scoring" of respiratory system compliance, chest radiographic findings, and the positive end expiratory pressure (PEEP) score. ARDS is defined if any of the daily lung injury scores are higher than >2.5 in the absence of clinical evidence of cardiogenic pulmonary edema. The concordance between this method and AECC criteria have varied in different clinical trials [5, 6].

Note that the cumulative evidence may indicate a need to redefine the diagnostic criteria of ALI/ARDS, especially considering the role that damage from hypoxia/hyperoxia may play in the pathogenesis of ALI/ARDS, which is one of the main objectives of this publication.

Numerous studies have demonstrated the direct injury or injury mediated by reactive oxygen species and the potential effects of these injuries on the development of MODS, which is especially important considering that oxygen therapy in ALI/ARDS would contribute to a greater imbalance in the redox state. Furthermore, redox state biomarkers must be identified in patients with ARDS, and should be included both in the diagnostic criteria and as potential prognostic markers.

Table 2. Murray's Lung Injury Score ARDS Criteria

Lung Injury Score Criteria for ARDS	
	Value
Chest x ray score	
No alveolar consolidation	0
Alveolar consolidation in one quadrant	1
Alveolar consolidation in two quadrants	2
Alveolar consolidation in three quadrants	3
Alveolar consolidation in four quadrants	4
Hypoxaemia score	
$PaO_2/FiO_2 > 300$	0
PaO_2/FiO_2 225–299	1
PaO_2/FiO_2 175–224	2
PaO_2/FiO_2 100–174	3
$PaO_2/FiO_2 < 100$	4
Positive end expiratory pressure score (when ventilated) (cm H_2O)	
< 5	0
6–8	1
9–11	2
12–14	3
> 15	4
Respiratory system compliance score (when ventilated) (ml/cm H_2O)	
> 80	0
60–79	1
40–59	2
20–39	3
< 19	4
Final score*	
No lung injury 0	0
Acute lung injury 0.1–2.5	0.1–2.5
Severe injury (ARDS) > 2.5	> 2.5

Etiology

ALI/ARDS has several causes. Classically, the disease has been classified into pulmonary and extrapulmonary sources. ARDS of primary pulmonary origin (also called direct lung injury) includes diseases of the upper airways, lower airways, pulmonary parenchyma or pulmonary circulation. Extrapulmonary causes (indirect lung injury) involve pathologies such as trauma, burns, transfusions, and pancreatitis. The literature does not make a major distinction between ARDS with a pulmonary or extrapulmonary origin (with pulmonary origin representing approximately 60-75% of cases) (6-8). The most common cause of pulmonary ARDS is pneumonia, and extrapulmonary ARDS most commonly results from sepsis and trauma with severe SIRS. These clinical situations may overlap in a given patient. Evidence showing increased mortality between those groups is controversial [6, 8-10], and clarification of some of differences in responses between groups is needed in terms of respiratory mechanics, radiographic and tomographic patterns, and specific treatment measures. Moreover, other variables of systemic failure in the extrapulmonary ARDS could be independent factors associated with mortality.

In children, ARDS occurs mainly as a result of pneumonia, pulmonary aspiration, sepsis, and near-drowning [11]. In particular, sepsis and pneumonia account for more than 50% of cases.

Epidemiology

Incidence

Because of the inadequacies of the disease definition, there is a broad range in the reported incidence of ALI/ARDS. In addition, there may be significant regional variations in incidence and outcomes due to a number of factors, including epidemiology, etiology, access to health care, management, differences in the overall structure of health care, the structure and implementation of intensive care and inaccuracies in the administrative coding of patients with the disease.

In 1999, Luhr *et al.* conducted a prospective survey among adult ICU patients in Sweden, Denmark and Iceland, estimating the prevalence of ALI and ARDS as 17.9 and 13.5 cases/ 100.000 person-years respectively, [8] according to the A-ECC Criteria. Interestingly, the authors obtained an incidence of 7.6 cases/100.000 person-years using the LIS score for ARDS. Other studies such as Bernsten and Arroliga in 2002 showed incidence rates of about 15-30 cases/100.000 person-years [6, 7].

Of particular interest is the data collected by Goss in 2003 [12]. This study used data from clinical trials conducted by the ARDS network [13] and the national American Hospital Association survey of hospitals, and then performed a series of sensitive analyses, obtaining an incidence of ALI of 64 cases/100.000 person-years.

The reported incidence in children is less than that in adults, with rates between 2.2 and 12 per 100.000 in the pediatric population [14, 15]. A population-based study performed in Cologne, Germany by Bindl *et al.* in 2005 showed an incidence of 3.2 cases/100.000 person-year, according to the A-ECC criteria [16].

Mortality

In the adult population, the overall mortality of ALI/ARDS is significant, with rates of about 35-50%. The largest population-based study, performed by Rubenfeld *et al.* in 2005, reported a mortality rate of 38.5% [17].

The literature contains conflicting data about the trend of mortality in ALI/ARDS; however, there seems to be a decreasing trend attributed to improved outcomes resulting from the adoption of low tidal volume ventilation [18], rational use of volume [19] and other strategies such as antioxidant treatment [20].

Mortality in the pediatric population is less than that reported in adults but still significant, with rates ranging from 22 to 35%, and is more frequently associated with multi-organ failure [11, 14-15]. In fact, patients who progress from ALI to ARDS double their death rate.

Despite the high rate of pneumonia as a cause of ARDS, this etiology does not account for the higher mortality in this group of patients. The most important factor is the role played by near-drowning, concomitant heart disease and sepsis [11, 21].

Predictors of Risk

In adults, the most important risk factors associated with mortality in ARDS include age, APACHE II score, the presence of sepsis and immunosuppression [17, 22, 23].

In children, in contrast with the adult population, the initial severity of hypoxemia as expressed by the $PaFiO_2$ ratio is an important prognostic factor, as well as the presence of nonpulmonary and non–central nervous system (CNS) organ dysfunction and CNS dysfunction [11, 24]. Interestingly, Flori et al. found that age was not a risk factor for mortality. The factors mentioned above are also associated with a longer duration of mechanical ventilation [11].

In a study performed in Australia and New Zealand in 2007, Erickson showed that factors such as the IO ratio, $PaFiO_2$ ratio, and non-pulmonary sepsis were causes of ARDS and that immunosuppression is associated with an increased risk of mortality. In addition, the study showed that children who survived were younger than those who did not [15].

4. Pathophysiology

Classically, the development of ALI/ARDS has been described to occur in two phases. The initial acute, exudative phase that typically occurs in the first week of the disease manifests as a rapid onset respiratory failure mediated by diffuse alveolar damage as well as the activation of cytokines, proinflammatory cells and protein-rich edema fluid in the alveolar spaces. We focus on this phase now, describing the redox imbalance that occurs during its development. This phase can be resolved completely in some patients, but in other patients, it progresses to the fibroproliferative phase, characterized by persistent hypoxemia, increased alveolar dead space and decreased pulmonary compliance. In addition, this stage refers to the initiation of the healing process, which occurs together with the organization of the abnormal exudate within the alveolus and interstitium.

Finally, a recovery or fibrosis phase, which is characterized by the gradual resolution of hypoxemia, improved lung compliance, resolution of radiographic abnormalities and a variable degree of resolution of pulmonary fibrosis, occurs.

Although the objective of this chapter is to explain the pathophysiological mechanisms that are associated with redox imbalance and the consequent oxidative stress produced during the development of ARDS, it is necessary to provide a brief general overview of all the mechanisms involved in the development of ALI /ARDS.

In detail, ALI/ARDS is characterized by an initial insult that triggers cell-mediated mechanisms releasing a cascade of a variety of mediators, which are illustrated in Figure 1 and discussed in detail below.

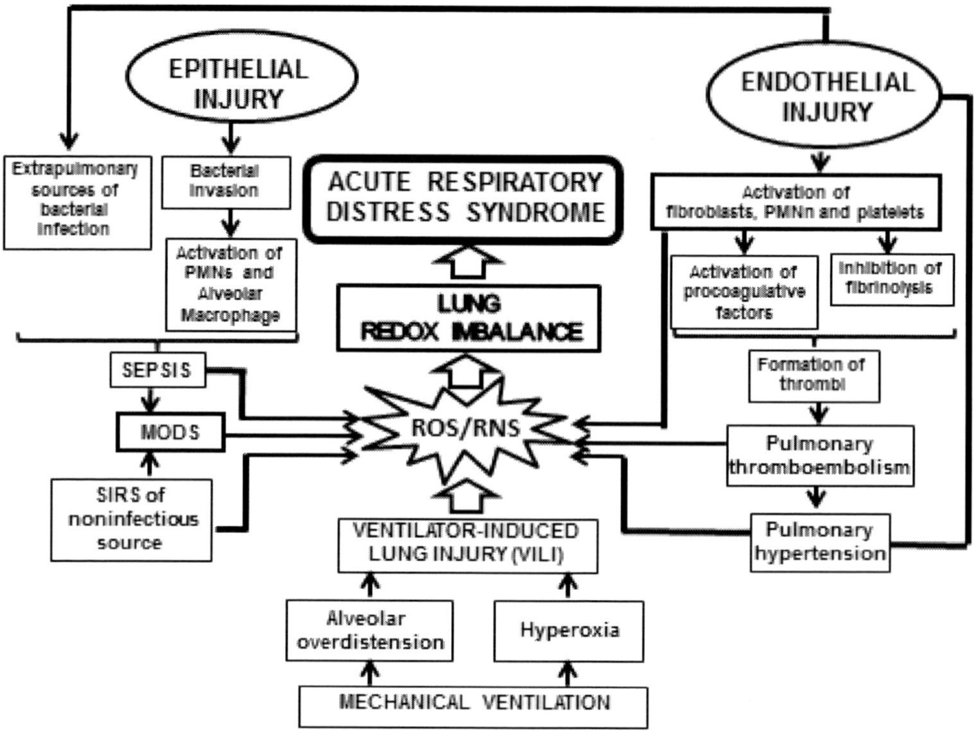

Figure 1. Pathophysiology of Acute Respiratory Distress Syndrome. The imbalance of the redox state has a fundamental role in the generation, development, perpetuation and progression of ARDS. The sources of reactive species (ROS or RNS) are multiple and can be grouped in agents causing endothelial or epithelial injury. 1) Agents that locally generate an epithelial injury, and usually are caused by pulmonary infectious agents, locally activating PMNs and alveolar macrophages, producing a local septic process that generates ROS/RNS. 2) Extrapulmonary infectious agents that cause endothelial injury, which also activate PMNs, fibroblasts, and platelets, generating ROS/RNS, leading to activation of procoagulant factors and inhibition of fibrinolysis. This causes the subsequent formation of thrombi causing pulmonary embolism which causes the generation of more reactive species in direct form and indirectly through induced pulmonary hypertension. In addition, reactive species generation and endothelial injury can be produced by other processes of non-infectious SIRS, which as well as those of infectious origin can evolve into a MODS. 3) Mechanical ventilation also contributes by alveolar overdistension and hyperoxia, the development of VILI, damage that is mediated also by the generation of reactive oxygen species. ROS, reactive oxygen species; RNS, reactive nitrogen species; MODS, Multiple Organ Dysfunction Score ; PMNs, poly-morphonuclear cells; VILI, ventilator-induced lung injury.

a) Endothelial damage. In the acute or exudative phase of ALI/ARDS, protein-rich edema fluid enters the air space as a result of the increased permeability of the alveolar-capillary barrier. This increased permeability leads to the formation of pulmonary edema. In addition, serum proteins precipitate with cellular debris in the alveolar spaces, forming the characteristic hyaline membranes.
b) Epithelial cell damage. The loss of epithelial integrity induces alveolar flooding and impedes the removal of fluids from the alveolar space. Injury of cuboidal type II cells alters ion transport, fluid removal capacity and surfactant production, and triggers the release of various mediators, including proinflammatory cytokines, leading to the activation of neutrophils and

stimulating chemotaxis. In addition, damage at this level can induce and facilitate bacterial invasion leading to sepsis and septic shock.

c) Activation of cytokines, neutrophils and macrophages. Triggering of cytokines initiates and amplifies the inflammatory response. The inflammatory process may originate from a direct insult, such as pneumonia, aspiration, or inhalation of substances, or secondarily as part of a systemic inflammatory response, such as in sepsis or trauma.

The role of cytokines in ALI/ARDS is known. The cytokine response, known as a "cytokine storm," is triggered and amplified by myeloid and lymphoid cells, as well as by others, such as epithelial cells.

The roles of proinflammatory cytokines such as tumor necrosis factor and interleukins 6 and 8 have been extensively studied, and these cytokines have been associated with the development of ALI/ARDS in several models, with complex relationships of induction and regulation elucidated with other substances, such as endotoxins and the nuclear factor kappa B. In addition, cytokine production has been shown to vary according to the origin of ARDS (e.g., in trauma versus sepsis).

The presence and activation of neutrophils in ALI/ARDS is well established, given the presence of neutrophils and their products, such as lysosomal enzymes in bronchoalveolar lavage from patients with ARDS, although lung injury can develop in the absence of neutrophils, such as in neutropenic patients.

d) Activation of platelets and interaction with the hemostatic system. In ALI/ARDS, a close relationship exists between inflammatory mediators and the coagulation cascade, with the activation of pro-coagulates factors and the inhibition of fibrinolysis leading to the production of platelet-fibrin thrombi in small pulmonary vessels. Platelet activation and consumption have been observed in ARDS, as well as the local activation of the coagulation system, altered clearance of thrombin and thrombomodulin and increased tissue plasminogen inhibitor-1. These activities leads to the formation of microthrombi and pulmonary thromboembolism that, together with the pulmonary vasoconstriction seen in patients with ARDS, may lead to pulmonary hypertension, which can become irreversible as it leads to pulmonary arterial muscularization and fibrous obliteration of the microcirculation.
e) Role of surfactant. Surfactant is a lipoprotein complex composed of phospholipids and apoproteins that plays an important role in normal lung function, decreasing alveolar surface tension and reducing alveolar collapse, especially during the low lung volumes of exhalation. Surfactant is produced by type II pneumocytes in response to alveolar stretch. In ARDS, the production and composition of surfactant is altered by the direct damage to type II pneumocytes in conjunction with the effect of ROS and proteins released by neutrophils in the alveolar space.
f) Effects on lung mechanics and gas exchange. In terms of alveolar exchange, the hallmark of ARDS is severe hypoxemia refractory to oxygen administration. This severe hypoxemia is due to the left-to-right intrapulmonary shunt, which can reach 25-50% of cardiac output. This can be explained by atelectatic and

fluid-filled alveoli that impede the alveolar exchange and are refractory to treatment with oxygen.

From the works of Gattinoni, we now know that ARDS does not result from a uniform increase in the elastic recoil of lung tissue but instead that it is caused by a reduction in the volume of the aerated lung. The remaining portion of the lung is nonaerated and does not participate in ventilation. The compliance of the aerated lung can be normal but a smaller volume (defined as a “baby lung”). Another important phenomenon is the distribution of water in the lungs, which accumulates in the gravity-dependent areas (defined as "sponge lung").

The differences in the distribution of lung injury in ARDS between pulmonary and extrapulmonary origin have been described, but whether this distribution plays some role in lung mechanics has not been established [10].

g) Healing phase. After the exudative phase of lung injury, the proliferative phase begins, characterized by the hyperplasia of type II pneumocytes, the migration of fibroblasts and collagen deposition in the lung tissue. The speed of this process can be highly variable, which could play a role in predicting short and long term outcomes.

The magnitude and severity of pulmonary fibrosis depends on the collagen deposition, the apoptosis and the persistence of proinflammatory cytokines and growth factors, and these factors can also interact with each other.

h) Oxidants and Lung Injury. These mechanisms are the focus of the present chapter. Since the original description of ARDS more than 30 years ago, investigators have endeavored to elucidate the mechanisms that regulate the pathways leading to lung injury, with the ultimate goal of developing therapeutic tools to ameliorate or prevent lung and multi-organ injury in at-risk patients. One of the aspects of ALI/ARDS that has not been well studied is the pathophysiological mechanisms related to a redox imbalance. Oxidative injury to the lung is mediated by ROS, partly reduced derivatives of molecular oxygen. Biologically important ROS include superoxide anion radical (O_2^-), hydrogen peroxide (H_2O_2), hydroxyl radical (OH^-), and hypohalous acids such as HOCl. Reactive nitrogen species, derivatives of nitric oxide (NO) including peroxynitrate ($ONOO^-$), have also been implicated in the oxidation (nitration) of proteins and lipids. Reactive oxygen (ROS) and nitrogen species (RNS) can lead to cell injury by various mechanisms, including (i) direct damage to DNA resulting in strand breaks and point mutations; (ii) lipid peroxidation with the formation of vasoactive and pro-inflammatory molecules, such as thromboxane; (iii) oxidation of proteins (primarily at sulfhydryl groups) that alter protein activity, leading to the release of proteases and the inactivation of antioxidant and antiprotease enzymes; and (iv) alteration of transcription factors such as activator protein-1 and nuclear factor kappa-β (NF)-κB, leading to enhanced expression of proinflammatory genes.

To neutralize free radicals and counteract the detrimental effects of ROS generated during normal metabolism, cells express a number of endogenous antioxidants such as superoxide dismutase, catalase, and glutathione peroxidase. However, these antioxidants are rapidly overwhelmed during an acute inflammatory response.

The following chapters will provide a more detailed discussion of the relationship between the pathophysiology of ARDS and oxidative stress.

5. Role of Oxidants and Redox Imbalance in the Pathogenesis of ARDS

General characteristics of the redox balance and effects of its disruption

ALI/ARDS is characterized by an initial insult that triggers cell-mediated mechanisms releasing a cascade of a variety of mediators, resulting in a redox imbalance among other outcomes. This imbalance is manifested as oxidative stress, and it plays an important role in the development, modulation and perpetuation of the local and systemic inflammatory responses.

Although some events during the development of inflammation are common to several organs, the pulmonary parenchyma exhibits special performance with unique features that require a different sort of analysis for the pathophysiology of ARDS/ALI.

The alveolar compartment is permanently exposed to reactive oxygen (ROS) and nitrogen species (RNS) derived from inhaled air pollutants. The antioxidant defense system of the epithelial lining fluid consists of several low molecular weight compounds, such as reduced glutathione (GSH), ascorbic acid (vitamin C) and uric acid; lipophilic antioxidants, such as α-tocopherol (vitamin E), retinol (vitamin A) and plasmalogens (1-alkenyl-phospholipids); and antioxidant enzymes, such as superoxide dismutase, catalase and glutathione peroxidase. Under normal conditions in the lung, complex and coordinated interactions occur among all these antioxidant compounds to provide protection of the distal lung structures from the damaging effects of oxidative attack [25].

As we noted, regardless of the underlying illness, the clinical and pathologic manifestations of ALI/ARDS have similar features, indicating the existence of common final pathways. Therefore, a severe injury caused by an initiating event can lead to dysfunction and a compromise of the barrier properties of the pulmonary endothelium and epithelium as a consequence of an unregulated acute inflammatory response. The earliest events are characterized by the activation of the pulmonary endothelium and macrophages (alveolar and interstitial), up-regulation of adhesion molecules, and production of cytokines and chemokines that induce a massive sequestration of neutrophils within the pulmonary microvasculature [26].

These cells transmigrate across the endothelium and epithelium into the alveolar space and release a variety of cytotoxic and pro-inflammatory compounds, including proteolytic enzymes, cationic proteins, lipid mediators, additional inflammatory cytokines and the compounds of interest here: reactive oxygen species (ROS) and nitrogen species (RNS).

This increase in the generation of reactive species (ROS and RNS) perpetuates a vicious cycle by recruiting additional inflammatory cells that in turn produce more cytotoxic mediators, ultimately leading to an increase in the severity of the injury to the alveolar-capillary membrane and resulting in an increase in respiratory failure. Furthermore, although the changes in the inflammatory cascade and oxidative injury mainly affect the lungs at first, generating respiratory system dysfunction, ALI/ARDS are part of a systemic process involving micro-vascular dysfunction in diverse organs, finally resulting in multi-organ dysfunction [26].

Characteristics of Injury Resulting from Oxidative Stress and Inflammation at the Pulmonary Level

In the lungs, one of the earliest events in ALI/ARDS, are the alterations in vascular permeability. Recent animal studies have revealed that endothelial injury appears within minutes to hours after ALI induction and results in the formation of intercellular gaps in the endothelium, which can be regarded as the basis for increased micro-vascular permeability [27]. In addition, the contribution of epithelial injury to the progression of ALI/ARDS has become increasingly obvious. Decreases in the function of the epithelial cell barrier facilitate the influx of protein-rich fluid and other macromolecules into the alveolar space. Furthermore, epithelial injury leads to impaired cell fluid transport and reduced production of surfactant [28].

Lung edema is added to endothelial and epithelial injury, which is then accompanied by an influx of neutrophils into the interstitium and broncheo-alveolar space. Innate immunity in general and neutrophils in particular are considered to play key roles in the progression of ALI and ARDS [29], because the activation and transmigration of neutrophils is a hallmark event in the progression of ALI and ARDS. Proof of the importance of neutrophils in ALI comes from both clinical evidence and animal models. For example, in patients with ARDS, the concentration of neutrophils in the broncho-alveolar lavage (BAL) fluid correlates with the severity and outcome of ARDS [30, 31], while the severity of lung injury can be reduced by neutrophil depletion in mice [32]. Furthermore, after blocking interleukin-8 (IL-8), a major chemoattractant for neutrophils, rabbits have been protected from acid aspiration-induced lung injury [33]. Although neutrophils can migrate into the alveolar space without damaging the alveolar-capillary barrier [34], recruitment of neutrophils into the lung is an important step in ALI. In addition, ALI/ARDS can occur in children and adults with neutropenia [35, 36], indicating that under specific conditions, neutrophil-independent mechanisms alone allow for the development of ALI. Nevertheless, a multitude of experimental and clinical data point at the causative role of neutrophils in lung injury. Although neutrophil activation is vital for the host defense, overzealous activation leads to tissue damage through the release of cytotoxic and immune cell–activating agents, such as proteinases, cationic polypeptides, cytokines, and reactive oxygen species (ROS). This review aims to highlight the mechanisms by which neutrophils are recruited into the lung, and by which neutrophils contribute to the onset and progression of ALI by means of infiltrating the lung tissue and releasing preformed granule proteins or vast amounts of ROS. The majority of this review is based on experimental data derived from various animal models of ALI. When examining the role of individual proteins in a complex pathophysiological process such as ALI, it is important to keep in mind that there is likely a publication bias against studies with negative outcomes.

Evaluation of Inflammation and Redox State by Broncho-Alveolar Lavage

Inflammation of the lung may be result from the activation of macrophages and neutrophils, and simultaneously, they could lead to increased inflammation, releasing free radicals due to a respiratory burst. In addition, commonly used high inspiratory concentrations of oxygen may contribute to the generation of more free radicals [37]. Accordingly, a large number of authors have provided evidence that oxidative degradation products are elevated in acute respiratory distress syndrome (ARDS) patients, both in bronchoalveolar lavage fluid (BALF) and in exhaled breath condensate [38]. This imbalance between newly generated oxidative compounds and the local antioxidant systems may also contribute to lung injury, resulting in increased capillary leakage [39], altered surfactant metabolism [40] and diminished surfactant function [41]. This may further enhance alveolar edema and collapse, frequently encountered in ARDS and acute lung injury (ALI).

Since ARDS/ALI are associated with elevated levels of reactive oxidants in BALF, and considering findings that blood antioxidant concentrations are reduced [42], it has long been hypothesized that alveolar antioxidants may be decreased in the BALF of these patients [43]. Data regarding the low molecular weight antioxidant compounds are conflicting and scarce. For example, GSH has been suggested to be reduced in the BALF of ARDS patients [44]. The analysis of single compounds may be complicated by the low overall levels of these substances in BALF due to the 100- to 200-fold dilution of epithelial lining fluid (ELF) during the lavage procedure. Thus, highly sensitive and selective analytical procedures seem to be prerequisites for such analyses.

Influence of the Etiology and the Patient's Immune Response in the Development of ALI/ARDS

To understand the role of oxidative stress in the development of ALI/ARDS, we must first understand that this stress has multiple sources and that the amount of reactive species generated depends on the cause of ALI/ARDS and other factors that depend on the patient's immune response.

With respect to the etiology, whereas pneumonia or sepsis can undoubtedly cause ALI and ARDS, several noninfectious causes also may trigger ALI/ARDS, such as acid aspiration, hyperoxia, high pressure ventilation, pulmonary contusion, reperfusion or bleomycin [45].

The causative factors of ALI can be grouped broadly into direct and indirect factors. Direct factors include bacterial and viral infections in the lungs and aspiration of gastric contents, all of which cause direct injury to the airway and alveolar epithelium and other structures in the airspaces. Indirect factors include systemic infections that cause sepsis syndrome, blood transfusions, and the effects of systemic medications and illicit drugs. This dual paradigm is plausible, even though clinical studies do not show major differences in outcomes between patients with direct versus indirect ALI [46].

While these agents induce lung damage by direct exposure to the lung, similar lung damage can arise indirectly. In particular, trauma, pancreatitis or transfusion can initiate an inflammatory response called systemic inflammatory response syndrome (SIRS) that may lead to ALI or ARDS.

Note that while some mechanisms are common to all causes, the severity and development of ALI/ARDS will depend on the etiology and clinical characteristics of the patient, especially on the characteristics of their immune response.

The major theme emerging from clinical studies is that humans are inherently variable in their responses to the stimuli that cause ALI. Although investigators planning clinical trials strive to enroll uniform patient populations, clinicians recognize that patients with seemingly similar stimuli, for example, pneumococcal bacteremia, vary considerably in the clinical severity of their disease. Studies of how normal people respond to the common bacterial stimulus gram-negative lipopolysaccharide (LPS) show differences of more than 2 orders of magnitude in cytokine responses in the whole blood. Studies of normal humans who were high or low responders to bacterial products identified a polymorphism in the Toll-like receptor (TLR)1 that marked high cytokine responses to gram-positive bacterial peptidoglycan. This polymorphism was more common in critically ill patients with gram-positive sepsis who died. Thus, studying the variability in innate immune responses in the normal population can provide important insights about disease susceptibility in critically ill patients [47, 48].

Animal Models

Modeling the acute and chronic pathologic changes of ALI to understand cellular and molecular pathogenesis has been a significant challenge from the time that ARDS was first described in humans [49]. Many different animal models have been used, and each model has advantages and disadvantages.

Animal models have been useful in studying individual pathways involved in pathogenesis and new ideas for treatment. No single animal model mimics all of the clinical features of ALI in humans, and each animal model has unique features that affect responses to treatment. Nevertheless, many themes have emerged from animal models that provide valuable insight about lung injury in humans. Studies of innate immunity have shown that innate immunity is triggered not only by microbial products but also by endogenous products of tissue damage and inflammation that can drive inflammation even in the absence of microbial products in tissue.

Variability in host innate immune responses accounts for a great deal of variability in the clinical manifestations of ALI. Innate immunity and mechanical stretch have important synergistic interactions in adults that accentuate ALI, and these synergistic interactions seem to be acquired with age and are much less pronounced in juvenile animals. Therefore, these interactions are important factors to take into account to enable an adequate interpretation of the results obtained from these models.

Apoptosis pathways are important in the clearance of bacteria from the lungs and in causing injury and death to alveolar epithelial cells, enhancing permeability edema. Stem cell biology has been extended to ALI, finding unexpected paracrine effects of MSC in reducing the severity of ALI. New ideas about the resolution of ALI have been derived from studies of the clearance of apoptotic cells in the lungs and the role of regulatory lymphocytes in recovery from lung inflammation and injury [50].

Progress is being made, but strong links between the laboratory and the critical care bedside are still needed to translate new ideas from laboratory studies into clinical treatments that will lessen the severity and improve outcomes for ALI patients [50].

Oxidants can be generated by lung macrophages and recruited PMNs. Although certain chemicals are metabolized into highly toxic products in the lung, we will restrict our comments to oxidants generated by phagocytic cells in the lung or by enzyme/substrate combinations delivered to the lung. Toxic oxygen products can be generated when macrophages or PMNs undergo stimulation by factors such as bacterial LPS or IgG immune complexes (IgGIC). Toxic oxygen products (superoxide, O2 •; hydrogen peroxide, H_2O_2 or its peroxidative products) can be intercepted by naturally occurring or induced antioxidants, such as superoxide dismutase (SOD) or catalase. Those antioxidant enzymes are present naturally in the lung, but the intrapulmonary levels of these enzymes can be greatly elevated when the lung faces a large burden of oxidants (such as hyperoxia) that compromise the redox balance of the lung. Phorbol myristate acetate (PMA) can powerfully activate lung macrophages, overwhelming the antioxidant reserves of the lung and resulting in catastrophic parenchymal damage, as described below. In the case of LPS- or IgGIC-induced injury, lung damage is limited and reversible, and the lung architecture is restored to normal in a matter of a few days [51].

In the case of PMA, the damage is so intense as to overwhelm the repair and regenerative abilities of the lung, leading to pulmonary fibrosis. Under such conditions, extensive damage/destruction of alveolar epithelial cells and vascular endothelial cells occurs, resulting in intense alveolar edema ("alveolar flooding") and intraalveolar hemorrhage. The reversibility or irreversibility of ALI seems to result from the extent of damage/destruction of vascular endothelial and alveolar epithelial cells. In the latter case, stem cells resident in the lung or borne by the blood may enhance the regenerative capacity of the lung. If this capacity is overwhelmed, alveolar collapse and the development of dense cross-linked collagen will occur, which will ablate local gas exchange between the alveolar compartment and the capillaries.

Neutrophils produce vast quantities of reactive oxygen (ROS) and nitrogen (RNS) species, such as O2 •– and NO•, through their oxidant-generating systems, such as the phagocyte NADPH oxidase and nitric oxide synthase (NOS), respectively.

The controlled enzymatic generation of ROS, which includes superoxide anion, hydrogen peroxide, hydroxyl radical and others by neutrophils, is an integral component of the innate immune system. During the ingestion of invading pathogens into phagosomes, ROS generated at the phagosome membrane are released directly into the phagosome. In addition to the well-known antimicrobial function of ROS during phagocytosis, low-level formation of ROS acts as an intracellular signal, also called "redox signaling". ROS are released into the cytosol where they alter the redox state of the cell and modify other cell contents, such as proteins and lipids by oxidation. The membrane-bound multicomponent NADPH oxidase enzyme complex, which is dormant in resting cells and can be activated rapidly by chemoattractant peptides or chemokines, generates a significant amount of ROS after activation. The oxidase of the catalytic subunit gp91phox (otherwise known as NOX2), which is found predominately in phagocytes, belongs to the family of NOX and dual oxidases (DUOX). In vivo, NOX-1–/– mice but not NOX-2–/– mice are protected from the hyperoxia induced by ALI. Therefore, these results reveal that NADPH oxidase 1 plays a crucial role in the hyperoxia induced by ALI. A previous study with NADPH oxidase–/– mice revealed no protection from CVF-induced ALI, indicating that oxygen radical production and lung injury may occur through alternative pathways in mice with genetic deletion of NADPH oxidase. Furthermore, the inhibition of NADPH or nitric oxide synthase (NOS) has decreased sepsis-induced ALI or LPS-induced ALI, respectively. ROS may prolong inflammation by modulating neutrophil function. Consequently, neutrophil-derived oxidants are considered to have a major role in neutrophil-mediated tissue injury, including in ALI/ARDS [52].

In summary, the activation and migration of neutrophils into the lung is one of the key events in ALI, with their secreted products exerting both direct and indirect effects. Until now, no pharmacological therapy has emerged for the treatment of all patients with ALI/ARDS, because the patients and the causes underlying the disease are highly heterogeneous. Whereas the inhibition of adhesion molecules has reduced the incidence of ALI in several animal models, reproducing similar findings in clinical trials has proven difficult because of the redundancy of the molecules involved. Hence, the inflammatory response induced by neutrophils can be controlled by the inhibition of degranulation to avoid host tissue damage. Furthermore, antioxidants may reduce ROS-related tissue damage in acute lung injury. Although neutrophil recruitment into the lung is necessary for the host defense in the case of bacterial infection, regulation of neutrophil activity might be one possible therapeutic approach [52].

6. Ventilator-Induced Lung Injury (VILI)

Oxidative Stress and VILI

Mechanical ventilation (MV) by itself has been established to damage the lungs, a concept known as ventilator-induced lung injury (VILI) [53,54]. This susceptibility depends on the heterogeneous distribution of lung damage, which promotes anisotropic inflation of the phase alveolar opening and the collapse of the expiratory end, promotes lung damage, triggers a systemic inflammatory response, and may result in the development of multiple organ dysfunction syndrome (MODS).

For this reason, a great deal of ARDS research has been directed toward identifying a ventilation strategy that respects the capacity of the diseased lung aeration, exploring the potential for recruitment (RPP) and the adjustment of positive end-expiratory pressure (PEEP) but preventing the development of VILI and MODS. Clinical studies have shown that mortality associated with ALI/ARDS may be reduced by ventilation strategies that prevent excessive stretching of the lung tissue. Ventilatory strategies and open lung approaches for this purpose have been widely disseminated by the ARDS Network (ARDSNet) [55].

Although several potential causes of VILI exist, VILI has been primarily linked to two phenomena: The first phenomenon occurs at the end of inspiration and is associated with the use of a high inspiratory oppression of tidal volume (VT) that promotes alveolar over-distension, a process related to the risk of rupture of the airway and alveolar walls in the non-dependent (R-ND) area of the lung. The second phenomenon unfolds in a regions dependent (RD), which are exposed to significant stress when the airway and alveoli open on inspiration and collapse on expiration (tidal recruitment). This phenomenon is mainly associated with the use of insufficient PEEP to prevent alveolar collapse and cyclical reopening.

The two phenomena may overlap, since unnecessarily high PEEP may lead to overdistension, and the reduction of VT could limit cyclic alveolar collapse and reopening. In this sense, the benefits observed in the low VT ARDSNet study might not result from the control of distension alone.

There is a lack of consensus about the precise contribution, kinetics and primary role of each of these mechanisms. The hypothesis that lung collapse is detrimental during ALI/ARDS is still controversial. However, experimental studies show that the collapse of the airspace and the cyclical recruitment are crucial in the development of VILI. Moreover, about 10-20% of patients receiving MV without an initial diagnosis of ALI/ARDS are exposed to VILI [55].

In this context, allowing the airway and alveoli to remain collapsed or filled with liquid, hindering extensive ventilation of lung regions ("permissive" atelectasis), has not proven superior to the application of lung recruitment maneuvers (MRP). Furthermore, permissive areas of atelectasis are unable to clear secretions, whose confinement is known to cause inflammation.

Pathophysiology of VILI

One of the features of ALI/ARDS is the loss of airway epithelial and endothelial integrity, resulting in pulmonary edema. Mechanical ventilation (MV) with high tidal volumes causes excessive alveolar distention, resulting in lung epithelial injury and increased vascular permeability, with the subsequent exit of content-rich proteins into the alveolar space [56].

On the other hand, the MV causes a systemic inflammatory response because of the cyclic recruitment of unstable overdistended alveolar regions [57], which ultimately can lead to severe MODS. Cytokines and chemokines are potential effector molecules that modulate and regulate VILI initial mechanisms. The accumulation of neutrophils in the lung tissue can also lead to increased levels of inflammatory cytokines, which play a fundamental role in the development of VILI [58]. KC (human homologue of CXCL1) and the chemokine MIP-2 are two potent neutrophil chemotactic factors that play significant roles in the lung inflammatory responses induced by MV [59]. Elevated IL-6 levels have been detected in various experimental models of VILI [60] and in the serum and bronchoalveolar lavage fluid of patients with ARDS under MV [57]. Recently, the determination of expression profiles using libelous and protective forms of MV in the presence and absence of inflammatory stimuli revealed the involvement of a complex network of genes that encode proteins involved in extracellular matrix remodeling, pro-inflammatory cytokines and transcription factors in VILI [61]. The exact molecular mechanisms that control the expression levels of these genes in response to MV and its contribution to the development or susceptibility to the development of VILI are unclear and remain the focus of ongoing research.

In vitro studies have used cyclic strain to mimic the physical forces of the MV. These studies demonstrate that the deformation of the endothelial and epithelial cells and the physical alteration of the membrane integrity lead to an alteration in the structure and function of these essential components of the alveolar-capillary membrane, resulting in the activation of pro-inflammatory and pro-oxidant pathways [62]. Plasma concentrations of lipid peroxidation products are higher in patients with ALI/ARDS, and the plasma levels of endogenous antioxidants are concomitantly decreased [63]. The concentrations of oxidized glutathione (GSSG) resulting from the consumption of reduced glutathione (GSH) by free radicals are higher in the alveolar fluid of patients with ARDS [64]. Together, these studies suggest that some redox imbalance exists in the lungs for the production of reactive oxygen species (ROS) in the pathophysiology of ALI/ARDS. Free radicals are known to activate non-phagocytic and phagocytic cells in the lung, which in turn generate high levels of reactive oxygen species (ROS) and nitrogen (ERN) and other toxic metabolites.

The Relationship between VILI and the Occurrence of Oxidative Stress

The mechanisms by which conventional MV exacerbates lung injury and local inflammation are of considerable clinical importance. In this context, the redox imbalance has been postulated as one of several mechanisms that could promote and perpetuate susceptibility to VILI. A better understanding of these mechanisms would not only help to mitigate the side effects of mechanical injury but also aid in the development of new therapeutic strategies.

The contribution of ROS generated by lung fibroblasts, epithelial cells and endothelial cells (which are directly affected by the elastic strain associated with mechanical ventilation) to the development or perpetuation of VILI is of increasing interest. Experimental evidence obtained from cell culture studies indicates that cyclic strain increased ROS production in approximately 30 minutes after the exposure of lung epithelial and endothelial cells [65], suggesting that these ROS could contribute to the development of lung injury induced by the MV. Moreover, ROS generation, measured by fluorophores that detect ROS generation such as DCFDA, was significantly higher in cells exposed to pathologically relevant cyclic stretch (15-18%) than in those exposed to a physiological rate (5%) and was correlated with the duration of exposure. On the other hand, larger cyclic stretching is known to reduce the levels of reduced glutathione (GSH), the main intracellular antioxidant [66], and increase the generation of oxidized glutathione (GSSG) [67]. These observations suggest that the in vitro pro-oxidant imbalance caused by cyclic stress can be an important factor in perpetuating or contributing to the development of VILI.

Molecular Mechanisms Associated with the Occurrence of VILI and the Generation of Oxidative Stress

Several studies on cyclic strain associated with conventional methods with a high tidal volume MV have provided an idea of ROS generation by pulmonary epithelial and endothelial cells, fibroblasts, and vascular smooth muscle cells [68]. Exposure to cyclic strain increases the activity of NADPH oxidase, an enzyme that produces ROS, whereas pharmacological inhibition of this enzyme reduces the amount of ROS generated. The system consists of NADPH oxidases belonging to various members of the NOX family, which are transmembrane and cytosolic proteins. Both the transfer and assembly of these oxidases in the plasma membrane are essential for electron transport through the membrane into the extracellular space. Deficiencies in the ROS production of NADPH oxidase subunits alter and generally confer protection against oxidant and toxin-induced lung injury [69]. Moreover, cyclic strain induces the recruitment of the p47phox subunit to the complex in the membrane NADPH [70]. These studies demonstrate that cyclic strain does not stimulate the production of ROS in pulmonary artery endothelial cells and vascular smooth muscle cells lacking the p47phox gene. Activation of adhesion molecules and cytokine expression are also decreased in p47phox-deficient cells. Therefore, the p47phox subunit appears to play a key role in the generation of ROS and the activation of NADPH oxidase in lung epithelial cells in response to cyclic strain. The expression, regulation and the role of various isoforms of NOX, such as DUOX1 and DUOX2, in epithelial cells in response to outside stimuli and inflammatory cytokines have recently been documented [71], but the role of these factors in VILI remains unclear.

Furthermore, nitrosative stress produced by the nitration of proteins by RNA generated by nitric oxide products have recently been postulated in the pathogenesis of IPA on the basis of the formation of nitrotyrosine residues in lung tissue samples from these patients [72]. These RNA have also been found in the bronchoalveolar lavage fluid from patients with suspected sepsis or trauma (at risk or ARDS) and have been associated with increased mortality [73]. Experimentally, the use of inhibitors of nitric oxide synthase (NOS) have attenuated lung injury and inflammation induced by MV, supporting the role of NO and its metabolites in VILI [74, 75].

Biomarkers of Oxidative Stress in VILI

Because VILI is an important factor in the initiation and propagation of a systemic inflammatory response and because ROS and RNS are mediators of crucial importance, biomarkers of oxidative damage and antioxidant depletion might be expected to increase during the pathophysiological events that lead to VILI.

In vivo results confirm this expectation, with induced lung distension leading to not only increased local oxidative stress levels (LBA) but also a system characterized by a depletion of antioxidants, such as GSH, and increased non-enzymatic lipid peroxidation products, such as 8-isoprostane. In vitro, cells permeable to some forms of GSH and its precursor N-acetylcysteine (NAC) were used to increase intracellular GSH. A dose-dependent increase of intracellular GSH occurred with these cycles of relaxation. Increasing intracellular GSH inhibited stretch-induced oxidative stress, as measured by 8-isoprostane levels, and IL-8 production [76]. In vitro, the lung epithelium only caused a small increase in intracellular GSH, but this increase was not sufficient to inhibit the induced strain.

However, the intracellular GSH increased over the homeostatic range, allowing for the pharmacological manipulation of the production of some cytokines. At present, in vivo experiments have demonstrated that the NAC also increases the amount of total GSH and inhibits pulmonary inflammation induced by MV [77].

References

[1] de Hemptinne Q, Remmelink M, Brimioulle S, Salmon I, Vincent JL. ARDS: a clinicopathological confrontation. *Chest* 2009; 135:944-949

[2] Ashbaugh DG, Boyd Bigelow D, Petty TL, Levine LE. Acute Respiratory Distress in Adults. *The Lancet* 1967; 290:319-323

[3] Bernard G, Artigas A, Brigham K, Carlet J, Falke K, Hudson L, Lamy M, LeGall JR, Morris A, Spragg R. The American-European Consensus Conference on ARDS. Definitions, mechanisms, relevant outcomes, and clinical trial coordination. *Am J Respir Crit Care Med* 1994; 149:818-824

[4] Murray J, Matthay M, Luce J, Flick MR. An expanded definition of the adult respiratory distress syndrome. *Am Rev Respir Dis* 1988; 138:720-723

[5] Meade MO, Guyatt GH, Cook RJ, Groll R, Kachura JR, Wigg M, Cook DJ, Slutsky AS, Stewart TE. Agreement between Alternative Classifications of Acute Respiratory Distress Syndrome. *Am J Respir Crit Care Med* 2001; 163:490-493

[6] Bernsten AD, Edibam C, Hunt T, Moran J. Incidence and Mortality of Acute Lung Injury and the Acute Respiratory Distress Syndrome in Three Australian States. *Am J Respir Crit Care Med* 2002; 165:443-448

[7] Arroliga AC, Ghamra ZW, Perez Trepichio A, Perez Trepichio P, Komara JJ Jr, Smith A, Wiedemann HP. Incidence of ARDS in an Adult Population of Northeast Ohio. *Chest* 2002; 121:1972-1976

[8] Luhr OR, Antonsen K, Karlsson M, Aardal S, Thorsteinsson A, Frostell CG, Bonde J. Incidence and Mortality after Acute Respiratory Failure and Acute Respiratory Distress Syndrome in Sweden, Denmark, and Iceland. *Am J Respir Crit Care Med* 1999; 159:1849-1861

[9] Agarwal R, Srinivas R, Nath A, Jindal SK. Is the Mortality Higher in the Pulmonary vs the Extrapulmonary ARDS?. *Chest* 2008; 133:1463-1473

[10] Pelosi P, Caironi P, Gattinoni L. Pulmonary and Extrapulmonary Forms of Acute Respiratory Distress Syndrome. *Semin Respir Crit Care Med* 2001; 22:259,268

[11] Flori HR, Glidden DV, Rutherford GW, Matthay MA. Pediatric Acute Lung Injury: Prospective Evaluation of Risk Factors Associated with Mortality. *Am J Respir Crit Care Med* 2005; 171:995-1001

[12] Goss CH, Brower RG, Hudson LD, Rubenfeld GD; ARDS Network. Incidence of acute lung injury in the United States. *Crit Care Medicine* 2003; 31:1607-1611

[13] Ventilation with Lower Tidal Volumes as Compared with Traditional Tidal Volumes for Acute Lung Injury and the Acute Respiratory Distress Syndrome. The Acute Respiratory Distress Syndrome Network. *N Engl J Med* 2000; 342:1301-1308

[14] Dahlem P, van Aalderen WM, Hamaker ME, Dijkgraaf MG, Bos AP. Incidence and short-term outcome of acute lung injury in mechanically ventilated children. *Eur Respir J* 2003; 22:980-985

[15] Erickson S, Schibler A, Numa A, Nuthall G, Yung M, Pascoe E, Wilkins B; Paediatric Study Group; Australian and New Zealand Intensive Care Society. Acute lung injury in pediatric intensive care in Australia and New Zealand-A prospective, multicenter, observational study. *Pediatr Crit Care Med* 2007; 8:317-323

[16] Bindl L, Dresbach K, Lentze MJ. Incidence of acute respiratory distress syndrome in German children and adolescents: A population-based study. *Crit Care Med* 2005; 33:209-312

[17] Rubenfeld GD, Caldwell E, Peabody E, Weaver J, Martin DP, Neff M, Stern EJ, Hudson LD. Incidence and Outcomes of Acute Lung Injury. *N Engl J Med* 2005; 353:1685-1693

[18] Kallet RH, Jasmer RM, Pittet JF, Tang JF, Campbell AR, Dicker R, Hemphill C, Luce JM. Clinical implementation of the ARDS network protocol is associated with reduced hospital mortality compared with historical controls. *Crit Care Med* 2005; 33:925-929

[19] National Heart, Lung, and Blood Institute Acute Respiratory Distress Syndrome (ARDS) Clinical Trials Network, Wiedemann HP, Wheeler AP, Bernard GR, Thompson BT, Hayden D, deBoisblanc B, Connors AF Jr, Hite RD, Harabin AL. Comparison of Two Fluid-Management Strategies in Acute Lung Injury. *N Engl J Med* 2006; 354:2564-2575

[20] Spragg RG, Bernard GR, Checkley W, Curtis JR, Gajic O, Guyatt G, Hall J, Israel E, Jain M, Needham DM, Randolph AG, Rubenfeld GD, Schoenfeld D, Thompson BT, Ware LB, Young D, Harabin AL. Beyond Mortality: Future Clinical Research in Acute Lung Injury. *Am J Respir Crit Care Med* 2010; 181:1121-1127

[21] Sheu CC, Gong MN, Zhai R, Chen F, Bajwa EK, Clardy PF, Gallagher DC, Thompson BT, Christiani DC. Clinical Characteristics and Outcomes of Sepsis-Related vs Non-Sepsis-Related ARDS. *Chest* 2010; 138:559-567

[22] Luecke T, Muench E, Roth H, Friess U, Paul T, Kleinhuber K, Quintel M. Predictors of mortality in ARDS patients referred to a tertiary care centre: a pilot study. *Eur J Anaesthesiol* 2006; 23:403-410

[23] Brun-Buisson C, Minelli C, Bertolini G, Brazzi L, Pimentel J, Lewandowski K, Bion J, Romand JA, Villar J, Thorsteinsson A, Damas P, Armaganidis A, Lemaire F; ALIVE Study Group. Epidemiology and outcome of acute lung injury in European intensive care units. *Intensive Care Med* 2004; 30:51-61

[24] Goh AY, Chan PW, Lum LC, Roziah M. Incidence of acute respiratory distress syndrome: a comparison of two definitions. *Arch Dis Child* 1998; 79:256-259

[25] Schmidt R, Luboeinski T, Markart P, Ruppert C, Daum C, Grimminger F, Seeger W, Günther A. Alveolar antioxidant status in patients with acute respiratory distress syndrome. *Eur Respir J* 2004; 24:994-9

[26] Chung-Wai Chow, Maria Teresa Herrera Abreu, Tomoko Suzuki, and Gregory P. Downey. Oxidative Stress and Acute Lung Injury. *Am J Respir Cell Mol Biol* 2003; 29: 427–431

[27] Ware LB. Pathophysiology of acute lung injury and the acute respiratory distress syndrome. *Semin Respir Crit Care Med* 2006;27: 337-349

[28] Manicone AM. Role of the pulmonary epithelium and inflammatory signals in acute lung injury. *Expert Rev Clin Immunol* 2009;5: 63-75

[29] Abraham E. Neutrophils and acute lung injury. *Crit Care Med* 2003;31: S195-S199

[30] Matthay MA, Eschenbacher WL, Goetzl EJ. Elevated concentrations of leukotriene D4 in pulmonary edema fluid of patients with the adult respiratory distress syndrome. *J Clin Immunol* 1984;4: 479-483

[31] Steinberg KP, Milberg JA, Martin TR, Maunder RJ, Cockrill BA, Hudson LD. Evolution of bronchoalveolar cell populations in the adult respiratory distress syndrome. *Am J Respir Crit Care Med* 1994;150: 113-122

[32] Abraham E, Carmody A, Shenkar R, Arcaroli J. Neutrophils as early immunologic effectors in hemorrhage- or endotoxemia-induced acute lung injury. *Am J Physiol Lung Cell Mol Physiol* 2000;279: L1137-1145

[33] Folkesson HG, Matthay MA, Hebert CA, Broaddus VC. Acid aspiration-induced lung injury in rabbits is mediated by interleukin-8-dependent mechanisms. *J Clin Invest* 1995;96: 107-116

[34] Martin TR, Pistorese BP, Chi EY, Goodman RB, Matthay MA. Effects of leukotriene B4 in the human lung. Recruitment of neutrophils into the alveolar spaces without a change in protein permeability. *J Clin Invest* 1989;84: 1609-1619

[35] Ognibene FP, Martin SE, Parker MM, Schlesinger T, Roach P, Burch C, Shelhamer JH, Parrillo JE. Adult respiratory distress syndrome in patients with severe neutropenia. *N Engl J Med* 1986;315: 547-551

[36] Sivan Y, Mor C, al-Jundi S, Newth CJ. Adult respiratory distress syndrome in severely neutropenic children. *Pediatr Pulmonol* 1990;8: 104-108

[37] Lang JD, McArdle PJ, O9Reilly PJ, Matalon S. Oxidantantioxidant balance in acute lung injury. *Chest* 2002; 122: 314S–320S

[38] Lamb NJ, Gutteridge JM, Baker C, Evans TW, Quinlan GJ. Oxidative damage to proteins of bronchoalveolar lavage fluid in patients with acute respiratory distress syndrome: evidence for neutrophil-mediated hydroxylation, nitration, and chlorination. *Crit Care Med* 1999; 27: 2028–2030

[39] Messent M, Sinclair DG, Quinlan GJ, Mumby SE, Gutteridge JM, Evans TW. Pulmonary vascular permeability after cardiopulmonary bypass and its relationship to oxidative stress. *Crit Care Med* 1997; 25: 425–429

[40] Putman E, van Golde LM, Haagsman HP. Toxic oxidant species and their impact on the pulmonary surfactant system. *Lung* 1997; 175: 75–103

[41] Gilliard N, Heldt GP, Loredo J, Redl H, Merritt TA, Spragg RG. Exposure of the hydrophobic components of porcine lung surfactant to oxidant stress alters surface tension properties. *J Clin Invest* 1994; 93: 2608–2615

[42] Leff JA, Parsons PE, Day CE, Taniguchi N, Jochum M, Fritz H, Moore FA, Moore EE, McCord JM, Repine JE. Serum antioxidants as predictors of adult respiratory distress syndrome in patients with sepsis. *Lancet* 1993; 341: 777–780

[43] Comhair SA, Erzurum SC. Antioxidant responses to oxidant-mediated lung diseases. *Am J Physiol* 2002; 283:L246–L255

[44] Pacht ER, Timerman AP, Lykens MG, Merola AJ. Deficiency of alveolar fluid glutathione in patients with sepsis and the adult respiratory distress syndrome. *Chest* 1991; 100: 1397–1403

[45] Matute-Bello G, Frevert CW, Martin TR. Animal models of acute lung injury. *Am J Physiol Lung Cell Mol Physiol* 2008; 295:L379–99.

[46] Martin TR, Matute-Bello G. Experimental models and emerging hypotheses for acute lung injury. *Crit Care Clin* 2011;27:735-52

[47] Wurfel MM, Park WY, Radella F, et al. Identification of high and low responders to lipopolysaccharide in normal subjects: an unbiased approach to identify modulators of innate immunity. *J Immunol* 2005;175:2570–8

[48] Wurfel MM, Gordon AC, Holden TD, et al. Toll-like receptor 1 polymorphisms affect innate immune responses and outcomes in sepsis. *Am J Respir Crit Care Med* 2008;178:710–20

[49] Matute-Bello G, Frevert CW, Martin TR. Animal models of acute lung injury. *Am J Physiol Lung Cell Mol Physiol* 2008;295:L379–99

[50] Martin TR, Matute-Bello G. Experimental models and emerging hypotheses for acute lung injury. *Crit Care Clin* 2011;27:735-52

[51] Ward PA. Oxidative stress: acute and progressive lung injury. *Ann N Y Acad Sci* 2010;1203:53-9

[52] Grommes J, Soehnlein O. Contribution of neutrophils to acute lung injury. *Mol Med* 2011;17:293-307.

[53] Bove PF and van der Vliet A. Nitric oxide and reactive nitrogen species in airway epithelial signaling and inflammation. *Free Radic Biol Med* 2006;41: 515–527.

[54] Brower RG, Lanken PN, MacIntyre N, Matthay MA, Morris A, Ancukiewicz M, Schoenfeld D, and Thompson BT. Higher versus lower positive end-expiratory pressures in patients with the acute respiratory distress syndrome. *N Engl J Med* 2004; 351: 327–336.

[55] ARDSnet1. Ventilation with lower tidal volumes as compared with traditional tidal volumes for acute lung injury and the acute respiratory distress syndrome: the Acute Respiratory Distress Syndrome Network. *N Engl J Med* 2000; 342: 1301–1308.

[56] Ware LB and Matthay MA. The acute respiratory distress syndrome. *N Engl J Med* 2000; 42: 1334–1349.

[57] Ranieri VM, Suter PM, Tortorella C, De Tullio R, Dayer JM, Brienza A, Bruno F, and Slutsky AS. Effect of mechanical ventilation on inflammatory mediators in patients with acute respiratory distress syndrome: a randomized controlled trial. *JAMA* 1999; 282: 54–61.

[58] Goodman RB, Pugin J, Lee JS, and Matthay MA. Cytokine-mediated inflammation in acute lung injury. *Cytokine Growth Factor Rev* 2003; 14: 523–535.

[59] Belperio JA, Keane MP, Lynch JP 3rd, and Strieter RM. The role of cytokines during the pathogenesis of ventilator-associated and ventilator-induced lung injury. *Semin Respir Crit Care Med* 2006; 27: 350–364.

[60] Steinberg JM, Schiller HJ, Halter JM, Gatto LA, Lee HM, Pavone LA, and Nieman GF. Alveolar instability causes early ventilatorinduced lung injury independent of neutrophils. *Am J Respir Crit Care Med* 2004; 169: 57–63.

[61] Gharib SA, Liles WC, Matute-Bello G, Glenny RW, Martin TR, and Altemeier WA. Computational identification of key biological modules and transcription factors in acute lung injury. *Am J Respir Crit Care Med* 2006; 173: 653–658.

[62] Vlahakis NE and Hubmayr RD. Cellular stress failure in ventilator-injured lungs. *Am J Respir Crit Care Med* 2005; 171: 1328–1342.

[63] Metnitz PG, Bartens C, Fischer M, Fridrich P, Steltzer H, and Druml W. Antioxidant status in patients with acute respiratory distress syndrome. *Intensive Care Med* 1999; 25: 180–185.

[64] Bunnell E and Pacht ER. Oxidized glutathione is increased in the alveolar fluid of patients with the adult respiratory distress syndrome. *Am Rev Respir Dis* 1993; 148: 174–1178.

[65] Chapman KE, Sinclair SE, Zhuang D, Hassid A, Desai LP, and Waters CM. Cyclic mechanical strain increases reactive oxygen species production in pulmonary epithelial cells. *Am J Physiol Lung Cell Mol Physiol* 2005; 289: L834–L841.

[66] Jafari B, Ouyang B, Li LF, Hales CA, and Quinn DA. Intracellular glutathione in stretch-induced cytokine release from alveolar type-2 like cells. *Respirology* 2004; 9: 43–53.

[67] Papaiahgari S, Yerrapureddy A, Hassoun PM, Garcia JG, Birukov KG, and Reddy SP. EGFR-activated signaling and actin remodeling regulate cyclic stretch-induced Nrf2–ARE activation. *Am J Respir Cell Mol Biol* 2006; 36: 304–312.

[68] Mata-Greenwood E, Grobe A, Kumar S, Noskina Y, and Black SM. Cyclic stretch increases VEGF expression in pulmonary arterial smooth muscle cells via TGF-beta1 and reactive oxygen species: a requirement for NAD(P)H oxidase. *Am J Physiol Lung Cell Mol Physiol* 2005; 289: L288–L289.

[69] Bedard K and Krause KH. The NOX family of ROS-generating NADPH oxidases: physiology and pathophysiology. *Physiol Rev* 2007; 87: 245–313.

[70] Grote K, Flach I, Luchtefeld M, Akin E, Holland SM, Drexler H, and Schieffer B. Mechanical stretch enhances mRNA expression and proenzyme release of matrix metalloproteinase-2 (MMP-2) via NAD(P)H oxidase-derived reactive oxygen species. *Circ Res* 2003; 92: e80–e86.

[71] Wesley UV, Bove PF, Hristova M, McCarthy S, and van der Vliet A. Airway epithelial cell migration and wound repair by ATPmediated activation of dual oxidase 1. *J Biol Chem* 2007; 282: 3213–3220.

[72] Haddad IY, Pataki G, Hu P, Galliani C, Beckman JS, and Matalon S. Quantitation of nitrotyrosine levels in lung sections of patients and animals with acute lung injury. *J Clin Invest* 1994; 94: 2407–2413.

[73] Sittipunt C, Steinberg KP, Ruzinski JT, Myles C, Zhu S, Goodman RB, Hudson LD, Matalon S, and Martin TR. Nitric oxide and nitrotyrosine in the lungs of patients with acute respiratory distress syndrome. *Am J Respir Crit Care Med* 2001; 163: 503–510.

[74] McVerry BJ, Peng X, Hassoun PM, Sammani S, Simon BA, and Garcia JG. Sphingosine 1–phosphate reduces vascular leak in murine and canine models of acute lung injury. *Am J Respir Crit Care Med* 2004; 170: 987–993.

[75] Reddy SP, Hassoun PM, Brower R. Redox imbalance and ventilator-induced lung injury. *Antioxid Redox Signal* 2007; 9(11):2003-12.

[76] Bove PF and van der Vliet A. Nitric oxide and reactive nitrogen species in airway epithelial signaling and inflammation. *Free Radic Biol Med* 2006; 41: 515–527.

[77] Reddy NM, Kleeberger SR, Cho HY, Yamamoto M, Kensler TW, Biswal S, and Reddy SP. Deficiency in Nrf2–GSH signaling impairs type II cell growth and enhances sensitivity to oxidants *Am J Respir Cell Mol Biol* 2007; 37: 3–8.

In: Oxidative Stress and the Critically Ill Patient
Editors: Ramón Rodrigo and Bettina von Dessauer
ISBN: 978-1-62081-576-2

Chapter X

OXYGEN THERAPY AND OXIDATIVE STRESS

Bettina von Dessauer[1] and Jazmina Bongain[2]
[1]Director of the Pediatric Intensive Care Unit, Doctor Roberto del Río Children's Hospital, Santiago de Chile, Ass Prof. of Pediatrics and Intensive Care, University of Chile
[2]Staff member of the Pediatric Intensive Care Unit, Doctor Roberto del Río Children's Hospital, Santiago de Chile, Ass Prof of Pediatrics and Intensive Care, University of Chile

1. ABSTRACT

Aerobic metabolism of the human being requires oxygen (O_2) and produces carbon dioxide (CO_2) in the process of combustion of nutrients to release energy. Primary goal in any critically ill patient is to maintain adequate tissue oxygenation, caring for microcirculation and adequate oxygen cell utilization trying to sustain this aerobic metabolism. Clear endpoints to achieve this goal, in relation to specific requirements and the amount of additional therapeutic O_2, are till now unknown. Overuse may be the rule, causing added damage in critically ill patients, more in infants, where oxidative stress (OS) occurs easily and earlier.

Hypoxia, dysoxia and hyperoxia, all of them part of frequent clinical situations, may have different consequences if they occur in a previously healthy person with a normal functional reserve or in a critically ill acute or chronic patient with an ongoing inflammatory response. First in experimental studies, it was demonstrated that oxygen supply is not innocuous and may damage tissues by his by-products of metabolism, the reactive oxygen species or free radicals. Overproduction of these, and an insufficient antioxidant response to counterbalance its effect, leads to oxidative stress (OS) and finally multiple organ dysfunction syndrome (MODS) if the process continues.

Not only from the patients-security view, but also considering the cost/effectiveness of a high-cost oxygen-therapy in any clinical situation requires clear endpoints, standards and guidelines to be developed, for an adequate and better utilization in the future.

Abbreviations

ALI	Acute lung injury
ATA	Atmosphere
CaO_2	arterial O2 content
CO_2	Carbon dioxide
CO	Carbon monoxide
DO_2	O_2 delivery
FR	Free radicals
HBO_2	Hyperbaric oxygen
HbO_2	Hemoglobin binded oxygen
IFO_2	Inspired Fraction of O_2
MODS	Multiple organ dysfunction syndrome
O_2	Oxygen
O_2ER	Oxygen extraction ratio
OS	Oxidative stress
PaO_2	Partial arterial oxygen pressure
ROS	Reactive oxygen species
RNS	Reactive nitrogen species
SMSR	Systemic metabolic stress response
SpO_2	Peripheral oxygen saturation
VO_2	Oxygen uptake

2. Introduction and Epidemiology

Aerobic metabolism of the human being requires oxygen (O_2) and produces carbon dioxide (CO_2) for the combustion of nutrients to release energy. The utilization of oxygen to produce energy is not without risks because the respiratory chain works within a narrow range of cell O_2 concentration. That means that hypoxia and hyperoxia induce a fast overproduction of toxic reactive oxygen species with possible cell death.

Oxygen homeostasis is a central objective in metazoan organisms. The respiratory and cardiovascular systems are in charge to deliver an adequate oxygen amount to every system, organ and cell. For acute alterations of basic oxygenation fast compensatory mechanisms exist. Humans in industrialized countries today are less exposed to acute diseases and more to ageing and his consequences, another cause of oxidative stress (OS). Adaptive phenomena for the maintenance of enough oxygenation occur also in these circumstances. New therapeutic strategies are being explored in this context [1]. Hypoxia is a relative term with a wide spectrum of definitions: it can be continuous or intermittent, acute or chronic, systemic or local, depending on the trigger. The adaptive processes to restore oxygen homeostasis will include different biological cellular pathways depending on the underlying condition and also a varying clinical systemic response [2].

Primary goal in any critically ill patient, mostly in sepsis and septic shock, has been for long to maintain adequate tissue oxygenation: this includes caring for adequate circulation, ventilation, maintenance of microcirculation and adequate oxygen cell utilization trying to sustain this aerobic metabolism [3]. Oxygen supply in clinical settings today is perceived as a basic easy available service, with poor consciousness about risks, costs and limits of benefits. Normobaric medical oxygen supplement applied through different techniques, invasive and non-invasive ones, is part of any treatment when respiratory or hemodynamic failure occurs. Given that sepsis, shock, respiratory diseases and trauma are huge problems worldwide requiring hospitalization, the rate of O_2-therapy in hospitalized patients is known to be high.

In the last years, emphasis in critically ill patients has been on avoidance of hypotension and hypoxia, with less caring about eventual hyperoxia and his consequences, at least as important as the former. Volume replacement has been a cornerstone in any guideline, but the documented exact need of O_2 to sustain the normal aerobic process under different clinical conditions and requirements is unclear, in part because tissue oxygenation and peripheral oxygen utilization is not accurately directly measurable in clinical settings [4]. PaO_2 is mostly utilized in daily clinical practice as the indicator of oxygen blood content in spite of the known fact that oxygen bound to hemoglobin is the principal determinant.

Clear endpoints and limits (measurable optimal values) for the need, amount, concentration and duration of oxygen-therapy in different pathologies are still lacking, with poor related research. Guidelines are being developed to clear the panorama.

Clinicians are responsible for titrating this support maximizing his eventual benefits and minimizing the risks. Compliance with this is still insufficient. Mentioned involved factors are de-emphasis on staff education of oxygen-therapy-risks, nursing shortage, slower than expected changes of physician-indicated treatment, staffing issues including de-sensibilization of the team [5]. Additional therapeutic oxygen-supply induces by definition a hyperoxic condition, enhances the production of more reactive oxygen species (ROS), and may induce OS when these are in excess for the antioxidant response capacity, and the physiologic balance is lost.

Hypoxia, dysoxia and hyperoxia differ in the involved mechanism inducing damage, but all of them influence ROS and RNS (reactive nitrogen species) production and eventually the development of OS. The risk of any additional oxygen support is higher in the youth, mostly in newborns, when immaturity facilitates damage in hyperoxic tissues. On the other hand these small patients are prone to respiratory depression and diseases in which early hypoxia and later hyperoxia, due to medical therapy, may occur [6]. The goal continues to be to use therapeutic oxygen supply as soon as needed, at the lowest possible concentration to achieve the desired result avoiding tissue hypoxia, and during the shortest period of time necessary to stabilize the patient. Research is still lacking to bring this into practice.

In this chapter we will try to explain why O_2 has to be used carefully, avoiding hypoxia or hyperoxia, restoring oxygen homeostasis as soon as possible, considering that enough information is available arguing about the risks and still unclear clinical endpoints to achieve in each clinical condition [7]. In modern clinical settings safety of the patients, expertise of involved professionals, but also the cost/effectiveness of this therapy has to be taken into account [8].

3. Physiology and Pathophysiology

3.1 Physiology of Oxygenation

Normoxia is defined as the tissue oxygenation necessary to maintain aerobic metabolism with a maximum inspired natural FIO_2 of 160 Torr (21% O_2 x 760 Torr at sea level = 160 Torr O_2 = 0,21 ATA O_2), minimizing the generation of free radicals (FR). During normoxia cells are exposed to oxygen concentrations as low as 1% (3-35 Torr) [2]. Oxygen enters the body through the lungs and is transported via the vascular system to the metabolizing tissues. It does not readily dissolve in water, so hemoglobin as a specialized oxygen-binding molecule is needed for the transport (HbO_2). When oxygen reaches the systemic capillaries, dissociation of HbO_2 and entrance of O_2 to the tissues occurs, called oxygen uptake (VO_2). This, equivalent to oxygen consumption, is the amount of oxygen leaving the capillaries effectively, stated that tissues do not store oxygen. Arterial oxygen content (CaO_2) is the sum of hemoglobin-bound (98%) and plasma dissolved oxygen (1,5-2%), so hemoglobin is mostly the determining factor for the transport. Oxygen extraction ratio ($O_2ER = VO_2 / DO_2$) is the ratio between uptake and delivery and an index of efficiency. It ranges around 25%, so that 75% of HbO_2 remains in the circulation, able to be adjusted according to physiologic needs.

Adequate tissue oxygenation requires a balance between VO_2 and metabolic tissue requirement for O_2 (MRO_2). If balanced, glucose is completely oxidized to 36 ATP molecules/mole of glucose/6 moles of O_2 producing 673 kcal. If not, part of the glucose forms lactate with less metabolic energy production (47 kcal/mole of glucose) and dysoxia occurs. Shock is the clinical expression of that physiologic disorder differing in the trigger: deficit of organ perfusion and oxygen supply in hypovolemic or cardiogenic shock or mitochondrial misuse in distributive or septic shock [9].

When DO_2 declines, due to relative or absolute hypovolemia, VO_2 initially remains constant by an enhanced O_2ER, up to 50-60%. After that point is reached, VO_2 goes down and hypoxia ensues. The critical DO_2 is the point at which VO_2 becomes supply-dependent to maintain aerobic metabolism. If this is not achieved ATP production falls and shock and progressive MODS occurs as a clinical manifestation [10]. VO_2 is a measure of oxygen uptake and consumption due to the absence of a tissue O_2 reserve. A low value may be due to dysoxia or hypometabolism (thought to be rare in critical patients). Consequently it can be interpreted as impaired tissue oxygenation. The cumulative deficit is called oxygen debt, which is related to an eventual development and progression to MODS [11].

Hypoxia can be a continuous or an intermittent event depending on the cause. When a patient is subjected to hypoxia, a prompt hyperventilation is an expectable physiologic reaction with the goal of a fast normalization of tissue oxygenation by enhancing minute ventilation, maximizing perfusion, oxygen transport and delivery to the cell. If inadequate oxygen delivery persists, other mechanisms are activated, including oxygen-sensing prolyl-hydroxilases (PHDs), which act in the alpha subunit of the hypoxia-inducible transcription factor (HIF-1). As a consequence of hypoxia an inflammatory response arises, inducing between other phenomena, a capillary leak. This leads to a volume shift from the intravascular to the interstitial space in different organs and systems reducing the intravascular compartment and than tissue perfusion. Hypoxia is proposed to be a contributor to this process by regulating the oxygen-dependent gene expression [12].

Interestingly HIF-1 is also inducible in normoxic states as an anticipatory response to the presence of bacterial lipopolysaccharides, between other causes (refer to Chapter 2). HIF-1is the master regulator of oxygen homeostasis in normal individuals controlling the delivery and utilization of oxygen, but in genetic disorders, ageing and some chronic disorders this action is impaired. A counter-inflammatory process tries to reduce the injury in impaired tissues by activating HIF-1 and anti-inflammatory molecules, including adenosine. This should lead to a reduction of vascular fluid leakage and of inflammatory cells in injured tissues [13]. Occult hypoxia is reported to be present in tumor tissues worsening the outcome. In presence of bacterial infections the HIF-pathway is also involved influencing the physiologic response and further evolution, as different studies report.

In sepsis VO_2 has to be carefully interpreted. Activation of neutrophils and macrophages due to inflammation enhances the cell oxygen consumption (respiratory burst), used for the production of FR. This contributes to a higher VO_2 but not to aerobic metabolism. Tissue oxygenation may be normal but the utilization by the mitochondria is reduced. So the real peripheral tissue need of O_2 has still to be elucidated in abnormal disease states like sepsis to allow a specific accurate supply. Additional oxygen supply in this context may not reduce dysoxia, increase the ROS and RNS production, enhance the imbalance between oxidant and antioxidant response and finally induce OS, pathway to MODS.

The total body oxygen blood reserve to sustain aerobic metabolism lasts around 3-4 minutes, which leaves a short time in emergency situations to begin rescue maneuvers. This small reserve may be part of a natural cell protection mechanism, avoiding the risk of the potentially deleterious effect of oxygen derived toxic metabolites due to unnecessary excess oxygen presence. So if we, in a near future, would be able to measure VO_2 or related biomarkers of real tissue oxygenation and cell utilization, probably it would help to prevent dysoxia, oxidative stress and its consequences for the patient.

Normobaric hyperoxia by definition occurs at any point above IFO_2 (inspired fraction of O_2) of 0,21, with tissue PO_2 over 35 Torr. For others (from the clinical point of view) with IFO_2 of 50% or higher, or when oxygen supply is reflected on PaO_2 above 90 mmHg or SpO_2 (peripheral oxygen saturation) over 98% [14]. In experimental models, alveolar hyperoxia in the lung produces free radicals, inflammation, genetic overexpression, cell damage with necrosis and possible caspase-induced apoptosis, alveolar de-recruitment and final atelectasis [15]. The transcription factor HIF-1 is inactive in this situation.

Hyperoxia induces a biphasic response on the central nervous respiratory control system: a transient reduction of minute ventilation by inhibition of peripheral chemoreceptors and than a central paradox hyperventilation. The physiologic objective is to modulate central reduction-oxidation reactions, oxidative enzymes and ROS production with the aim to optimize the balance between O_2 demand and supply [16]. Central CO_2 chemoreceptors are directly stimulated by ROS [17]. In experimental studies it has been demonstrated that normobaric hyperoxia has damaging effects on neuronal function in the immature and modulating influence in the mature central nervous system [18].

Hyperbaric oxygen (HBO_2) is O_2 at more than 1 ATA (atmosphere) of pressure. The clinical effect is attributable mostly to the concentration of oxygen, not the pressure, and its anti-inflammatory action. Available literature indicates that oxidative stress does not occur below 2 ATA and even can reduce it [19]. Clinical supply may be as high as 2280 Torr (equivalent to 3 ATA) or even more. The mechanism of action of HBO_2 is based on an increase of PaO_2 and the hydrostatic pressure, reducing the volume of gas-filled spaces (decompression in divers, reduction of gas in infected wounds). In the patient with a systemic metabolic stress response (SMSR), the supply of HBO_2 together with an increase in tissue oxygenation produces an acceleration of tissue repair, neovascularization by angiogenesis and vasculogenesis, reduction of pro-inflammatory cytokines and increase of growth factors and collagen formation. This does not occur in the healthy person. Organ reperfusion damage is reduced by inhibition of neutrophil β_2-integrin adhesion in injured patients but also in carbon monoxide (CO) intoxication. Other functions of neutrophils are maintained, so that immune-depression is not an expectable consequence.

The emergence of an oxidative stress response is time dependent (time exposed to HBO_2), inducing a positive or negative physiologic consequence depending on the intensity and the balancing counter-reaction of the antioxidant response [20].

3.2 Oxygen, Free Radicals and Oxidative Stress

Free radicals are always present in human nature due to the constant production of partially reduced forms of oxygen in the cells. While maintained in balance with the counter-regulatory antioxidant response system, no harm and different positive physiologic functions are expectable, an antibacterial activity between others. If the balance is lost OS occurs.

Infants and mostly newborns are at a higher risk of oxidative stress due to an increased production of free radicals and an immaturity derived lower antioxidant reserve [21]. ROS are constantly generated as natural by-products of metabolism, including superoxide (O_2•), hydrogen peroxide (H_2O_2), and hydroxyl (HO•). Production of energy as ATP takes place via a flow of electrons passing along the five molecular complexes of the electron transport chain. As part of this process, ROS are generated as by-products of the incomplete four-electron reduction of molecular oxygen to water, the final electron acceptor in the process of ATP production. RNS include nitric oxide (NO) and peroxynitrite (ONOO), which is the product of a reaction between O_2• and NO [22].

Scavenging antioxidants combat the overproduction of reactive species. In normal physiologic conditions, enzymes and antioxidants maintain a balance between production and elimination of ROS. When this capacity is overwhelmed by overproduction of FR and/or deficit of antioxidants, oxidative stress occurs and cell destruction begins with significant damage of lipids, proteins, and nucleic acids [23].

Not only mayor pro-inflammatory states are accompanied by overproduction of free radicals and oxidative stress. Hypoxia and hyperoxia in peripheral tissues are also responsible for this process. Hypoxia induces oxidative stress via an over-generation of ROS. Cellular hypoxia is generally characterized by a reductive state and has been described as a form of "reductive stress" [24]. During hypoxia mitochondrial electron transport slows, enhancing the reduction state of electron carriers by elevations in reducing equivalents mostly NADH and FADH2. This accumulation of reducing equivalents favors superoxide production by increasing the electrical potential for single electron reduction of oxygen to superoxide. For the ROS production in hypoxia it requires at least a persistent minimum oxygen supply to be present above the hypoxia level [25]. In fact, the data support the role of mitochondria as a potential ROS source and also as a specific oxidative target under severe hypoxic conditions.

Changes in O_2 concentration in the cell can be sensed and modulate the activity of HIF-1. Studies in humans corroborated the previous in vitro findings demonstrating that ROS are involved in HIF-1 alpha transcription (hypoxia inducible factor alpha) [26], which is associated with transcriptional targets that participate in adaptive responses to hypoxia.

(A more detailed description on mitochondrial phenomena is available in chapter 4). The electron transport chain of mitochondria is the mayor source of intracellular ROS. Hyper-inflammatory states, such as sepsis, increases the production of mitochondrial ROS, nitric oxide and peroxynitrite. This organelle is not only the producer but also the main target of ROS. The peroxidation of the mitochondrial lipid cardiolipin, which is present in the inner mitochondrial membrane and important for energy metabolism, leads to the dissociation of cytochrome c and causes reduced ATP production, and even more ROS production. Oxidative stress-mediated damage to mtDNA can lead to a vicious cycle of ROS production and further mtDNA damage. In other words, a perpetual cycle of ROS production facilitated by ROS-induced ROS release can occur [27]. As a result of the decrease in energy production tissue oxygen consumption also decreases, in spite of the recovering of an adequate supply of oxygen. This situation has been called cytopathic hypoxia [28].

Exposure to a hyperoxic environment leads to toxic phenomena. The severity of these depends on the magnitude of the hyperoxia and the duration of the exposure. Again hyperoxic toxicity is due to the production of ROS in excess for the capacity of the cellular defense mechanisms to inactivate these toxic species. Thus the sensitivity to oxygen toxicity could be expected to vary depending on the cell defense mechanisms.

In the decades of 1970 and 1980 different studies were realized with cell cultures and in experimental models with small animals submitted to prolonged hyperoxia. These provided direct evidence of the increased production of ROS in this condition [29]. In humans it could be established that the use of high IFO_2 may produce a local oxidative environment, which may aggravate lung injury induced by mechanical ventilator [15]. When therapeutic concentrated oxygen is supplied to normal healthy individuals without inflammatory phenomena, the adaptive antioxidant response is enhanced, more reactive species are produced transiently, but no oxidative stress occurs [30]. In the context of hospitalized sick patients requiring oxygen-therapy, the O_2 homeostatic balance is disrupted as a consequence of both the underlying pathology and the treatment. While immediate clinical needs must be achieved, additional oxygen-therapy can exacerbate the production and accumulation of excessive ROS.

Children and infants, mostly very low birth weight babies, are particularly sensitive to oxygen toxicity. Oxidative stress is generated as a consequence of many different clinical conditions in pediatrics leading to inflammation and SMSR, imbalance of oxygen homeostasis and in the induced context of hyperoxia [31]. It is assumed that lung damage caused by hyperoxia is mediated by excess production of reactive oxygen intermediates (ROIs) either through direct damage to tissue constituents or via altered oxidative signaling [32]. The mitochondrial electron transport chain can generate·O2 − by the transfer of an electron to molecular O2 at Complex I, II, or III, *in lieu* of complete transfer to Complex IV where O_2 is reduced to water. Under conditions of hyperoxia, the generation of ROS from mitochondria increases linearly with oxygen tension [33].

Using knockout mice, Carnesecchi et al [34] demonstrated that NOX1, but not NOX2, was an important mediator of hyperoxia-induced acute lung injury (ALI). The cellular damage and death takes place through activation of kinases (via intracellular ROS signal) in neutrophils and monocytes, which accumulate within the pulmonary circulation, interstitial and air spaces under hyperoxic conditions. This represents an additional source of ROS [35]. Overwhelming production of ROS from these sources can lead to oxidative modifications of macromolecules, leading to pulmonary cell death, characteristic for hyperoxic lung injury [36].

Diagram of oxidative stress pathways in oxygen disturbance:

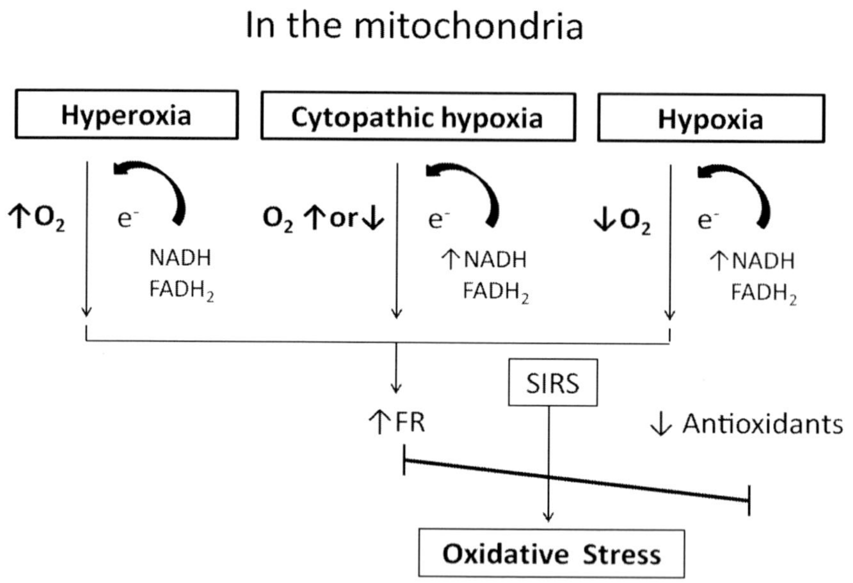

Figure 1. Aumento en la producción de RL mitocondrial en hiperoxia por mayor disponibilidad de O2, en hipoxia por stress reductivo e hipoxia citopatica por bloqueo de la cadena respiratoria mitocondrial en presencia de citoquinas inflamatorias The increase in the release of mitochondrial FR in hyperoxia is due to higher availability of O_2, in hypoxia due to reductive stress and in cytopathic hypoxia due to a blockade of the respiratory chain in presence of inflammatory cytokines.

Apoptosis results from activation of the mitochondrial cell death pathway. This leads to the activation of caspase-9 or the receptor-mediated death pathway, an extrinsic pathway leading to activation of caspase-8. Both pathways converge to caspase-3. Activation of caspase-3, caspase-8, and caspase-9, has all been described following hyperoxic exposure suggesting that both mitochondrial and receptor-mediated pathways are active [32].

In summary all clinical situations in the critically ill patient leading to an imbalance of oxygen homeostasis and misuse of oxygen in the mitochondria are able to increase ROS and RNS production and OS when the antioxidant response system fails to counterbalance this process.

In all three situations the final result is an increase of FR production: in hyperoxia due to an excess of O_2 reacting with free electrons, in cytopathic hypoxia due to an increase of NADH and consequently more available free electrons and in hypoxia an increase of NADH together with less O_2. This last one only leads to ROS production in presence of at least a few residual oxygen cell supply.

4. CLINICAL ASPECTS AND STUDIES

Oxygen is the basic element allowing human life on earth, but the almost liberal use as a therapeutic concentrated drug in clinical settings has received less attention than required for an avoidance of additional harm in critically ill patients. Any condition which leads to respiratory and/or hemodynamic failure, imbalances oxygenation of the human organism and may need external supply. Oxygen-therapy from IFO_2 22% up to 100% is possible using different applications, from external masks up to endotracheal tubes when mechanical ventilation is necessary.

Available clinical bedside empiric endpoints for oxygenation are certain values of peripheral SpO_2, arterial or venous PO_2, central mixed venous blood saturation and indirect parameters of gas exchange including end tidal CO_2 or volumetric capnography when the patient is ventilated with modern microprocessors. None of these has an evidence-based real precise value to be met as an endpoint for cell oxygenation in a specific clinical condition and particular patient balancing benefits and avoiding additional harm of additional oxygen supply. The difference or coincidence between normal values established for healthy individuals and expectable values in sick organisms with adaptive responses has to be elucidated. In the past skin color, respiratory rate and breathing work, heart rate and neurologic improvement were the guiders. A gap between abundant available basic science research showing the risks of a too late initiated or excess oxygen supply and a consequent clinical behavior in praxis exists till now.

More emphasis has been put on avoidance of hypoxia than hyperoxia in clinics, the first known to promote an inflammatory response with in part easy recognizable clinical symptoms and signs when significant. In hypoxic peripheral tissues of obese patients additionally this fact could contribute to insulin resistance and a metabolic syndrome. This knowledge may be important to take into account in ICUs in relation to the increasing rate of obese children.

Hypoxic systemic consequences will depend on the underlying disease: in adults with a chronic obstructive lung disease it leads to pulmonary hypertension and right heart failure and in children first to apneas and later right ventricular hypertrophy and cor pulmonale when prolonged on time. In intermittent hypoxia due to sleep apnea systemic hypertension is expectable when prolonged. Altitude-induced chronic hypoxemia produces polycythemia and also cor pulmonale. Local hypoxia as seen in atherosclerosis, huge problem in industrialized countries, is the major cause of myocardial infarction. Enhanced metabolic myocardial oxygen needs and reduced supply due to obstruction leads to cell death. Intra-tumor hypoxia as seen in many cancers, worsens the outcome by an over-activation of the HIF-1 pathway [37]. Inflammatory phenomena in injured tissues also may aggravate hypoxia in a vicious cycle. Ischemia, thrombosis, tissue loss or compression in trauma and local edema may reduce the access of energy substrates in spite of increased needs of the cells.

Studies showed that hypoxia induced by altitudes (above 3400 m) increased the blood level of inflammatory biomarkers as C-reactive protein, interleukin-6 and cytokines. Low PaO_2, ischemia, vascular leakage and pulmonary edema were the clinical evidences [38]. In neonatal resuscitation special emphasis has been put on conservative targets with no more than 30-40% of IFO_2 to achieve SpO_2 of 85-93%, very different than in the past. The developmental stage and prematurity influence what could be considered the optimal oxygen exposure and the risk of harm. Tight control of the targets is necessary using health team education and protocols to reach the goal. This is based on the knowledge that at more immaturity more ROS and less antioxidants are present, and that many of the persistent or chronic clinical conditions in premature neonates are associated to OS [21].

Many studies proceed from neonatal settings because premature babies are particularly sensible to oxygen toxicity with early and delayed consequences. Higher incidence of recurrent wheezing at 3 years of age has been associated to neonatal exposure of O_2 [39]. Respiratory morbidity may not only be associated to the exposure but also to the cumulative dose of oxygen supply in VLBW (very low birth weight) babies without bronchopulmonar dysplasia (BPD), as stated by Stevens. Using an area under the curve analysis of exposure (integration of the concentration over time) he showed that this was more predictive of later respiratory symptoms than the exposure in number of days alone [40].

A growing number of prematurely born infants, surviving with chronic respiratory failure, are a challenge in pediatric critical care units. BPD is associated to oxidative stress in newborns with respiratory failure. Great efforts currently have been done to reduce the rate of BPD in these patients. Strategies include oxygen control but also enhancement of the antioxidant response [31]. Also retinopathy and blindness, added to the presence of neonatal sepsis and low gestational age is an expectable consequence of oxygen excess. An Indian report of higher than expected incidence of retinopathy in big babies was related to unmonitored supplemental oxygen [41]. In infants with congenital heart disease management with $O_{2,}$ while waiting for transport or soon surgery, has to be goal-directed for each anatomic condition, with clear targets to fulfill, avoiding major hemodynamic disturbances and harm [42]. Hyperoxia in infants presenting with repetitive apneas or ALTE (Apparent Life-Threatening Event) destabilizes the breathing pattern, similar to experimental studies in rats were an enhanced incidence of sleep-related apneas and periodic breathing have been reported [43].

Prolonged hypoxemia and hypoxia in infants and children include failure to thrive, together with cardiovascular and respiratory adaptive conditions, in part similar to adults. In healthy adult divers submitted to 100% O_2 intermittently during 12 weeks of training, total antioxidant capacity showed an initial decline and recovery in the last week, evidencing an adaptive process to hyperoxia and non-significant oxidative stress [30]. Similar results were observed in other studies [44].

Hyperbaric oxygen exposure at a PO_2 approximately of 120 kPa(a) for 3,5 hours induced in healthy divers lipid peroxidation, increased fragility of red blood cells and insufficient endogenous antioxidant capacity, requiring eventually exogenous supplementation to reduce oxidative stress, as a proposal [45]. In children with autism treated with HBO_2 at 1,5 atm (1142 mmHg) to improve cerebral perfusion, this did not increase intracellular oxidative stress known to exist in this clinical condition [19].

In summary oxygen homeostasis in the critically ill patient is the goal but difficult to reach o recover, with still lacking evidence-based clear targets, clinical available precise tools and measurable endpoints. Free radicals, ROS and RNS, are constantly present in nature, contributing to maintain homeostasis and an antibacterial activity between other roles. While in balance with the antioxidant response syndrome no harm is expectable from them.

5. Management of Supplemental Oxygen

In relation to O_2 supply, the potential risk of unlimited, endpoints-lacking oxygen-therapy is a major topic for the clinician. Education of health teams working in clinical settings is the basics [46]. Clinical pilot trials managing patients with automated adjustment of inspired oxygen fraction has been done, intending to avoid excessive exposure with tight control of FiO_2 in relation to preestablished limits of PaO_2 or SpO_2 values [47].

Lower oxygenation targets in the neonatal- resuscitation setting were defined considering the higher potential excess of free radical production and antioxidant deficit in this babies, associated to later morbidity [21]. In elder children and adults also the target of SpO_2 today should be lower than in the past, adapted to and in the context of the clinical condition, around 88-92%, with few exceptions, and PaO_2 of up to 90 mmHg. Central mixed venous blood oxygenation is used in critical care settings but again it is an index of the arterial-venous oxygen extraction rate, but not of tissue and cell oxygenation. Accurate measurement is via a co-oximeter and not as a difference between venous and arterial blood gases.

Hyperbaric oxygen therapy with 2-4 ATA has been reported to be beneficial in different clinical situations, some of them still in research settings. HBO_2 has been used in diabetic wounds, general wound healing, skin graft survival, extremity re-implantation, delayed radiation injuries, CO intoxication, necrotizing fasceitis, myonecrosis and many others. [20].

In summary therapeutic oxygen supply is in constant review, lifesaving but also can be harmfull inducing oxidative stress, and needs further related research. The monitoring of oxygenation and CO_2 production and elimination is essential in clinical settings as part of many other parameters to be measured. In almost all critically ill patients blood gases are part of the basics. Arterial or venous, isolated values or with continuous measurement, invasive or non-invasive techniques, are part of available monitoring methods of oxygenation. No one measures cell oxygenation.

Different technologies are available: gas analyzers measure blood dissolved pO_2, pCO_2 and pH and calculate many other parameters including base excess, bicarbonate and saturation. Errors may occur at any point of the process, including room temperature. Results are different in arterial, mixed venous, venous or capillary blood. The last both have little relation with PaO_2 and may not be considered for therapy-adjustment. Pulse-oximeters measure saturation of arterial HbO_2 (SpO_2) by pulse wave via spectrophotometry. In presence of carbon monoxide intoxication, methemoglobinemia, intravenous organic colorants (methylene blue, indocyanin green) and nail onicomycosis, measured values may be inaccurate. Arterial pulse wave has to be present and detectable when the oximeter is used with any critically ill patient, factor to be taken into account when hypothermia, hypovolemia, overall hemodynamic compromise or even shock is present. Also hyperoxia and severe hypoxia, both in the extremes of the HbO_2-dissociation -curve, cannot be measured accurately by this way. In as normal defined ranges of PaO_2 correlation with SpO_2 exists. Other methods exist like transcutaneous pO_2, depending on the arterial oxygen content and blood flow, mostly utilized in newborns to detect hypoxia and prevent hyperoxia [48,49].

In summary oxygen homeostasis for the maintenance of aerobic metabolism is the goal but difficult to achieve in intensive care settings while endpoints for desirable and expectable tissue and cell oxygenation values are still being investigated. Markers for oxygen stress are being developed pretending an easier access for clinicians in the near future (See chapter 11).

Conclusions and Future Goals

In spite of the known benefits and risks of oxygen-therapy research is lacking and endpoints are not clear. Oxygen homeostasis is still a challenge in critical care. Early detection of clinical situations in which hypoxia, dysoxia or hyperoxia may occur, and insufficient or excess supplemental oxygenation for the physiologic needs may be supplied, has to be identified.

What "adequate management of O_2 therapy" means has to be elucidated for every clinical situation and diagnosis, requiring a specific goal-directed-therapy. Prevention of additional complications, including the maintainance of an inflammatory response syndrome, oxidative stress, tissue destruction and secondary functional damage in acute critically ill and in chronic patients, has to be in the center of the attention.

Available endpoints and precise diagnostic tools trying to maintain tissue perfusion and cell oxygenation for a normal oxygen homeostasis must be part of clinical and basic science research in the future.

References

[1] Semenza G. Life with oxygen. *Science* 2007;318:62-64.

[2] Semenza G. Oxygen homeostasis. *WIREs Syst Biol Med* 2010;2:336–361.

[3] Sakr Y, Dubois MJ, De Backer D, Creteur Vincent JL. Persistent microcirculatory alterations are associated with organ failure and death in patients with septic shock. *Crit Care Med* 2004;32:1825-1831.

[4] Rivers E, Nguyen B, Havstad S, Ressler J, Muzzin A, Knoblich B, Peterson E, Tomlanovich M. Early Goal- Directed Therapy Collaborative Group. Early goal-.directed therapy in the treatment of severe sepsis and septic shock. *N Engl J Med* 2011;345:1825-1831.

[5] Johnson K, Scott SD, Fraser KD. Oxygen use for preterm infants: factors that may influence clinical decisions surrounding oxygen titration. *Adv Neonatal Care* 2011;1:8-17.

[6] Walsh BK, Brooks T, Grenier B. Oxygen therapy in neonatal care environment. *Resp Care* 2009;54:1193-1199.

[7] Zimmerman J. Defining the role of oxyradicals in the pathogenesis in sepsis. *Crit Care Med* 1995;23:616-617.

[8] Porter M, Olmsted E. Redefining competence in health care. *Harvard Business Review* 2004;57-64.

[9] Fink MP. Impaired cellular use of oxygen in critically ill. *J Crit Illness* 2001;16:28-32.

[10] Shoemaker WC, Appel P, Kram HB. Role of oxygen debt in the development of organ failure, sepsis, and death in high-risk surgical patients. *Chest* 1992;102:208-215.

[11] Dunham CM, Seigel JH, Weireter L et al. Oxygen debt and metabolic acidemia as quantitative predictors of mortality and the severity of the isquemic insult in hemorrhagic shock. *Crit Care Med* 1991;19:231-243.

[12] Eltzschig H, Carmeliet P. Hypoxia and Inflammation. *N Engl J Med* 2011;17:656-665.

[13] Taylor CT, Colgan SP. Hypoxia and gastrointestinal disease. *J Mol Med* 2007;85:1295-1300.

[14] Visner G, Fogg S, Nick H. Hyperoxia-responsive proteins in rat pulmonary microvascular endothelial cells. *American Journal of Physiology* 1996;270: 1517-1525.

[15] Gordo-Vidal F, Calco-Herranz E, Abella-Alvarez A, Salinas-Gabiña I. Toxicidad pulmonar por hiperoxia. *Med Intensiva* 2010;34:134-138.

[16] Dean JB, Mulkey DK, Henderson RA, Potter SJ, Putnam R. Hyperoxia, reactive oxygen species and hyperventilation: oxygen sensitivity of brain stem neurons. *J Appl Physiol* 2004;96:784-791.

[17] Mulkey DK, Henderson RA, Putman R, Dean JB. Hyperbaric oxygen and chemical oxidants stimulate CO_2/H^+ sensitive neurons in rat brainstem slices. *J Appl Physiol* 2003;95: 910-921.

[18] Ahdab-Barmada J, Moossy J, Painter M. Pontosubicular necrosis and hyperoxemia. *Pediatrics* 1980;66:840-847.

[19] Rossignol D, Rossignol L, James S, Melnyk S, Mumper E. The effects of hyperbaric oxygen therapy on oxidative stress, inflammation, and symptoms in children with autism: an open-label pilot study. *BMC Pediatrics* 2007;7:36 doi:10.1186/1471-2431-7-36.

[20] Thom S. Oxidative stress is fundamental to hyperbaric oxygen therapy. *J Appl Physiol* 2009;106:988-995.

[21] Finer N, Leone T. Oxygen saturation monitoring for the preterm infant: the evidence basis for current practice. *Pediatr Res* 2009;65:375-380.

[22] Valko M, Leibfritz D, Moncola J, Cronin M, Mazura M, Telser J. Free radicals and antioxidants in normal physiological functions and human disease. *The International Journal of Biochemistry & Cell Biology* 2007;39:448-484.

[23] Crimi E, Sica V, Williams-Ignarro S, Zhang H, Slutsky A, Ignarro LJ, Napoli C. The role of oxidative stress in adult critical care. *Free Radical Biology & Medicine* 2006;40:398-406.

[24] Clanton TL. Hypoxia-induced reactive oxygen species formation in skeletal muscle. *J Appl Physiol 2007;*102:2379-2388.

[25] Dawson T, Gores GJ, Nieminen AL, Herman B, Lemasters JJ. Mitochondria as a source of reactive oxygen species during reductive stress in rat hepatocytes. *Am J Physiol Cell Physiol 1993;*264:961-967.

[26] Pialoux V, Mounier R, Brown AD, Steinback CD, Rawling JM, Poulin MJ. Relationship between oxidative stress and HIF-1 alpha mRNA during sustained hypoxia in humans. *Free Radic Biol Med* 2009;15:321-326.

[27] Galley HF. Oxidative stress and mitochondrial dysfunction in sepsis. *British Journal of Anaesthesia* 2011;20:1-8.

[28] Fink Mitchel P. Bench-to-bedside review: Cytopathic hypoxia. *Critical Care* 2002;6:491-499.

[29] Jamieson D, Chance B, Cadenas E, Boveris A. The relation of free radical production to hyperoxia. *Ann Rev Physiol* 1986;48:703-719.

[30] Alvarez-García MJ, Albaladejo MD, Acevedo C, Olea A, Zamora S, Martinez P, Parra S. Effects of hyperoxia on biomarkers of oxidative stress in closed-circuit oxygen military divers. *J Physiol Biochem* 2008;64:135-142.

[31] Saugstad OD. Oxygen and oxidative stress in bronchopulmonar dysplasia. *J Perinat Med*;38:571-577.

[32] Altemeier WA, Sinclair SE. Hyperoxia in the intensive care unit: why more is not always better. *Curr Opin Crit Care* 2007;13:73-78.

[33] Turrens JF. Mitochondrial formation of reactive oxygen species. *J Physiol* 2003;52:335-344.

[34] Carnesecchi S, Deffert C, Pagano A, Garrido-Urbani S, Métrailler- Ruchonnet I, Schäppi, M, Donati, Y, Matthay, M.A, Krause KH, Barazzone A. NADPH oxidase-1 plays a crucial role in hyperoxia-induced acute lung injury in mice. *Am J Respir Crit Care Med 2009;*180:972–981.

[35] Chollet-Martin S, Jourdain B, Gibert C, Elbim C, Chastre J, Gougerot- Pocidalo MA. Interactions between neutrophils and cytokines in blood and alveolar spaces during ARDS. *Am J Respir Crit Care Med 1996;*154:594–601.

[36] Mantell LL, Horowitz S, Davis JM, Kazzaz JA. Hyperoxia-induced cell death in the lung – the correlation of apoptosis, necrosis, and inflammation. *Ann N Y Acad Sci 1999;*887:171–180.

[37] Semenza G. Oxygen sensing, homeostasis and disease. *N Engl J Med* 2011; 365:537-547.

[38] Hartmann G, Tschöp M, Fischer R et al. High-altitude increases circulating interleukin-6, interleukin-1 receptor antagonist and C-reactive protein. *Cytokine* 2009;12:246-252.

[39] Escobar GJ, Ragins A, Li SX, Prager L, Masaquel AS, Kipnis P. Recurrent wheezing in the third year of life among children born at 32 weeks`gestation or later: relationship to laboratory-confirmed, medically attended infection with respiratory syncytial virus during the first year of life. *Arch Pediatr Adolesc Med* 2010;164:915-922.

[40] Stevens TP, Dylag A, Pantaghani I, Pryhuber G, Halterman J. Effect of cumulative oxygen exposure on respiratory symptoms during infancy among VLBW infants without bronchopulmonary dysplasia. *Pediatr Pulmunol* 2010;45:371-379.

[41] Shah PK, Narendran V, Kalpana N, Gilbert C. Severe retinopathy of premature in big babies in India: history repeating itself? *Indian J Pediatr* 2009;76:801-804.

[42] Shivananda S, Kirsh J, Whyte HE, Muthalally K, McNamara PJ. Impact of oxygen saturation targets and oxygen therapy during the transport of neonates with clinically suspected congenital heart disease. *Neonatology* 2010; 97:154-162.

[43] Berger PJ, Brodecky V, Margaret C, Adamson TM, Wilkinson MH. Unusual respiratory response to oxygen in an infant with repetitive cyanotic episodes. *Am J Respir Crit Care Med* 2000;161:2107-2111.

[44] Lushchak V, Bagnyukova T, Husak V, Luzhnak O, Storey K. Hyperoxia results in transient oxidative stress and an adaptative response by antioxidant enzymes in goldfish tissues. *The International Journal of Biochemistry & Cell Biology* 2005;1670-1680.

[45] Bearden SE, Cheuvront SN, Ring TA, Haymes EM. Oxidative stress during 3.5-hour exposure to 120 kPa(a)PO_2 in human divers. *Undersea & Hyperbaric Medicine* 1999;26:159-164.

[46] Higgins RD, Bancalari E, Willinger M, Raju TN. Executive summary of the workshop on oxygen in neonatal therapies: controversies and opportunities for research. *Pediatrics* 2007;119:790-796.

[47] Claure N, D` Ugard C, Bancalari E. Automated adjustment of inspired oxygen in preterm infants with frequent fluctuations in oxygenation: a pilot clinical trial. *J Pediatr* 2009;155:640-645.

[48] Casado Flores J, Martínez de Azagra A, Serrano A. *Mechanical Ventilation in neonates, infants and children.* Textbook in Spanish. Edit Ergon Madrid,Spain. Second edition 2011 Chapter 5:41-47.

[49] Moyle JT. Use and abuse of pulse oxymetry. *Arch Dis Child* 1996;74:77-80.

In: Oxidative Stress and the Critically Ill Patient
Editors: Ramón Rodrigo and Bettina von Dessauer
ISBN: 978-1-62081-576-2

Chapter XI

BIOMARKERS OF OXIDATIVE STRESS

Rodrigo Castillo
Pathophysiology Program, Institute of Biomedical Sciences, Faculty of Medicine, University of Chile

1. ABSTRACT

In the absence of an adequate gold standard for diagnosing sepsis, there has been considerable and growing interest in identifying suitable biomarkers. Several studies in adults confirm the occurrence of severe oxidative stress in patients with SIRS, which is demonstrated by reduced values in the antioxidant capacity of plasma and its components (i.e., uric acid, protein SH groups, unconjugated bilirubin, vitamin C, vitamin E, and unidentified antioxidants in plasma). Furthermore, elevated markers of lipid and protein oxidation damage, such as malondialdehyde, F2-isoprostane, and total carbonyls, have been observed in septic patients, and some of these markers have been associated with mortality. In addition, it has been reported that an increased plasma concentration of NO products occurs (e.g., peroxynitrite) in patients with septic shock; and novel, molecular biomarkers that are related to genes involved in the immune response, which includes genes related to the innate and adaptive immune responses, cell cycling, differentiation, extracellular remodeling, and immune modulation, have been used in longitudinal, pre-clinical trials of this disease. The current trend is to find more sensitive biomarkers for acute pathologies, such as SIRS and septic shock, that are associated with high mortality. Identifying children who could benefit from specific therapeutic approaches that target the occurrence of oxidative stress will only be achieved by early diagnosis.

ABBREVIATIONS

EPR:	Electron paramagnetic resonance
$DCFH_2$:	Dichlorodihydrofluorescein
DCF:	Dichlorofluorescein
$CO_3^{\bullet}$:	Carbonate radical

$NO_2^\bullet$:	Nitrogen dioxide radical
RhH_2:	Dihydrorhodamine
$LC^{2+:}$	bis-N-methylacridinium dinitrate
$LC^{\bullet:}$	lucigenin
LH:	luminol
DMPO:	1-pyrroline N-oxide
DPPH:	2,2-diphenyl-1-picrylhydrazyl
ABTS:	2,2'-azinobis(3-ethylbenzthiazoline-6-sulfonic acid) cation radical
ORAC:	Oxygen radical absorbance capacity,
TRAP:	Total radical antioxidant parameter
TEAC:	Trolox equivalent antioxidant capacity
FRAP:	Ferric Reducing Antioxidant Power
CUPRAC:	Cupric Reducing Antioxidant Power
$LOO^\bullet$	Lipid peroxyl radical
MDA:	Malondialdehyde
4-HNE:	4-hydroxy-2-nonenal
IsoPs:	Isoprostanes
TBA:	Thiobarbituric acid
PAR:	Poly-ADP ribose
ALI:	Acute lung injury
$ONOO^-$:	Peroxynitrite
HPLC:	High performance liquid chromatography
MS:	Mass spectrometry
3-NT:	3-nitrotyrosine
Nrf2:	Nuclear factor erythroid 2-related factor 2
HUVEC:	Human umbilical vein endothelial cells
FABP1:	Fatty acid-binding protein 1
PMX-F:	Polymyxin B-immobilized fiber hemoperfusion
PON1:	Serum paraoxonase 1
8-OHdG:	8-deoxyguanosine

2. Introduction

Regardless of how oxidative stress is defined, a persistent pro-oxidant environment in cells can modify redox-sensitive molecules. A common approach to assess oxidative stress in biological systems involves the measurement of the increase or decrease in a redox-sensitive molecule that responds to oxidative stress. In general, reliable markers of oxidative stress possess the following qualities: i) chemically unique and detectable, ii) increase or decrease during periods of oxidative stress, iii) possessing relatively long half-lives, and iv) not influenced by other cellular processes (e.g., cell cycle, energy metabolism, etc.).

3. General Concepts of Oxidative Stress Biomarkers

Plasma antioxidant potential in septic patients has been shown to be lower than that in healthy subjects at the beginning of the disease, later increasing to normal or even supranormal levels in septic patients who survived, but not in patients who died [1]. Lipid peroxidation products levels are higher, as shown by increased levels of thiobarbituric acid-reactive substances, in septic patients who develop MODS. In addition, increased levels of malondialdehyde, another marker of lipid peroxidation, have been reported in survivors in relation to nonsurvivors [2]. Xanthine oxidase is an enzymatic source of ROS that has been shown to be activated in sepsis, pointing to a failure of microvasculature control that leads to underperfusion and ischemia. In children, a potential association between markers of oxidative modifications and intensive care disease severity scores, such as PIM 2 (Paediatric Index of Mortality 2), PELOD (Paediatric Logistic Organ Dysfunction) and PELODd (Paediatric Logistic Organ Dysfunction daily) [3], has not been established.

3.1 Detection of Free Radicals

Free radicals play a relevant role in the functioning of multiple biological systems. Our understanding of their particular role in certain physiological or pathophysiological processes—that is, whether under certain circumstances they are friends, foes, or both—is based on our ability to perform a reliable measurement of free radicals under conditions pertinent to the normal functioning of biological systems. Ideally, that would require in vivo measurements of free radicals. Although some progress along this view has been achieved we are still confronted with many methodological obstacles even when measuring free radicals in rather simple systems, such as isolated cell membranes. The most important difficulty in detecting free radicals is their exceptionally short lifetime, which practically impedes their direct measurement (it is technically possible to directly detect the existence of some free radicals in real time, but not in biological systems). Hence, it is necessary to introduce into the system under investigation a compound (scavenging or trapping agents) that reacts with radicals, forming producing a more stable compound, which can be detected by conventional techniques. Various methods have been applied and EPR (Electron paramagnetic resonance) spin trapping has proven to be the best [4].

3.1.1 Spectrophotometric versus EPR Techniques in the Detection of Free Radicals

Detection of short-life free radicals is a difficult task, even in pure free radical generating chemical systems. The half-life of an $OH^{\bullet}$ radical is the a few nanoseconds, while the half-life of superoxide is typically on the order of tenths of microseconds. Any substance that scavenges short-lived radicals and transforms them into long-lived ones which can be subsequently detected using, for example, the spectrophotometry can be used in vitro. However, detection is more cumbersome in biological systems, since these regularly produce more than one free radical species and their presence produces some methodological limitations, since some of the substances used interact with the biological systems investigated. For example, most of the measurements of $O2^{\bullet}$ radicals were performed by coupling them to colored or chemiluminescent compounds, such as during the nitroblue tetrazolium reduction or stimulation of lucigenin luminescence. However, the lucigenin should not be used in the presence of flavoprotein reductases or other enzymatic reducing systems, since it has been shown that under these conditions lucigenin itself can generate $O2^{\bullet}$ [5]. The use of nitroblue tetrazolium reduction and cytochrome c reduction suffers from short comings of questionable specificity and low sensitivity. These problems are best illustrated in comparative methodological studies demonstrating that test reactions commonly used for the assay of $O2^{\bullet}$ production by eukaryotic cells or their components can lead to divergent results even when applied to the same experimental system. Such short comings can be bypassed by using EPR spin trapping, a technique based on a reaction in which the transient radical species reacts with specific nitrone or nitroso spin-traps to yield more persistent nitroxide spin adducts. These are readily detected by EPR spectroscopy qualitatively (different species can be distinguished) and with greater sensitivity. For example, detection of the superoxide radical with EPR spin trap DEPMPO (5-diethoxyphosphoryl-5-methyl-1-pyrroline-N-oxide) is 40 times more sensitive than spectrophotometric cytochrome c assay [6]. Despite this, the use of the EPR technique of spin trapping has an illustrious history in detecting •OH and $O2^{\bullet}$ in biology and chemistry.

The EPR spin trapping has a prominent, but not fully exploited role in detecting oxygen (as well as the other) radicals in some biological systems. The development of new spin traps with improved capabilities will certainly expand the range of application of EPR spin trapping. Technically this is not very complicated, but certain rules should be observed to obtain reliable results.

3.1.2 Chemical Probes

With the rapid growth of interest in free radicals in biology has come a need to identify radicals being produced, to measure either their integrated production rates or the steady-state (instantaneous) concentrations, and to visualize their spatial distribution. The ideal chemical probe for a free radical, or a non-radical product such as hydrogen peroxide, would be highly reactive at low concentrations; specific; sensitive; without other reactivity; nontoxic; well-characterized chemically; easy to load into organelles, cells, or tissues without subsequent leakage or unwanted diffusion, excretion, or metabolism; readily available; easy to use without too specialized apparatus; and cheap. No probe matches this challenging specification, but probes generating either a fluorescent product or inducing chemiluminescence offer high sensitivity and can be applied using a variety of analytical techniques, from “plate readers” with fluorescence detection, through high performance liquid chromatography, to sophisticated optical microscopy involving multiphoton excitation with the potential to create three-dimensional images of radical generation in tissue.

3.1.2.1 Dihydrofluoresceins

Dichlorodihydrofluorescein ($DCFH_2$) is by far the commonest probe; the main reaction pathways involved in its use in biology are outlined in figure 1(Fig. 1). We consider first the initial step, of oxidation of $DCFH_2$ to its radical $DCFH^{\bullet}$. Dichlorodihydrofluorescein has very low reactivity toward superoxide radicals, or the dismutation product, hydrogen peroxide—although the latter can facilitate oxidation indirectly via a catalyst as described below: any "background" oxidation of $DCFH_2$ by $O_2^{\bullet}$ or H_2O_2 probably reflects metal impurities in the buffer, etc. (Oxidation by Fenton chemistry ($Fe(II)/H_2O_2$) was characterized in Chapter 1.

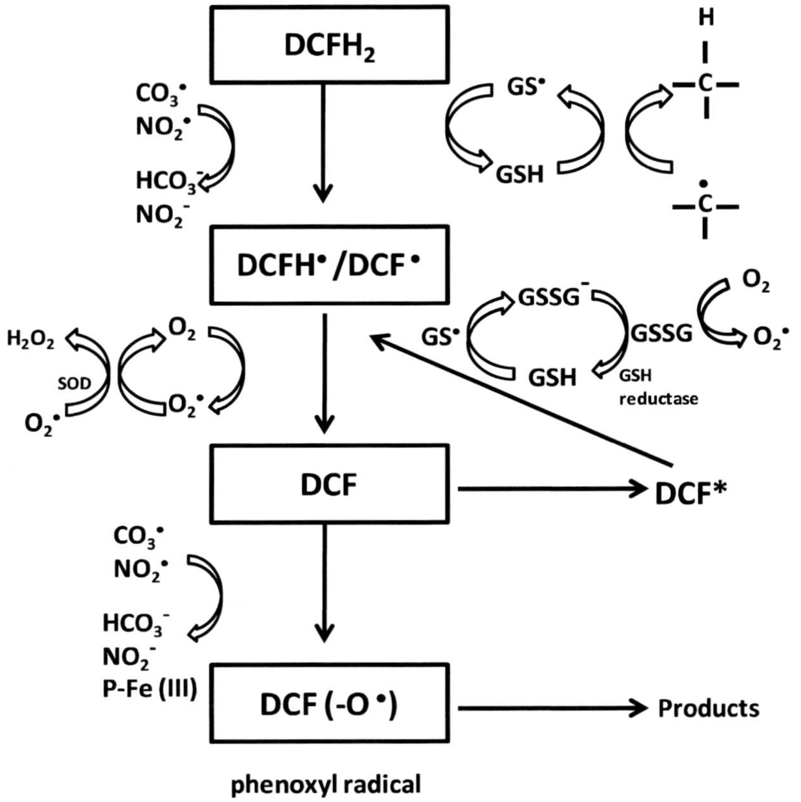

Figure 1. Main reaction pathways possible in the use of reduced fluorescein dyes such as dichlorodihydrofluorescein to measure reactive species in vitro. P, peroxidase-like catalysts. DCFH2:Dichlorodihydrofluorescein; CO3• : Carbonate radical; NO2•:Nitrogen dioxide radical; HCO3: bicarbonate; DCF• : Dichlorofluorescein radical; GSH: glutathione; GSSG: glutathione disulphide; H2O2: Hydrogen peroxide; Fe(III): Ferric ions.

Superoxide dismutase had no effect on $DCFH_2$ oxidation when $O_2^{\bullet}$ was generated enzymatically; exceedingly weak fluorescence was observed when $O_2^{\bullet}$ was generated by the radiolysis of oxygenated formate solutions (a highly specific, well-quantified and controllable source of superoxide) containing $DCFH_2$. Hence by itself (i.e., without a catalyst), $DCFH_2$ is not actually a useful probe for the two commonest "reactive oxygen species" in biology, despite still being widely viewed as such. It is also probably not effectively reactive directly with peroxynitrite, although several studies have shown oxidation initiated by peroxynitrite. However, efficient conversion of $DCFH_2$ to DCF was reported using $CO_3^{\bullet}$ and $NO_2^{\bullet}$ as oxidants, species that can be formed via peroxynitrite [7].

Comparable effort has not been directed toward other probes, but the comparison above of the reactivity of $CO_3^{\bullet}$ and $NO_2^{\bullet}$ toward $DCFH_2$ or RhH_2 with reactions of these radicals with phenol or aniline are important pointers suggestive that other reduced fluoresceins, Amplex Red, and dihydrocalcein will behave qualitatively similarly to $DCFH_2$; other reactions of rhodamines, too, can be predicted by appropriate comparison with aromatic amines [8].

While superoxide is unreactive toward the common probes based on fluorescein or rhodamine, its dismutation product, H_2O_2, can participate in catalyzed oxidation cycles. Catalysts can include trace iron and copper (e.g., buffer impurities) via Fenton chemistry, but the commonest catalysts are hemes. Peroxidase or hematin was used as a required component in early studies applying $DCFH_2$ to measure H_2O_2 (and a wide variety of organic hydroperoxides [9]), but this requirement seems to have been overlooked by many authors despite the importance of catalysts being demonstrated in these and several subsequent studies. Peroxidase-like catalysis of $DCFH_2$ and/or RhH_2 oxidation has been reported by the commonest peroxidase, from horseradish, but also with cytochrome c, which is a general catalyst for oxidation of a variety of organic molecules and nitrite by H_2O_2 [10].

3.1.2.2 Involvement of Antioxidants in Probe Chemistry

Four separate aspects of the involvement of antioxidants in probe chemistry must be considered: the direct competition between the probe and antioxidants for reactions with radicals such as $CO3^{\bullet}$ and $NO2^{\bullet}$; the reaction of antioxidant radicals, such as thiyl radicals, with the probes; the reactions of antioxidants with intermediates of catalyst chemistry such as peroxidases; and the "repair" of probe radicals by antioxidants. Rate constants for the reactions of oxidizing radicals with probes enable us to assess the possibility that the probe response might reflect changes in the levels of intracellular antioxidants rather than, or as well as, changes in the flux of "reactive oxygen/nitrogen" species. The key comparison is with the product of the rate constant and the concentration of the probe or antioxidant. The main problems in such a comparison are twofold: first, few users of the probes measure the intracellular concentrations of the probes; second, even if these concentrations were measured, the values usually reflect the average cytosolic concentrations; therefore, a comparison in a particular organelle may be more appropriate.

To illustrate this point, a representative concentration of DCFH2 of 0.3 mM was assumed. When using this value, if the intracellular GSH concentration is 5 mM, then approximately 67% of the $CO3^{\bullet}$ will be intercepted by the probe that is in competition with the reaction with GSH and only approximately 4% of the $NO2^{\bullet}$ radicals will be scavenged by the probe. Other antioxidants, e.g., urate (particularly in plasma) and ascorbate (in tissue samples), must also be considered. Both cysteine and urate inhibited the peroxynitrite-mediated oxidation of dihydrorhodamine. It was therefore stressed that many studies probably involve non-saturating concentrations of probes and that changes in probe loading or in antioxidant levels will result in a change in probe response, even at a constant oxidizing radical flux. Of course, if "oxidative stress" is defined as a disturbance of the pro-oxidant–antioxidant balance in favor of the former [11] then probe response might encompass this broad definition.

The simple competition for reaction is not the only factor in probe chemistry; the reaction of oxidizing radicals with thiols generates thiyl radicals, which are also reactive toward $DCFH_2$. The thiol and oxygen concentrations influence $DCFH_2$ oxidation by $GS^{\bullet}$, and the effects of GSH/GSSG on DCF formation in the presence of cytochrome c or HRP [12] have been reported, but these studies used lower concentrations of $DCFH_2$ than what is used in cellular systems. Thus, the oxidation of $DCFH_2$ by thiyl radicals would have been much less likely in these studies than under more biomimetic conditions because other pathways for thiyl radical reactions would be favored at such low $DCFH_2$ levels. The vitamin E analog Trolox enhanced DCF formation in a cell-free system [13], although the kinetics of radical transfer between the two phenols have not been reported.

3.1.2.3 Probes Reactive toward Peroxynitrite and Peroxyl Radicals

In somewhat related studies having potentially wider applicability but less selectivity, fluorescein esters with oxidizable phenolic or anilinyl substituents have been shown to react with OH•, ONOO–, and ClO– to release free fluorescein. While this concept is, in fact, based on oxidation, it is a substituent in fluorescein that is oxidized, and not dihydrofluorescein, and thus the approach shares some conceptual basis with the above probes based on nucleophilic release of a leaving group. The work extends from earlier related studies on probes for OH• [14].

From observations of cyclization reactions of some ketones on treatment with peroxynitrite, a probe was developed which is based on oxidation modifying a ketone substituent to release the free fluorescein derivative [15]. Selectivity toward peroxynitrite, and fluorescence from neuronal cells treated with the peroxynitrite donor, was reported although whether reaction is actually via NO2• and/or CO3• is unknown. A probe reactive toward peroxyl radicals has been recently described [16]. Oxidation of a phenol/fluorescein conjugate by peroxyl radicals stimulated release of free fluorescein in a related probe. These studies illustrate both current interest in developing new probes which avoid some of the pitfalls of the reduced dyes, and the elegance of new rationally designed probes, but further studies are needed to characterize reactivity as well as the potential of interference by biomolecules.

3.1.2.3.1 Chemiluminescent ProbesfFor Superoxide: Lucigenin

Chemiluminescence can be an extremely sensitive detection method for radical production. Lucigenin, i.e., bis-N-methylacridinium dinitrate (LC^{2+}), has been used in over a thousand studies as a luminescent indicator of superoxide production. However, there is no doubt that, like $DCFH_2$, this probe has the potential to generate superoxide radicals. Luminescence occurs via the addition of superoxide to the free radical that is obtained upon the reduction of lucigenin ($LC^{\bullet}$), which forms an unstable dioxetane (Fig. 2).

The dioxetane cleaves spontaneously to produce N-methylacridone in an excited state, and this substance emits light. Lucigenin is not specific for superoxide; numerous nucleophiles and reducing agents can also induce luminescence (including alkaline H_2O_2) [17]. This occurrence is not surprising because reducing agents can generate the radical $LC^{\bullet}$, which generates a superoxide via a reaction, which can be observed either indirectly, e.g., by cytochrome c reduction, more specifically by spin trapping the superoxide that is produced [18], or directly by real-time observation of the absorbance of the $LC^{\bullet}$.

Several articles have defended the use of lucigenin as a probe for superoxide and have suggested the use of very low concentrations of lucigenin to reduce the effects of redox cycling. While redox cycling to generate $O2^{\bullet}$ will always occur with lucigenin, if low concentrations of the probe are used, additional superoxide will be formed via the following reaction: $LC^{\bullet} + O_2 \leftrightarrow LC^{2+} + O_2^{\bullet}$, which is a reaction that may become insignificant when compared to basal or otherwise stimulated levels.

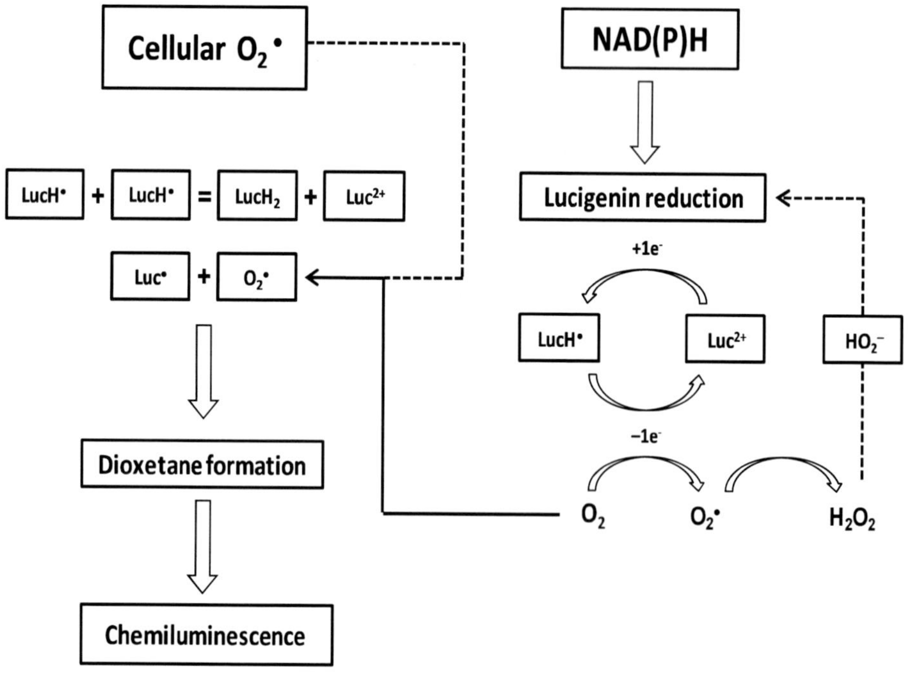

Figure 2. Schematic representation of the underlying chemistry of lucigenin chemiluminescence. Luc2+ = lucigenin; LH• = a lucigenin radical created by the one electron reduction of Luc2+. The reaction of LH• with oxygen generates O2•. The latter then participates in an oxygenation reaction with LH• generating a dioxetane that decomposes with the generation of chemiluminescence. Any entity that can bring about the one electron reduction of lucigenin can potentially create a redox cycle in the presence of oxygen that produces high levels of O2• and chemiluminescence. It is impossible to distinguish the relative contribution of such probe-dependent and cell-dependent chemiluminescence.

How low the concentration of probe must be to effectively eliminate this problem is likely to vary between biological systems and will reflect differences in reductase activity. In one study involving vascular homogenates, 5 μM LC^{2+} was sufficient to induce a doubling of superoxide that was trapped by 1-pyrroline N-oxide (DMPO) in a spin trap. [19], and the same concentration of LC^{2+} exhibited effects on endothelium-dependent relaxation of aortic endothelial cells [20].

However, even with the use of low probe concentrations to reduce the effects of redox cycling, any reagent, including superoxide, which can change the steady-state concentration of $LC^{\bullet}$ has the potential to influence the probe response. In this regard, an obvious contender would be, in some applications, quinones, which are used as tools to stimulate superoxide generation [21].

3.1.2.3.2 Luminol

The chemistry of this probe has been studied rather extensively. Luminol is known to illicit chemiluminescence under a nearly unlimited variety of conditions [22], which should caution us to its use in biology. Additionally, some authors concluded that "luminol-dependent chemiluminescence gives at present very little ability to discriminate between individual oxygen and radical species Furthermore, luminol-dependent chemiluminescence used in biological systems is extremely prone to much interference, which is very difficult to control. [23,24]."

Despite these cautions, the luminol probe remains in widespread use. It is therefore important to outline the basis for its limitations. Luminol emits chemiluminescence via a two-step process that begins with a precursor of the emitting species, and the initial step is oxidative, which is in contrast to lucigenin. However, the luminal radical that is obtained upon oxidation reacts with oxygen to generate $O2^{\bullet}$; therefore, some parallels between the two probes exist. The initial oxidation step, where luminol (LH^{-}) is converted to the radical ($LH^{\bullet}$), cannot be achieved by superoxide, but most other biologically relevant oxidants react with luminol.

Chemiluminescence occurs with luminol and peroxynitrite, which is modulated by bicarbonate/CO2 [25], but the rate constant for the reaction of peroxynitrite decay in the presence of luminal has not been reported. Therefore, it is not clear whether a similar situation, as with peroxynitrite and $DCFH_2$ and RhH_2, i.e., homolysis to $NO2^{\bullet}$ and/or reaction with CO2, occurs faster than peroxynitrite can oxidize luminol.

Antioxidants could compete with radicals and lead to the oxidation of luminol to LH, and they could react directly with this key intermediate; indeed, the effects on luminescence have been used to assay antioxidants, such as urate and ascorbate, in biological fluids [26]. The (hypo)xanthine/xanthine oxidase system is a popular and convenient source of superoxide in model systems. The by-product, urate, has a marked inhibitory effect on luminal chemiluminescence [27], presumably because of the reaction of urate with $LH^{\bullet}$. In addition to thiyl radicals, ascorbate radicals have been observed during the oxidation of luminol by peroxidase, and probably via the interaction of ascorbate with $LH^{\bullet}$. A further complication in the biological applications of luminol is the possibility that the obligate intermediate radical, $LH^{\bullet}$, can be routed down a "dark" pathway by reacting with nitric oxide [28].

3.2 Assessment of Antioxidant Defense

Antioxidants may be defined as substances that, when present at lower concentrations than an oxidizable substrate, significantly delay, or inhibit, the oxidation of that substrate. Some antioxidants are proteins and enzymes, while others are small molecules. Mechanistically, antioxidants may be classified into the following groups: preventing antioxidants, scavenging antioxidants, and repair and de novo antioxidants. The preventing antioxidants function as the first line of defense against oxidants by suppressing the formation of reactive oxygen and nitrogen species (ROS and RNS, respectively) by reducing hydrogen peroxide and lipid hydroperoxides to water and lipid hydroxides, respectively, or by sequestering metal ions such as iron and copper. The scavenging antioxidants rapidly remove active species before they attack biologically essential molecules. Superoxide dismutase (SOD) converts superoxide to hydrogen peroxide, while carotenoids scavenge singlet oxygens, either physically or chemically. Many phenolic compounds and aromatic amines act as free radical-scavenging antioxidants. These scavenging antioxidants act as the second line of defense against oxidants in vivo. Various enzymes function in the third line of defense against oxidation by repairing damage, clearing wastes, and reconstituting lost functions. In addition, the adaptation mechanism functions as the fourth line of defense against oxidation and assures that appropriate antioxidants are generated at the correct time, are transferred to the right position, and are present in the correct concentrations. Furthermore, there is increasing evidence that shows that some antioxidants act as cellular signaling messengers that regulate the level of antioxidant compounds and enzymes. Various antioxidant compounds and enzymes play their roles at their respective sites and constitute a total defense network system in vivo. The term "antioxidant" is often used differently and may mean different things, which could cause inconsistency, ambiguity, and confusion. Often, the free radical-scavenging antioxidants are simply called antioxidants. Additionally, the critical oxidative modification of lipids, proteins, nucleic acids, and carbohydrates is induced and is mediated by free radicals and by non-radical mechanisms and, as such, various antioxidant compounds and enzymes with different functions are necessary for the defense network. The free radical-scavenging antioxidants serve as players in this defense system.

3.2.1 Factors that Determine the Radical Scavenging Capacity

Certain factors determine the antioxidant capacity for scavenging free radicals; therefore, understanding the mechanisms and dynamics of antioxidant action are essential for the proper selection of the assay method and interpretation of the resulting data. The quantitative structural activity is determined by the chemical structure of the antioxidant compound, but the actual free radical scavenging capacity of antioxidant compounds is determined by several factors shown below:

- i. the chemical reactivity toward free radicals and the stoichiometric number, that is, the rate of radical scavenging and the number of radical molecules that are scavenged;
- ii. the fate of antioxidant-derived radicals;
- iii. the interaction with other antioxidants;
- iv. the concentration and mobility of the antioxidant in the environment; and
- v. the absorption, distribution, retention, and metabolism of the antioxidant.

These factors determine the capacity and efficacy of an antioxidant. Various free radicals with different biological, chemical and physical properties may be involved in oxidative stress and include the following: $OH^{\bullet}$, alkoxyl, peroxyl, $O_2^{\bullet}$, $NO^{\bullet}$, and $S^{\bullet}$- and $N^{\bullet}$- centered radicals. It is unlikely that any antioxidant will scavenge hydroxyl and alkoxyl radicals efficiently in vivo because these radicals react predominantly with lipids, proteins, carbohydrates, and DNA, which are all less reactive but present in much higher concentrations than antioxidants. Superoxide and nitric oxide are too "unreactive" to attack biological molecules and induce their oxidation. Peroxyl radicals, i.e., the chain-carrying species of lipid peroxidation that have moderate reactivity toward biological molecules, are important targets for antioxidants. Therefore, it is important to assess the capacity of antioxidants for scavenging peroxyl radicals. It may be noted that the relative reactivities of antioxidants toward peroxyl and phenoxyl radicals, such as galvinoxyl, are similar. Another potentially important free radical is nitrogen dioxide, which adds to the double bond of a lipid to induce lipid peroxidation and results in nitro-fatty acids and other nitrogen-containing products [29].

3.2.2 Assessment of the Free Radical Scavenging Capacity of Antioxidants in Vitro

The free radical scavenging capacities of antioxidants in vitro have been evaluated by several different methods and under different conditions, and these capacities have been expressed using terms such as ability, activity, capacity, efficacy, parameter, potential, power, and reactivity. Unfortunately, in many reports, it was not clearly specified what was actually assessed. The "antioxidant capacity" often means different things at different occasions and to different people. This term may refer to the capacity of an antioxidant compound for scavenging free radicals or the capacity of "antioxidation", that is, how much and how long antioxidant compounds or the substances that contain antioxidants suppress oxidation. These refer to different things, and it is important to show which capacity is actually assessed.

3.2.2.1 The Reaction of an Antioxidant with a Stable Free Radical

The capacity of an antioxidant compound for scavenging free radicals should be assessed by two factors: the rate of scavenging radicals and the number of radicals each antioxidant molecule can scavenge, which are inherently determined by the chemical structure of the antioxidant compound and by the free radicals. These two parameters can be measured by following the reaction with a stable, reference-free radical, such as galvinoxyl and 2,2-diphenyl-1-picrylhydrazyl (DPPH) [30]. These radicals are commercially available, stable, easy to handle, and have strong visible absorptions with high molar extinction coefficients; hence, their reactions with an antioxidant can be followed easily using a conventional UV/visible absorption spectrophotometer. The 2,2'-azinobis(3-ethylbenzthiazoline-6-sulfonic acid) cation radical, $ABTS^{\bullet}$, is also stable and similarly used. In contrast to galvinoxyl and DPPH, which are stable free radicals, the ABTS radical cation must be generated from ABTS before measurement. The ABTS cation radical is soluble in water and organic solvent and can be applied similar to galvinoxyl and DPPH.

3.2.2.2 Assessment of an Antioxidant by the Competition Method

The capacity of an antioxidant and mixtures containing antioxidant compounds for scavenging free radicals has been widely assessed by a competition method using a reference compound, such as a probe. Various reference compounds have been applied as probes, and the capacity of antioxidants for scavenging free radicals has been assessed by measuring the extent of the suppression of probe consumption, which can be measured by UV/visible absorption, fluorescence, chemiluminescence, or EPR spectroscopy. Various methods have been developed and applied. Of these, the oxygen radical absorbance capacity (ORAC), total radical antioxidant parameter (TRAP), Trolox equivalent antioxidant capacity (TEAC), and total oxyradical scavenging capacity (TOSC) have been used most frequently [31]. The TRAP method was first applied for human plasma by measuring oxygen absorption with an oxygen electrode and then by measuring the decrease in fluorescence by R-phycoerythrin [32].

ORAC is one of the most widely used methods. In the typical ORAC assay, the loss of fluorescence of a probe, such as phycoerythrin or fluorescein, is followed over time in the absence and presence of antioxidant. The area under the fluorescence decay curve (AUC) is calculated, and the net increase in the AUC (i.e., (the AUC in the presence of antioxidant) – (the AUC in the absence of antioxidant)), is used to evaluate the antioxidant capacity (Fig. 3).

ORAC values are usually expressed as a Trolox equivalent, and the ORAC assay has been adapted to measure lipophilic and hydrophilic antioxidants using a solution of 50% acetone/50% water (v/v) that contains 7% randomly methylated beta-cyclodextrin to solubilize the antioxidants [33]. The capacity of antioxidants may also be assessed using heterogeneous aqueous suspensions such as micelles, liposomal membranes, low-density lipoprotein or plasma. It is essential that, in kinetic analyses, free radicals are generated at a constant and controlled rate and that the site and lipophilic and hydrophilic azo-initiators be used as a convenient source of free radicals.

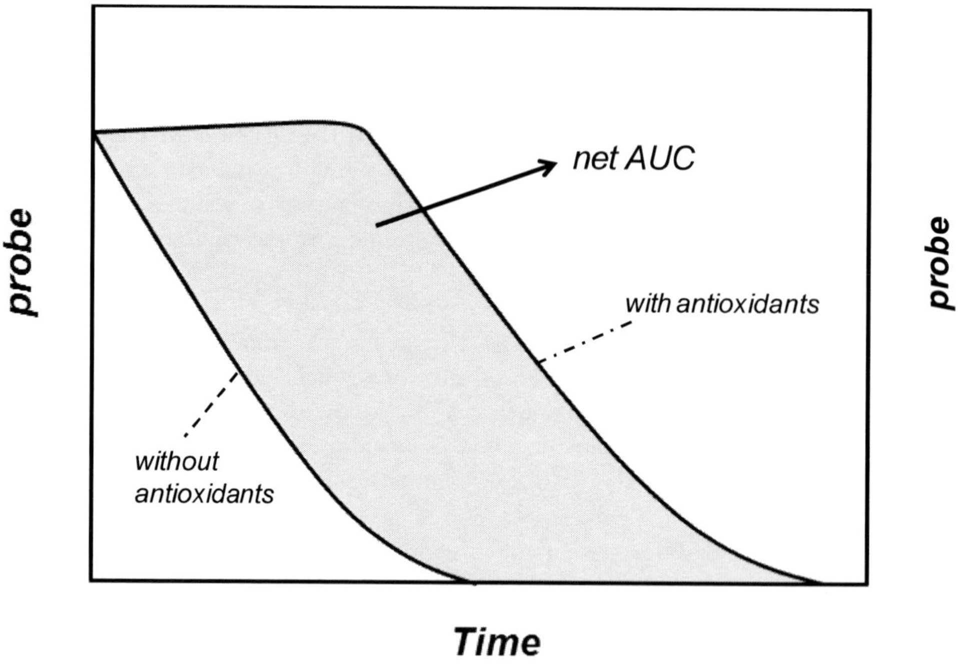

Figure 3. Assessment of radical scavenging capacity by competition method such as ORAC method. The consumption of a probe is followed in the absence and presence of tested sample and the capacity is assessed from the net area under the curve (AUC).

3.2.2.3 Assessment of Antioxidants by the Reduction of Metal Ions

A potent radical scavenging antioxidant often acts as a potent reductant. The FRAP (Ferric Reducing Antioxidant Power) [34] and CUPRAC (Cupric Reducing Antioxidant Power) [35] methods measure the ability of an antioxidant to reduce ferric [Fe(III)] and cupric [Cu(II)] ions to their respective lower valency states. The capacity that is measured by the FRAP or CUPRAC methods does not always correlate well with that for radical scavenging, which is measured by a competitive method such as ORAC. Interestingly, it was found that α-tocopherol and α-tocotrienol reduced cupric sulfate, but β, γ, and δ tocopherols and tocotrienols did not [36]. The separation and assessment of the reducing capacity of antioxidant compounds that were present in the mixtures have been performed using high-performance liquid chromatography that was coupled with electrochemical detection [37]. Additionally, because Fe(II) and Cu(I) are more reactive than Fe(III) and Cu(II) in decomposing hydrogen peroxide and hydroperoxides, the antioxidants that reduce metal ions may exert pro-oxidant effects under certain conditions. A typical example of this reaction is the combination of ascorbic acid and iron, which is known and used to induce free radical-mediated oxidation in vitro. However, iron and copper are sequestered by proteins in vivo, they are not readily reduced by ascorbate, and it was reported that ascorbic acid does not act as a pro-oxidant *in vivo* [38]. Polyphenols may also bind to metal ions and form a complex, which may be another antioxidant function of polyphenolic compounds.

3.2.3 Antioxidant Capacity in Vivo

The capacity of antioxidants in vivo is determined by many factors and should be taken into consideration during assessment. One of these factors is bioavailability. Antioxidants should be absorbed, transported, distributed, and retained properly in biological fluids, cells and tissues. The bioavailability of various antioxidants and the effects of dosage and duration have been studied by analyzing biological fluids and tissues of humans and experimental animals after being administered antioxidants. The time-course change in the concentrations of metabolites and the parent antioxidants have been analyzed. For some antioxidants, a different capacity is observed in vitro and in vivo. For example, 2,2,5,7,8-pentamethyl-6-chromanol (PMC) exerts a more potent activity than α-tocopherol against the lipid peroxidation of membranes, oxidative modification of LDL, and oxidative hemolysis of erythrocytes in vitro [39], but the efficacy of PMC in vivo is small because it is not retained in the cell but is excreted rapidly. Metabolism also affects the antioxidant capacity *in vivo*. Some antioxidants may undergo biotransformation through enzymatic conjugation with sulfate, methyl, or glucuronide groups [40]. Probucol, i.e., 4,4'-(isopropylidenedithio) bis(2,6-di-tert-butylphenol), is an anti-atherogenic drug that has antioxidant and lipid-lowering capacities. An interesting feature of probucol is the different pattern of metabolite or oxidation products between species. Diphenoquinone, bisphenol, and their precursor spiroquinone have been found in the sera of probucol-treated rabbits and mice. However, neither bisphenol nor diphenoquinone was detected in humans who were administered 500 mg/day of probucol for more than two months and whose LDL contained 6.1 +/- 2.0 molecules of probucol per LDL particle (n=12) [41,42]. These results suggested that the results of animal experiments should be treated with caution.

It should be noted that the role of antioxidants in the gastrointestinal tract might also be important. Diets contain various prooxidants, which include metals such as iron, copper, and heme, lipid hydroperoxides, aldehydes, and nitrite. Elevated levels of lipid peroxides have been observed in the postprandial state [43], and the activation of phagocytes in the gut may also increase ROS/RNS. These pro-oxidants may induce oxidative stress in the gastrointestinal tract, which could induce stomach ulcers that could develop into stomach, colon, or rectal cancer. The antioxidants that are contained in foods may suppress these oxidative stressors and their related diseases in the gastrointestinal tract before they are absorbed [44]. The capacity and efficacy of antioxidants *in vivo* may be assessed most accurately by the effect of antioxidant compounds and materials on the level of oxidation in biological fluids and tissues, such as plasma, erythrocytes, urine, and cerebrospinal fluids, from humans and experimental animals. Additionally, saliva and tears may be used. Reliable biomarkers are essential for this purpose, and many biomarkers for oxidative stress have been applied to measure the level of oxidation *in vivo*. The oxidation products of lipids, oxidative modification and expression of proteins and sugars, strand breaks of DNA and oxidation products of DNA bases have been used as oxidative stress biomarkers [45].

The effects of various antioxidants on the levels of biomarkers of oxidative stress have been evaluated in many studies on humans and experimental animals under normal and oxidative stress conditions. The effects of antioxidants have also been assessed in some clinical intervention studies and model animals for specific diseases. Some studies confirmed the positive effects of antioxidants and antioxidant-rich diets to reduce the level of oxidative stress *in vivo*, while others did not show any significant effects, in spite of an increase in the levels of those antioxidants. In contrast to cultured cells, which are often antioxidant-deficient and respond well to added antioxidants, the beneficial effects of antioxidants are difficult to observe in normal healthy subjects who have sufficient amounts of antioxidants, although high doses of vitamin E were found to decrease the plasma level of F2-isoprostanes [46]. Current evidence suggests that antioxidant intake does not reduce oxidative stress biomarkers appreciably in healthy individuals who have sufficient amounts of antioxidants under normal conditions, but antioxidants have been found to lower such biomarkers in subjects who were malnourished and had increased oxidative stress or in patients with diseases that were related to oxidative stress [47].

3.2.4 The GSH/GSSG Ratio

Here, we briefly describe the role of the major thiol antioxidant and redox buffer of the cell, the tripeptide glutathione (GSH) [48]. The oxidized form of glutathione is GSSG, glutathione disulfide. Glutathione is highly abundant in the cytosol (1–11 mM), nuclei (3–15 mM), and mitochondria (5–11 mM) and is the major soluble antioxidant in these cellular compartments. Because GSH is synthesized in the cytosol by the sequential actions of glutamate–cysteine ligase and glutathione synthetase, its mitochondrial presence requires inner membrane transport. Two mitochondrial electroneutral antiport carrier proteins have been shown to have the capacity to transport GSH: the dicarboxylate carrier protein and the 2-oxoglutarate carrier protein. Recently, it has been shown that externally added GSH is readily taken up by mitochondria, despite approximately 8 mM GSH being present in the mitochondrial matrix [49]. It therefore appears that GSH is taken up against a concentration gradient.

The main protective roles of glutathione against oxidative stress are the following: (i) glutathione is a cofactor of several detoxifying enzymes that act against oxidative stress, e.g., glutathione peroxidase (GPx) and glutathionetransferase; (ii) GSH participates in amino acid transport through the plasma membrane; (iii) GSH directly scavenges hydroxyl radicals and singlet oxygens, which detoxify hydrogen peroxide and lipid peroxides by the catalytic action of glutathionperoxidase; and (iv) glutathione is able to regenerate the most important antioxidants, Vitamins C and E, back to their active forms. Glutathione can reduce the tocopherol radical of Vitamin E directly or indirectly via the reduction of semidehydroascorbate to ascorbate [50]. The capacity of glutathione to regenerate the most important antioxidants is linked with the redox state of the glutathione disulfide-glutathione couple (GSSG/2GSH) [51].

Reduced glutathione in the nucleus maintains the redox state of critical protein sulfhydryls that are necessary for DNA repair and expression. Oxidized glutathione accumulates inside cells, and the ratio of GSH/GSSG is a good measure of the oxidative stress of an organism [52]. Normally, GSSG represents less than 1% of the total GSH pool. When H_2O_2 or $ONOO^{\bullet}$ is transiently elevated, an elevation in GSSG, which is also transient, can occur if a mechanism for signaling by means of thiol-disulfide exchange occurs. In this scenario, signaling is indirectly dependent upon ROS generation. Nonetheless, because this mechanism requires a change in GSSG that is usually only observed during oxidative stress, such signaling is more likely an oxidative stress response rather than one of physiologic redox signaling. In a recent study, pro- and anti-oxidant disturbances in sepsis and non-sepsis burn patients with systemic SIRS were evaluated. Pro-oxidant parameters were significantly elevated in sepsis patients at admission, and the intensity of ROS increased in burn patients until the 5th day. The decreased contents of erythrocyte GSH and plasma SH groups in sepsis patients indicated that the depletion of anti-oxidant resources upon admission was caused by prolonged oxidative stress, while acute-burn patients gradually developed oxidative stress during the study period [53]. However, in this and other studies, the oxidized component was not measured, which could be more sensitive to acute oxidative stress. Therefore, it is very important, when estimating the occurrence of oxidative stress in vivo, to measure both components that account for the factors that determine the intracellular redox potential.

3.3 Lipid Peroxides

3.3.1 The Lipid Peroxidation Process

Oxidative stress causes injury to biomolecules such as nucleic acids, proteins, structural carbohydrates, and lipids. Among these targets, the peroxidation of lipids is damaging because the formation of lipid peroxidation products leads to the spread of free radical reactions. The general process of lipid peroxidation consists of three stages: initiation, propagation, and termination [54]. The initiation phase includes hydrogen-atom abstraction. Several species can abstract the first hydrogen atom, and these species include the following radicals: $OH^•$, alkoxyl ($RO^•$), peroxyl ($ROO^•$), and possibly $HO2^•$ but not H_2O_2 or $O_2^•$. The membrane lipids, mainly phospholipids containing polyunsaturated fatty acids, are predominantly susceptible to peroxidation because of the abstraction of a hydrogen atom from a methylene (–CH2–) group, which contains only one electron, and leaves an unpaired electron on the carbon, –•CH–. The presence of a double bond in the fatty acid weakens the C–H bonds on the carbon atom, which are near the double bond, and thus facilitates $H^•$ subtraction. The initial reaction of $OH^•$ with polyunsaturated fatty acids produces a lipid radical (L•), which reacts with molecular oxygen to form a lipid peroxyl radical ($LOO^•$). The $LOO^•$ can abstract hydrogen from an adjacent fatty acid to produce a lipid hydroperoxide (LOOH) and a second lipid radical [54]. The LOOH that is formed can suffer reductive cleavage by reduced metals, such as Fe^{2+}, which produces a lipid alkoxyl radical (LO•). Both alkoxyl and peroxyl radicals stimulate the chain reaction of lipid peroxidation by abstracting additional hydrogen atoms. Peroxidation of lipids can disturb the assembly of the membrane, causing changes in fluidity and permeability, alterations in ion transport, and the inhibition of metabolic processes. Injury to mitochondria that is induced by lipid peroxidation can direct further ROS generation [55]. In addition, LOOH can break down, frequently in the presence of reduced metals or ascorbate, to reactive aldehyde products, which include malondialdehyde (MDA), 4-hydroxy-2-nonenal (HNE), 4-hydroxy-2-hexenal (4-HHE) and acrolein [56]. In fact, these oxidation products have been detected by a simple mass spectrometry method and by the production of a series of hydroxyl-alkenals that are generated from low-density lipoproteins that have undergone oxidation by a copper ion. In addition, some recent publications reported novel results regarding the oxidative products that are derived from the oxidation of erythrocyte membranes *in vitro* [57].

3.3.2 Compounds formed during Lipid Peroxidation

3.3.2.1 F2-Isoprostane

Lipid peroxidation is one of the major outcomes of free radical-mediated injury to tissue. The peroxidation of fatty acyl groups occurs mostly in membrane phospholipids, and peroxidation of lipids can greatly alter the physicochemical properties of membrane lipid bilayers, which results in severe cellular dysfunction. In addition, a variety of lipid byproducts are produced because of lipid peroxidation, some of which can exert adverse and/or beneficial biological effects on a cell. Several in vitro markers of oxidative stress are available, but most of these markers are of limited value in vivo because they lack sensitivity and/or specificity or require invasive methods. Isoprostanes (IsoPs) are prostaglandin (PG)-like compounds that are produced in vivo independently of cyclooxygenase enzymes, i.e., primarily by free radical-induced peroxidation of arachidonic acid. F(2)-IsoPs are members of a group of 64 compounds that are isomeric in structure to cyclooxygenase-derived PGF(2 alpha). Other products of the IsoP pathway are also formed in vivo by rearrangement of labile PGH(2)-like IsoP intermediates, which include E(2)-,D(2)-IsoPs,cyclopentenone-A(2)-,J(2)-IsoPs and highly reactive acyclic-ketoaldehydes (isoketals). The measurement of F-(2)-IsoPs is the most reliable approach to assess oxidative stress status *in vivo* and is an important tool for exploring the role of oxidative stress in the pathogenesis of human disease. Moreover, F-(2)-IsoPs and other products of the IsoP pathway exert potent biological actions via receptor-dependent and -independent mechanisms and may therefore be pathophysiological mediators of disease. The formation of highly reactive cyclopentenone isoprostane compounds (A3/J3isoprostanes) *in vivo* from eicosapentaenoic acid has been described recently [58]. Oxidation of docosahexaenoic acid, an abundant unsaturated fatty acid that is found in the central nervous system, results in the formation of IsoP-like compounds, termed neuroprostanes.

3.3.2.2 Malondialdehyde

Lipid oxidation can be measured in many ways, but commonly used methods, such as diene conjugation and the use of thiobarbituric acid (TBA)-reactive materials, are of questionable validity. In particular, the simple TBA test should be considered unacceptable in modern research because most TBA-reactive materials in human body fluids are not related to lipid peroxidation. A significant improvement to the TBA test can be made using HPLC to isolate the malondialdehyde (MDA)-TBA chromogen before analysis [61]. One can also assay MDA directly, but MDA is only one of many aldehydes that are formed during lipid peroxidation and can arise from a free radical attack on sialic acid and deoxyribose [62]. Unsaturated aldehydes such as 4-hydroxynonenal and acrolein may cause considerably more cytotoxicity in vivo than MDA; therefore, measuring these molecules is perhaps more logical [63]. Lipid hydroperoxides and aldehydes can also be absorbed from the diet. For example, some foods contain MDA–amino-acid adducts that can be absorbed through the gut and then excreted in the urine [64]. Therefore, it follows that measurements of urinary MDA can be confounded by diet and should not be used as an index of whole-body lipid peroxidation unless the diet is controlled.

3.4 Nitrosative Stress and Nitrotyrosine Detection

Previous studies have revealed the important roles of the different isoforms of nitric oxide (NO) synthases (NOS), peroxynitrite (ONOO-), and poly-ADP ribose (PAR) in the pathophysiology of cardiopulmonary derangement that is induced by acute lung injury (ALI) and sepsis, thereby offering potentially new treatment options, such as the inhibition of NOS, decomposition catalysis of $ONOO^-$, or inhibition of PAR polymerase (PARP) [65].

The pulmonary response to ALI and sepsis in sheep has been comprehensively studied. In vivo studies have shown that excessively produced NO may exert cytotoxic effects by reacting with superoxide radicals from activated neutrophils, thereby yielding reactive oxygen and nitrogen species such as $ONOO^-$. Peroxynitrite, in turn, may induce cell damage by oxidizing and nitrating/nitrosating proteins and lipids and by inducing the excessive activation of the nuclear repair enzyme poly(ADP-ribose) polymerase, which may cause ATP depletion and cell damage [66]. Together, these changes can induce endothelial damage, pulmonary capillary hyperpermeability, and pulmonary edema, which can result in severe deterioration of pulmonary gas exchange.

Nitrotyrosine is often thought to be a specific marker of attack of $ONOO^-$ upon proteins, but this molecule can also be formed from tyrosine by a range of reactive nitrogen species, and its production in vivo is often dependent on the production of such species as $NO2^{\bullet}$ by myeloperoxidase or other peroxidases. 3-Nitrotyrosine has been frequently measured by immunostaining, high performance liquid chromatography (HPLC) and mass spectrometry (MS) in human tissues, but we have been unable to detect it in human urine [43]. Nitrotyrosine is metabolized to 3-nitro-4-hydroxyphenylacetate (NHPA), which some groups have measured in urine as an estimate of nitrotyrosine production in vivo. However, some (and perhaps most) urinary NHPA arises through other mechanisms [67], which makes the assay questionable. Furthermore, simple HPLC-based assays for 3-nitrotyrosine are prone to artifacts; therefore, MS-based techniques are preferred.

Measurements based on MS-assays are used for the sensitive detection of nitro-, chloro- and ortho-tyrosines, which are useful as biomarkers of protein damage by RS and to determine how this damage can be modulated by antioxidant or other interventions. Proteomic methods can be used to separate proteins, followed by identification of the modified protein by blotting, and these techniques were used to identify targets of nitration in the muscle [68].

In a recent study, sheep were subjected to inhalation of 48 breaths of cotton smoke and the instillation of live *Pseudomonas aeruginosa* into both lungs. Lung tissue was obtained at the respective time points for the measurement of neuronal, endothelial, and inducible NOS (nNOS, eNOS, iNOS, respectively) mRNA and protein expression, calcium-dependent and -independent NOS activity, and 3-nitrotyrosine (3-NT) and poly(ADP-ribose) (PAR) protein expression. Changes in the injury-induced, severe pulmonary dysfunction, as indicated by a progressive decline in the oxygenation index and a concomitant increase in pulmonary shunt fraction, were associated with an early and transient increase in eNOS and an early and profound increase in iNOS expression, while the expression of nNOS remained unchanged.

Both 3-NT, a marker of protein nitration, and PAR, an indicator of DNA damage, increased early but only transiently [69].

The interrelation of plasma nitrotyrosine concentrations in septic shock patients and their prognoses were examined. Some studies have shown higher levels of plasma nitrotyrosine in non-survivors. Recently, concentrations of total nitric oxide were found to be stable within individuals, but marked inter-individual differences were only partly accounted for by illness severity or renal dysfunction [70].

The key points for the ideal biomarker of oxidative stress are shown in Table 1.

Table 1. Key points for the ideal biomarker of oxidative stress.

i.	This biomarker is predictive of the later development of disease.
ii.	The biomarker should detect a major part, or at least a fixed percentage, of total ongoing oxidative damage in vivo.
iii.	Its levels should not vary widely in the same subjects under the same conditions at different times.
iv.	It must employ chemically robust measurement technology.
v.	It should ideally be stable on storage, not being lost, or formed artifactually, in stored samples.

4. Pre-Clinical Evidence of the Assessment of Oxidative Stress Biomarkers in a Sepsis Model

Sepsis is a complex inflammatory syndrome with diverse etiology and a wide spectrum of severity. Several researchers have linked ROS and RNS with the onset, progression and outcome of sepsis in pre-clinical studies. Reactive oxygen and nitrogen species are important signaling molecules, but an organism must avoid the overproduction of these species; otherwise, oxidative stress will occur.

In various models of sepsis, such as cecal ligation and two-hole puncture [71], administration of live *Pseudomonas aeruginosa* [69], LPS [72] or the KO of an antioxidant gene, such as the nuclear factor erythroid 2-related factor 2 (Nrf2) [73], the occurrence of oxidative stress is evidenced by the detection of oxidation products of biomolecules or by the depletion of reduced antioxidants. However, studies to determine the causality between the occurrence of oxidative stress and the progression to multiple organ failure are not conclusive.

A recent study compared progressive sepsis that was induced by peritonitis or by continuous intravenous infusion of live *Pseudomonas aeruginosa* in pigs. This group found that only animals that developed renal failure exhibited an early progressive increase in sepsis, a remarkable inflammatory response (e.g., TNF-α, IL-6) and oxidative stress (e.g., lipid peroxidation). Indeed, in mice, endotoxin injection resulted in lipid peroxide formation and membrane damage in the livers of experimental animals, which caused decreased levels of scavengers or quenchers of free radicals [74]. Mitochondria are reported to play a crucial role in the development of sepsis. In this respect, the implication of the mitochondria and the role of oxygen availability in LPS-induced human umbilical vein endothelial cells

(HUVECs), which were used as an endothelial model of sepsis, was investigated. In particular, it was discovered that stimulation with LPS led to a decrease in mitochondrial oxygen consumption that was related to a specific inhibition of Complex I, enhanced ROS production and an altered redox state (i.e., decreased GSH content). These results support and expand previously published evidence regarding the presence of mitochondrial dysfunction, oxidative stress and/or GSH depletion in LPS-treated HUVECs [75] and HUVECs that were stimulated with plasma from patients with sepsis [76].

5. Clinical Evidence of Oxidative Stress Biomarkers in Critically Ill Patients

Several preclinical and clinical studies of sepsis focused on single-point inhibition (e.g., anti-tumor necrosis factor antibodies) or augmentation of specific key processes, but these studies failed to demonstrate therapeutic efficacy. Therefore, the use of biomarkers of oxidative stress and antioxidant status is particularly important in defining the optimal timing of intervention. Most researchers believe that higher levels of free radicals and lower antioxidant levels in patients with SIRS or septic shock lead to multiple organ failure. However, the total antioxidant capacity (TAC) of the serum is increased in critically surgical patients with septic shock [77]. Moreover, the endogenous peroxyl-radical scavenging ability in the plasma of SIRS patients was found to be elevated in non-survivors [78]. Therefore, the actual change in TAC in severe sepsis patients remains controversial.

Serum uric acid, like other antioxidants such as albumin, bilirubin, or vitamins A, C and E, is a powerful free-radical scavenger that increases in response to acute oxidative stress [79]. Uric acid formation may even provide a significant antioxidant defense mechanism against nitration by peroxynitrite in rat hearts during hypoxia. It is therefore postulated that the serum uric acid level is an important marker of oxidative stress. Recently, serum uric acid was identified as a strong predictor of mortality in patients with moderate-to-severe chronic heart failure [80], which brought up an interesting question about the actual pathophysiologic role of serum uric acid in critically ill patients.

In a recent study, the lipid peroxidation and antioxidant status, both enzymatic and non-enzymatic, in neonates with septicemia were evaluated. This prospective study included 44 septicemic babies as cases, and a group of 84 matched healthy babies formed the control group. Significantly elevated levels of MDA and depressed levels of uric acid were found in babies with late onset sepsis. Neonates who ultimately succumbed had significantly elevated levels of MDA, SOD, GSH-Px and CAT, whereas levels of uric acid and albumin were significantly depressed [81].

The mechanism of increased uric acid in patients with severe sepsis and septic shock is unknown, and increased production and decreased excretion may result in elevated serum levels of uric acid. Severe sepsis and septic shock may induce ischemia or hypoxia in multiple organs, which may further increase the change from xanthine/hypoxanthine to uric acid through the activation of xanthine oxidase in microvascular endothelium [82]. However, renal dysfunction that is induced by septic shock may reduce the secretion of uric acid from the kidneys, which may also increase serum uric acid and further elevate serum TAC [83].

6. Novel Molecular Biomarkers of Oxidative Stress in Critical Ill Patients

Based on the pre-clinical findings, a complete clinical research program was developed in order to establish the utility of the genetics biomarkers for the early diagnosis of sepsis. From these studies, 145 human white blood cell genes associated with acute infection and inflammation were identified as being abnormally expressed both in the equine and human contexts. Following, panels of 42 genes were identified a priori using pre-clinical research outcomes from the pre-clinical results. This panel of biomarkers has been primarily linked with innate and early adaptive immune function/activation pathways, including those governing cell cycling and growth, white blood cell differentiation, extracellular matrix remodelling, and immune modulation [84]. Based on the physiological response to infection, that is, monocytosis, neutrophil activation, monocyte-macrophage differentiation, extravasation, as well as cell-mediated responses, these patented markers appear to characterize a large cross-section of early immune behaviour.

In a recent study, 27 participants were enrolled to be assessed for sepsis and post surgical patients status using a gene expression biomarker test. These findings demonstrate that this novel gene expression biomarker test (SeptiCyte Lab) has the capability, based on diagnostic performance outcomes, to accurately detect early evidence of sepsis well before the availability of microbiology results. Current clinical research will further investigate the efficacy of this assay to provide guidance on the host immune response via the monitoring of severe sepsis patients, as well as to provide diagnostic information on other 'at risk' groups such as post-operatively following major surgery and patients with chronic immune incompetence [85].

6.1 Sepsis and Urinary FABP1

Fatty acid-binding protein 1 (FABP1) is expressed in renal proximal tubule cells and shed into urine in response to hypoxia caused by decreased peritubular capillary blood flow. Recently, urinary FABP1 was examined in septic shock patients. Urinary FABP1 levels in septic shock patients were significantly higher than those in healthy subjects. In a cohort of 145 septic shock patients, a logistic regression analysis including urinary FABP1, blood endotoxin level, C-reactive protein, peripheral white blood cell count, and serum creatinine revealed that only urinary FABP1 levels showed a significant association with patient survival. Forty septic shock patients in another cohort were treated by polymyxin B-immobilized fiber hemoperfusion (PMX-F). The high affinity of polymyxin B for endotoxin, the rationale underlying extracorporeal therapy would be to remove circulating endotoxin by adsorption, thus preventing progression of the biological cascade of sepsis. PMX-F treatment has been performed to treat severe sepsis in more than 30,000 patients in Japan since 1994, and a meta-analysis demonstrated its efficacy on septic shock treatment [86]. Of 40 septic patients, 28 survived and 12 died. Among the surviving patients, urinary FABP1 levels were reduced by treatment. However, the nonsurviving patients showed higher urinary FABP1 levels with smaller decrease after the treatment compared with the survivors. These results suggested that urinary FABP1 levels might be able to reflect the severity of sepsis, and also to monitor the effectiveness of treatment [87].

6.2 Paraoxonase 1

Serum paraoxonase 1 (PON1) has been demonstrated in multiple clinical and animal studies to protect against oxidative stress, but also to undergo inactivation upon that condition. It was found decreased plasma PON1 activity in patients with sepsis compared to healthy controls or critically ill patients without sepsis; furthermore, in sepsis patients PON1 activity was lower and remained lower in the course of sepsis in the non-survivors compared to the survivors. Plasma PON1 activity was positively correlated with high-density lipoprotein cholesterol and negatively correlated with markers of lipid peroxidation [88]. In an experimental animal model of sepsis, murine cecal ligation and puncture, the time course of plasma PON1 activity was very similar to that found in sepsis patients. Indeed, persistently low PON1 activity in plasma was associated with lethal outcome in human and murine sepsis [89].

Conclusions and Perspectives

The clinical trials that pretend show the relationship between oxidative stress occurrence and critically state such as SIRS and septic shock must be careful in selecting the correct oxidative damage biomarkers, the type of sample taken (plasma or urine), the marker measured, and when the sample is collected. Some biomarkers may be useful in measuring chronic damage (8-OHdG), some may be useful for both acute and chronic stages (isoprostanes), and some may be generated and rapidly cleared, so elevations could be seen only in acute studies. The selection of correct biomarkers and the times at which to measure them are critical in understanding the role of oxidative damage in human disease, nutrition, and toxicology.

Whatever method you use to trap radicals or measure oxidative damage, it is necessary to think carefully about how the method works, what is likely to confound it and how quantitative it can be (how, what and how much). With careful attention to understanding these points, erroneous interpretations can be minimized and the vibrant field of free radical research can continue to move forward.

References

[1] Doise J M, Aho L S, Quenot J P, Guilland J C, Zeller M, Vergely C, Aube H, Blettery B, Rochette L. Plasma antioxidant status in septic critically ill patients: a decrease over time. *Fundam Clin Pharmacol* 2008;22:203–209.

[2] von Dessauer B, Bongain J, Molina V, Quilodrán J, Castillo R, Rodrigo R. Oxidative stress as a novel target in pediatric sepsis management. *J Crit Care* 2011;26:103e1–103e7.

[3] Marcin J P, Pollack M M. Review of the acuity scoring systems for the pediatric intensive care unit and their use in quality improvement. *J Intensive Care Med* 2007;22:131–140.

[4] Villamena F A, Zweier J L. Detection of reactive oxygen and nitrogen species by EPR spin trapping. *Antioxid Redox Signal* 2004;6:619–629.

[5] Bacić G, Mojović M. EPR spin trapping of oxygen radicals in plants: a methodological overview. *Ann N Y Acad Sci* 2005;1048:230–243.

[6] Dikalov S I, Li W, Mehranpour P, Wang S S, Zafari A M. Production of extracellular superoxide by human lymphoblast cell lines: comparison of electron spin resonance techniques and cytochrome C reduction assay. *Biochem Pharmacol* 2007;73:972–980.

[7] Wrona M, Patel K B, Wardman P. Reactivity of 2`,7`-dichlorodihydrofluorescein and dihydrorhodamine 123 and their oxidized forms towards carbonate, nitrogen dioxide, and hydroxyl radicals. *Free Radic Biol Med* 2005;38:262–270.

[8] Zhao B, Ranguelova K, Jiang J, Mason R P. Studies on the photosensitized reduction of resorufin and implications for the detection of oxidative stress with Amplex Red. *Free Radic Biol Med* 2011;51:153–159.

[9] Cathcart R, Schwiers E, Ames B N. Detection of picomole levels of lipid hydroperoxides using a dichlorofluorescein fluorescent assay. *Methods Enzymol* 1984;105:352–358.

[10] Castro L, Eiserich J P, Sweeney S, Radi R, Freeman B A. Cytochrome c: a catalyst and target of nitrite-hydrogen peroxide-dependent protein nitration. *Arch Biochem. Biophys* 2004;421:99–107.

[11] Brenneisen P, Steinbrenner H, Sies H. Selenium, oxidative stress, and health aspects. *Mol Aspects Med* 2005;26:256–267.

[12] Jakubowski W, Bartosz G. 2,7-Dichlorofluorescin oxidation and reactive oxygen species: what does it measure? *Cell Biol Int* 2000;24:757–760.

[13] Huang D, Ou B, Prior R L. The chemistry behind antioxidant capacity assays. *J Agric Food Chem* 2005;53:1841–1856.

[14] Izumi S, Urano Y, Hanaoka K, Terai T, Nagano T. A simple and effective strategy to increase the sensitivity of fluorescence probes in living cells. *J Am Chem Soc.* 2009;131:10189–101200.

[15] Yang D, Wang H L, Sun Z N, Chung N W, Shen J G. A highly selective fluorescent probe for the detection and imaging of peroxynitrite in living cells. *J Am Chem Soc* 2006;128:6004–6005.

[16] Heyne B, Beddie C, Sciano, J C. Synthesis and characterization of a new fluorescent probe for reactive oxygen species. *Org Biomol Chem* 2007;5:1454–1458.

[17] Kuribayashi F, Tsuruta S, Yamazaki T, Nunoi H, Imajoh-Ohmi S, Kanegasaki S, Nakamura M. Cell adhesion markedly increases lucigenin-enhanced chemiluminescence of the phagocyte NADPH oxidase. *Genes Cells* 2008;13:1249–56.

[18] Afanasev I. Detection of superoxide in cells, tissues and whole organisms. *Front Biosci* 2009;1:153–160.

[19] Janiszewski M, Souza H P, Liu Z, Pedro M A, Zweier J L, Laurindo F R M. Overestimation of NADH-driven vascular oxidase activity due to lucigenin artifacts. *Free Radic Biol Med* 2002;32:446–453.

[20] Xu X, Arriaga EA. Qualitative determination of superoxide release at both sides of the mitochondrial inner membrane by capillary electrophoretic analysis of the oxidation

products of triphenylphosphonium hydroethidine. *Free Radic Biol Med* 2009;46:905–913.

[21] Watanabe N, Dickinson D A, Liu R M, Forman H J. Quinones and glutathione metabolism. *Methods Enzymol* 2004;378:319–340.

[22] Ashkenazi A, Marks R S. Luminol-dependent chemiluminescence of human phagocyte cell lines: comparison between DMSO differentiated PLB 985 and HL 60 cells. *Luminescence* 2009;24:171–177.

[23] Vilim V, Wilhelm J. What do we measure by a luminol-dependent chemiluminescence of phagocytes? *Free Radic Biol Med* 1989;6:623–629.

[24] Vladimirov Y A, Proskurnina E V. Free radicals and cell chemiluminescence. *Biochemistry* 2009;74:1545–1566.

[25] Turan N N, Ark M, Demiryurek A T. Comparison of spectrophotometric, HPLC and chemiluminescence methods for 3-nitrotyrosine and peroxynitrite interaction. *Arch Pharm Res* 2005;28:358–63.

[26] Waring W S, Mishra V, Maxwell S R. Comparison of spectrophotometric and enhanced chemiluminescent assays of serum antioxidant capacity. *Clin Chim Acta* 2003;338:67–71.

[27] Zhao S, Wang J, Ye F, Liu Y M. Determination of uric acid in human urine and serum by capillary electrophoresis with chemiluminescence detection. *Anal Biochem* 2008;378:127–31.

[28] Alvarez B, Radi R. Peroxynitrite reactivity with amino acids and proteins. *Amino Acids* 2003;25:295–311.

[29] Rubo H, Radi R. Protein and lipid nitration: Role in redox signaling and injury. *Biochim Biophys Acta* 2008;1780:1318–1324.

[30] Butkovic V, Klasinc L, Bors W. Kinetic study of flavonoid reactions with stable radicals. *J. Agric. Food Chem* 2004;52:2816–2820.

[31] Scalzo J, Mezzetti B, Battino M. Total antioxidant capacity evaluation: Critical steps for assaying berry antioxidant features. *BioFactors* 2005;23:221–227.

[32] De Mattia G, Bravi M C, Laurenti O, De Luca O, Palmeri A, Sabatucci A, Mendico G, Ghiselli A. Impairment of cell and plasma redox state in subjects professionally exposed to chromium. *Am J Ind Med* 2004;46:120-125.

[33] Ozyürek M, Bektaşoğlu B, Güçlü K, Güngör N, Apak R. Simultaneous total antioxidant capacity assay of lipophilic and hydrophilic antioxidants in the same acetone-water solution containing 2% methyl-beta-cyclodextrin using the cupric reducing antioxidant capacity (CUPRAC) method. *Anal Chim Acta* 2008;630:28–39.

[34] Benzie I F F, Strain J J. The ferric reducing ability of plasma (FRAP) as a measure of "antioxidant power": the FRAP assay. *Anal Biochem* 1996;239:70–76.

[35] Campos C, Guzman R, Lopez-Fernandez E, Casado A. Evaluation of the copper (II) reduction assay using bathocuproinedisulfonic acid disodium salt for the total antioxidant capacity assessment: The CUPRAC-BCS assay. *Anal Biochem* 2009;392:37–44.

[36] Wada S. Chemoprevention of tocotrienols: the mechanism of antiproliferative effects. *Forum Nutr* 2009;61:204–216.

[37] Niederlander H A G, van Beek T A, Bartasiute A, Koleva I I. Antioxidant activity assays on-line with liquid chromatography. *J Chromat A* 2008;1210:121–134.

[38] Valko M, Morris H, Cronin M T. Metals, toxicity and oxidative stress. *Curr Med Chem* 2005;12:1161–1208.

[39] Niki E, Noguchi N. Dynamics of antioxidant action of vitamin E. *Acc Chem Res* 2004;37:45–51

[40] Terao J. Dietary "avonoids as antioxidants. *Forum Nutr* 2009;61:87–94.

[41] Noguchi N, Niki E. Phenolic antioxidants: A rationale for design and evaluation of novel antioxidant drug for atherogenesis. *Free Radic. Biol Med* 2000;28:1538–1546.

[42] Ying Z, Kherada N, Kampfrath T, Mihai G, Simonetti O, Desikan R, Selvendiran K, Sun Q, Ziouzenkova O, Parthasarathy S, Rajagopalan S. A modified sesamol derivative inhibits progression of atherosclerosis. *Arterioscler Thromb Vasc Biol* 2011;31:536–42.

[43] Halliwell B, Whiteman M. Measuring reactive species and oxidative damage in vivo and in cell culture: how should you do it and what do the results mean? *Br J Pharmacol* 2004;142:231–255.

[44] Halliwell B, Rafter J, Jenner A. Health promotion by "avonoids, tocopherols, tocotrienols, and other phenols: direct or indirect effects? Antioxidant or not? *Am J Clin Nutr* 2005;81:268S–276S.

[45] Cadet J, Douki T, Ravanat J L. Measurement of oxidatively generated base damage in cellular DNA. *Mutat Res* 2011;711:3–12.

[46] Roberts L J I I, Oates J A, Linton M F, Fazio S, Meador B P, Gross M D, Shyr Y, Morrow J D. The relationship between dose of vitamin E and suppression of oxidative stress in humans. *Free Radic Biol Med* 2007;43:1388–1393.

[47] Finley J W, Kong A N, Hintze K J, Jeffery E H, Ji L L, Lei X G. Antioxidants in foods: state of the science important to the food industry. *J Agric Food Chem* 2011;59:6837–6846.

[48] Masella R, Di Benedetto R, Vari R, Filesi C, Giovannini C. Novel mechanisms of natural antioxidant compounds in biological systems: Involvement of glutathione and glutathionerelated enzymes. *J Nutr Biochem* 2005;16:577–586.

[49] Shen D, Dalton T P, Nebert D W, Shertzer H G. Glutathione redox state regulates mitochondrial reactive oxygen production. *J Biol Chem* 2005;280:25305–25312.

[50] Valko M, Leibfritz D, Moncol J, Cronin MT, Mazur M, Telser J. Free radicals and antioxidants in normal physiological functions and human disease. *Int J Biochem Cell Biol* 2007;39:44–84.

[51] Pickering G, Schneider E, Papet I, Pujos-Guillot E, Pereira B, Simen E, Dubray C, Schoeffler P. Acetaminophen metabolism after major surgery: a greater challenge with increasing age. *Clin Pharmacol Ther* 2011;90:707–711.

[52] Nogueira C W, Zeni G, Rocha J B T. Organoselenium and organotellurium compounds: Toxicology and pharmacology. *Chem Rev* 2004;104:6255–6285.

[53] Mühl D, Woth G, Drenkovics L, Varga A, Ghosh S, Csontos C, Bogár L, Wéber G, Lantos J. Comparison of oxidative stress & leukocyte activation in patients with severe sepsis & burn injury. *Indian J Med Res* 2011;134:69–78.

[54] Catalá A. Lipid peroxidation of membrane phospholipids generates hydroxy-alkenals and oxidized phospholipids active in physiological and/or pathological conditions. *Chem Phys Lipids* 2009;157:1-11.

[55] Paradies G, Petrosillo G, Paradies V, Ruggiero F M. Role of cardiolipin peroxidation and Ca^{2+} in mitochondrial dysfunction and disease. *Cell Calcium* 2009;45:643–650.

[56] Williams M V, Wishnok J S, Tannenbaum S R. Covalent adducts arising from the decomposition products of lipid hydroperoxides in the presence of cytochrome c. *Chem Res Toxicol* 2007;20:767–775.

[57] Liu Z Q, Shan H Y. Cholesterol, not polyunsaturated fatty acids, is target molecule in oxidation induced by reactive oxygen species in membrane of human erythrocytes. *Cell Biochem Biophys* 2006;45:185–193.

[58] Brooks JD, Milne G L, Yin H, Sanchez S C, Porter N A, Morrow J D. Formation of highly reactive cyclopentenone isoprostane compounds (A3/J3isoprostanes) in vivo from eicosapentaenoic acid. *J Biol Chem* 2008;283: 12043–12055.

[59] Hill B G, Dranka B P, Zou L, Chatham J C, Darley-Usmar V M. Importance of the bioenergetic reserve capacity in response to cardiomyocyte stress induced by 4-hydroxynonenal. *Biochem J* 2009;424:99–107.

[60] Stavrovskaya I G, Baranov S V, Guo X, Davies S S, Roberts L J, Kristal B S. Reactive gamma-ketoaldehydes formed via the isoprostane pathway disrupt mitochondrial respiration and calcium homeostasis. *Free Radic Biol Med* 2010;49:567–579.

[61] Young I S, Trimble E R. Measurement of malondialdehyde in plasma by high performance liquid chromatography with fluorimetric detection. *Ann Clin Biochem* 1991;28:504-508.

[62] Halliwell B. Antioxidant defence mechanisms: from the beginning to the end (of the beginning). *Free Radic Res* 1999;31:261–272.

[63] Uchida K. 4-Hydroxy-2-nonenal: a product and mediator of oxidative stress. *Prog Lipid Res* 2003;42:318–343.

[64] Spiteller G. The relation of lipid peroxidation processes with atherogenesis: a new theory on atherogenesis. *Mol Nutr Food Res* 2005;49:999–1013.

[65] Murakami K, Enkhbaatar P, Shimoda K, Cox R A, Burke A S, Hawkins H K, Traber L D, Schmalstieg F C, Salzman A L, Mabley J G, Komjati K, Pacher P, Zsengeller Z, Szabo C, Traber D L: Inhibition of poly (ADP-ribose) polymerase attenuates acute lung injury in an ovine model of sepsis. *Shock* 2004;21:126–133.

[66] Altmeyer M, Hottiger M O. Poly(ADP-ribose) polymerase 1 at the crossroad of metabolic stress and inflammation in aging. *Aging* 2009;20:458–469.

[67] Mani A R, Pannala A S, Orie N N, Ollosson R, Harry D, Rice-Evans C A, Moore KP. Nitration of endogenous para-hydroxyphenylacetic acid and the metabolism of nitrotyrosine. *Biochem J* 2003;374:521–527.

[68] Kanski K, Alterman M A, Schoneich C. Proteomic identification of age-dependent protein nitration in rat skeletal muscle. *Free Radic Biol Med* 2003;35:1229–1239.

[69] Lange M, Connelly R, Traber D L, Hamahata A, Nakano Y, Esechie A, Jonkam C, von Borzyskowski S, Traber L D, Schmalstieg F C, Herndon D N, Enkhbaatar P. Time course of nitric oxide synthases, nitrosative stress, and poly(ADP ribosylation) in an ovine sepsis model. *Crit Care* 2010;14:R129.

[70] Ho J T, Chapman M J, O'Connor S, Lam S, Edwards J, Ludbrook G, Lewis J G, Torpy D J. Characteristics of plasma NOx levels in severe sepsis: high interindividual variability and correlation with illness severity, but lack of correlation with cortisol levels. *Clin Endocrinol* 2010;73:413–420.

[71] Albayrak A, Uyanik M H, Odabasoglu F, Halici Z, Uyanik A, Bayir Y, Albayrak F, Albayrak Y, Polat B, Suleyman H. The effects of diabetes and/or polymicrobial sepsis

on the status of antioxidant enzymes and pro-inflammatory cytokines on heart, liver, and lung of ovariectomized rats. *J Surg Res* 2011;169:67–75.

[72] Shi D W, Zhang J, Jiang H N, Tong C Y, Gu G R, Ji Y, Summah H, Qu J M. LPS pretreatment ameliorates multiple organ injuries and improves survival in a murine model of polymicrobial sepsis. *Inflamm Res* 2011;60:841–849.

[73] Benes J, Chvojka J, Sykora R, Radej J, Krouzecky A, Novak I, Matejovic M. Searching for mechanisms that matter in early septic acute kidney injury: an experimental study. *Crit Care* 2011. *In press.*

[74] Sakaguchi S, Furusawa S. Oxidative stress and septic shock: metabolic aspects of oxygen-derived free radicals generated in the liver during endotoxemia. *FEMS Immunol Med Microbiol* 2006;47:167–177.

[75] Lowes D A, Thottakam B M, Webster N R, Murphy M P, Galley H F. The mitochondria-targeted antioxidant MitoQ protects against organ damage in a lipopolysaccharide-peptidoglycan model of sepsis. *Free Radic Biol Med* 2008;45:1559–1565.

[76] Huet O, Cherreau C, Nicco C, Dupic L, Conti M, Borderie D, Pene F, Vicaut E, Benhamou D, Mira J P, Duranteau J, Batteux F. Pivotal role of glutathione depletion in plasma-induced endothelial oxidative stress during sepsis. *Crit Care Med* 2008;36:2328–2334.

[77] Huet O, Obata R, Aubron C, Spraul-Davit A, Charpentier J, Laplace C, Nguyen-Khoa T, Conti M, Vicaut E, Mira J P, Duranteau J. Plasma-induced endothelial oxidative stress is related to the severity of septic shock. *Crit Care Med* 2007;35:821–826.

[78] Andresen M, Regueira T, Bruhn A, Perez D, Strobel P, Dougnac A, Marshall G, Leighton F. Lipoperoxidation and protein oxidative damage exhibit different kinetics during septic shock. *Mediators Inflamm* 2008;2008:168652.

[79] Teixeira de Lemos E, Pinto R, Oliveira J, Garrido P, Sereno J, Mascarenhas-Melo F, Páscoa-Pinheiro J, Teixeira F, Reis F. Differential effects of acute (extenuating) and chronic (training) exercise on inflammation and oxidative stress status in an animal model of type 2 diabetes mellitus. *Mediators Inflamm* 2011;2011:253061.

[80] Doehner W, Landmesser U. Xanthine oxidase and uric acid in cardiovascular disease: clinical impact and therapeutic options. *Semin Nephrol* 2011;31:433–440.

[81] Kapoor K, Basu S, Das B K, Bhatia B D. Lipid peroxidation and antioxidants in neonatal septicemia. *J Trop Pediatr* 2006;52:372–375.

[82] Gao X, Zhang H, Belmadani S, Wu J, Xu X, Elford H, Potter B J, Zhang C. Role of TNF-alpha-induced reactive oxygen species in endothelial dysfunction during reperfusion injury. *Am J Physiol Heart Circ Physiol* 2008;295:H2242-H2249.

[83] Ochiai M E, Barretto A C, Oliveira M T Jr, Munhoz R T, Morgado P C, Ramires J A. Uric acid renal excretion and renal insufficiency in decompensated severe heart failure. *Eur J Heart Fail* 2005;7:468-474.

[84] Purushothaman D, Sarin A. Cytokine-dependent regulation of NADPH oxidase activity and the consequences for activated T cell homeostasis. *J Exp Med* 2009;206:1515–1523.

[85] Sutherland A, Thomas M, Brandon R A, Brandon R B, Lipman J, Tang B, McLean A, Pascoe R, Price G, Nguyen T, Stone G, Venter D. Development and validation of a novel molecular biomarker diagnostic test for the early detection of sepsis. *Crit Care* 2011;15:R149.

[86] Cruz D N, Bellomo R, Ronco C. Clinical effects of polymyxin B-immobilized fiber column in septic patients. *Contrib Nephrol* 2007;156:444–451.

[87] Nakamura T, Sugaya T, Koide H. Urinary liver-type fatty acid-binding protein in septic shock: effect of polymyxin B-immobilized fiber hemoperfusion. *Shock* 2009;31:454–459.

[88] Draganov D, Teiber J, Watson C, Bisgaier C, Nemzek J, Remick D, Standiford T, La Du B. PON1 and oxidative stress in human sepsis and an animal model of sepsis. *Adv Exp Med Biol* 2010;660:89–97.

[89] Ozer E A, Pezzulo A, Shih D M, Chun C, Furlong C, Lusis A J, Greenberg E P, Zabner J. Human and murine paraoxonase 1 are host modulators of Pseudomonas aeruginosa quorum-sensing. *FEMS Microbiol Lett* 2005;253:29–37.

In: Oxidative Stress and the Critically Ill Patient
Editors: Ramón Rodrigo and Bettina von Dessauer
ISBN: 978-1-62081-576-2

Chapter XII

EXOGENOUS ANTIOXIDANTS AS POTENTIAL THERAPEUTIC AGENTS

Ramón Rodrigo*

Full Professor, Molecular and Clinical Pharmacology Program, Institute of Biomedical Sciences, Faculty of Medicine, University of Chile. Santiago, Chile

1. ABSTRACT

Critical illness and particularly sepsis are associated with a marked redox imbalance resulting from an increased production of oxidant species and a decrease in the endogenous antioxidant defense system. Plasma concentrations of antioxidant micronutrients are known to be depressed, as expected for the increased reactive oxygen (ROS) and nitrogen (RNS) species occurring in these settings. The body has an antioxidant defense system integrated by numerous endogenous agents, located at defined compartments, aimed to abrogate ROS and RNS effects through various complementary mechanisms such as free radical scavenging, chain-breaking, catalytic depuration, or metal chelation, among others. In addition, in the presence of oxidative stress the antioxidant system is capable to enhance its activity through a genomic survival response triggered by low to moderate concentrations of reactive species. However, as these compounds are normally available in limited amounts, their efficacy will be overwhelmed in clinical settings accompanied by increased production of reactive species. Consequently, oxidative damage will ensue due to a direct cellular injury and activation of intracellular signaling cascades leading to an inflammatory response, which might progress to multiple organ dysfunction syndrome. At the cell level, ROS irreversibly will damage lipids, proteins and nucleic acids, being the mitochondria an organelle of major vulnerability in the light of recent studies. Interventions with antioxidants, depending on the moment at which the support is instituted in the course of the disease, could have an impact in improving the prognosis and survival of these patients. The paradigm is based on the biological properties of antioxidant substances suitable to counteract the oxidative damage and its consequences. Experimental studies

*Address: Reyes Lavalle 3415, Depto. 71, Las Condes, C.P 7550164, Santiago, Región Metropolitana, Chile, Phone: 56-2-9786126, Email: rrodrigo@med.uchile.cl

and clinical trials regarding antioxidant therapy in critical illness provide increasing evidence in support of the beneficial effects of vitamins A, C and E, selenium, allopurinol, N-acetylcysteine, melatonin, polyphenols, and others. This chapter is devoted to present the evidence accounting for a protective role of opportune antioxidant supplementation in the critically ill patient.

Keywords: antioxidants, lipid peroxidation, oxidative stress, critically ill patients

Abbreviations

BH_4	tetrahydrobiopterin
eNOS	endothelial nitric oxide synthase
GSH	reduced glutathione
GSH-Px	glutathione peroxidase
ICU	intensive care unit
LPS	lipopolysaccharide
NADPH	reduced nicotinamide adenine dinucleotide
NF-κB	nuclear factor kappaB
NO	nitric oxide
ROS	reactive oxygen species
RNS	reactive nitrogen species
SePP	selenoprotein P
SOD	superoxide dismutase

2. Introduction

As discussed in previous chapters, the development of multiorgan failure in the critically ill patients caused by phenomena such as infections, autoimmune disease, fasting, anesthesia, hemorrhage, hypovolemia or ischemia-reperfusion, among others, is preceded by oxidative stress [1]. As occurs in sepsis, a complex inflammatory syndrome of diverse etiology and wide spectrum of severity, the propagation from organ to organ is a function of redox-depending constituents. There is cumulated evidence showing that reactive oxygen species (ROS) and reactive nitrogen species (RNS) are linked to the onset, progression and outcome of these settings, both in pre-clinical and in clinical studies. These reactive species behave as important signaling molecules in normal physiologic processes, giving rise to regulation of proteins that collectively favor cell survival [2]; however, if their overproduction overwhelm the antioxidant defense system of the organism, oxidative stress takes place.

In the pathophysiological underlying mechanisms of these processes, several factors interact in a long chain of events from pathogen recognition up to the overwhelming of host responses. Infection and endotoxemia provoke local and systemic responses, including increased massive free radical production, inflammatory cytokines and multiple mediators release [3]. The initiation involves the release of bacterial lipopolysaccharide (LPS) or other substances into the extracellular fluid during microbial lysis. Increased ROS and RNS allow explaining the mechanisms for the development of alterations found in critically ill patients.

In support of this view, it has been reported that treatments that reduce the generation or prevent or reverse the effects of ROS exert beneficial effects in a variety of models of endotoxic and septic shock. In addition, plasma concentrations of antioxidant micronutrients have been reported to be reduced in these patients [4]. The causes of the lower levels of these compounds could include losses with biological fluids, lower than needed intakes, dilution by abundant resuscitation fluids, as well as the systemic inflammatory response syndrome-mediated redistribution of micronutrients from plasma to tissues.

Concerning the generation of oxidative stress in sepsis (for more details see chapters 1 and 2), there has been a growing body of evidence suggesting that mitochondria are the major source of ROS. Studies aimed to improve the understanding of mitochondrial dysfunction, its involvement in the development of multiple organ failure and its role in the various phases throughout these pathophysiological processes has recently emerged (for more details see chapter 4). Mitochondria can be source and target of ROS. Furthermore, ROS are capable of increasing the inner mitochondrial membrane, thus giving rise to the opening of the transition pore, release of cytochrome c, caspase pathway activation and apoptosis. Peroxynitrite irreversibly inhibits enzyme complexes of the respiratory chain. Therefore, the generation of more knowledge in this field is fundamental before testing therapeutic strategies targeting mitochondria [5]. ROS react with various biological substrates, especially polyunsaturated fatty acids; induce membrane dysfunction, tissue damage, and organ injury. The amount of evidence supporting a role of oxidative stress in the pathogenesis of sepsis suggests that interventions consisting in the early and opportune supplementation of antioxidants could have an impact in improving the prognosis and survival of these patients.

Taking into account the major role of ROS and RNS in the pathophysiology of sepsis, septic shock and other related pathologies, as well as the associated reduction of of plasma antioxidant levels, it should be expected a beneficial effect of antioxidant supplementation against the worsening of these clinical settings. It has been recognized that exogenous antioxidants may be useful in sepsis [6]. The biological properties of naturally occurring exogenous compounds belonging to this group, such as α-tocopherol and ascorbic acid, have overwhelmed their antioxidant effects. The potential role for antioxidants acting specifically in mitochondria has been highlighted [7]. Despite the enormous interest in antioxidant vitamins as potential protective agents against the development of human disease, the real contributions of such compounds to health maintenance and the mechanisms whereby they act remain unclear. This chapter presents the pathophysiological bases supporting the potential therapeutic role of exogenous antioxidants in the management of the critically ill patient. An updated knowledge about the biological effects of various antioxidants, such as N-acetylcysteine, sellenium, melatonin, allopurinol, vitamin C, vitamin E, polyphenols, among others, is included in order to encourage the design and application of novel therapeutic schemes based on the supplementation of these easily available and low cost agents in appropriate doses, apparently innocuous, for the improvement of the clinical outcome of these patients.

2. Antioxidants against the Pathophysiological Events Occurring in the Critically Ill Patients

Antioxidants could play a key role in abrogating the pro-oxidant status occurring during critical illness and particularly sepsis. These settings are associated with a significant redox imbalance resulting from an increased production of oxidant species and a decrease in endogenous antioxidant defenses. It should be noted that available evidence supports the view that interventions with antioxidants could have an impact in improving the prognosis and survival of these patients, depending on the moment at which the support is instituted within the course of the disease.

Table 12-1. Summarized mechanisms supporting the beneficial effects of exogenous antioxidants in improving the clinical outcome of critically ill patients

Antioxidants	Mechanisms	Ref.
N-acetylcysteine	Hydroxyl free radical scavenging	[51]
	Reduction of macrophage cytokine release and of mitochondrial dysfunction	[53]
	Antiinflammatory effects	[55, 59]
	Improvement of clearance of infectious particles	[56]
	Decrease of platelet adhesion	[57]
	Reverse of inhibition of mitochondrial complexes I and II	[58]
	GSH replenishment	[60]
Allopurinol	Decreased superoxide production in response to LPS, decreased chemokine synthesis, reduced leukocyte adhesion	[73]
	Antiinflammatory effect by reduction of C5a accumulation	[71]
Vitamin C	Improvement of microcirculatory perfusion	[11]
	Increased capillary density and decreased stopped flow capillaries	[12, 13]
	iNOS and NADPH oxidase downregulation	[15, 13]
	Antiapoptotic effect	[16]
	Attenuation of proinflammatory and procoagulant states, prevention of superoxide and NO reaction	[17, 19]
	Improvement of microcirculatory perfusion	[20]
	Prevention of SOD activity impairment and increased MDA levels	[21]
	Down-regulation of NADPH oxidase and up-regulation of eNOS	[22]
	Prevention of eNOS uncoupling	[23]
	Prevention of endotoxin-induced renal damage	[26]
	Superoxide scavenging	[27]
	α-tocopherol recycling	[30]
Vitamin E	ROS and peroxyl scavenging	[28, 29]
	Amelioration of vasodilators expression	[31]
	Reduction of cytokine production in response to endotoxin	[32]
	Immunonutrition	[33]
	Abrogation of systemic inflammation	[37]
Melatonin	Regulation of sleep-wake cycle	[38]
	Antioxidant activity	[39, 41]
	Mitochondrial antioxidant effect	[7]
	ROS scavenging	[40]

Antioxidants	Mechanisms	Ref.
	Reduction of circulatory failure	[42]
	Reduction of oxidative stress biomarkers	[43, 44]
	Inhibition of proinflammatory cytokine production	[45]
	up-regulation of antioxidant enzymes activity and gene	
	expression	[46, 47]
	Restoration of ATP production in sepsis	[50]
Selenium	Increased GSH-Px activity	[64, 69]
	Modulation of immune and inflammatory responses	[66]
	Decreased risk of a new infection	[67]
	Lowering of incidence of hospital acquired pneumonia	[68]
Polyphenols	Antiinflammatory effect	[77]
	Reduction of LPS-induced nephrotoxicity	[82]
	Inhibition of neutrophil infiltration	[78]
	Peroxynitrite scavenging	[79]
	Protection of renal tubular epithelium	[80]
	Protective effect on LPS-induced acute phase response	[83]
	Inhibition of NF-κB/Rel-dependent transcription	[84]
Deferoxamine	Metal chelation, decreased oxidative stress and abrogation	
	of apoptosis	[91]
	Antiinflammatory effect	[53]
Vitamin A	Antiinflamatory effect through NF-κB inhibition	[87]
Statins	Maintenance of microvascular integrity	[85]

Despite the general occurrence of oxidative damage in different organs during sepsis development and a positive correlation between oxidative markers and organ injury, antioxidant effects seem to depend not only on the diminution of oxidative damage but also on its anti-inflammatory activity. The biological properties accounting for this effect for the main antioxidants will be analyzed below. The biological properties accounting for these effects for the main antioxidants will be analyzed below and are summarized in Table 12-1.

3.1 Vitamin C

In general, low ascorbate concentrations in plasma and leukocytes are common features of the critically ill patients [8]. Further, patients with advanced cancer are generally deficient in ascorbic acid. Once these patients develop septic symptoms, a further decrease in ascorbic acid levels occurs. Thus, the use of ascorbate has been suggested as adjuvant to existing modalities in the treatment and prevention of cancer-associated sepsis [9].The effect of vitamin C supplementation has been studied in relation to capillary blood flow, which is impaired in severe sepsis because of compromised microvascular responsiveness. Microcirculatory alterations may play an important role in the development of sepsis-related organ dysfunction; it was recently found that vitamin C can markedly improve the microcirculation in this setting [10]. Compared with healthy volunteers and ICU controls, patients with severe sepsis have a decrease in vascular density together with an increased number of capillaries with stopped or intermittent flow. Importantly, capillaries in which there is no flow at a given time may be well perfused a few minutes later, and perfused vessels may later have no flow. These alterations have been observed in different models of sepsis, including those created by administration of endotoxin or live bacteria and bacterial peritonitis in all organs investigated [11]. In rodents, administration of vitamin C improved microcirculatory perfusion, increasing capillary density and decreasing the number of stopped flow capillaries, beneficial results that persisted even when vitamin C was administered up to 24 h after the initiation of sepsis [12, 13].

When L-arginine pretreatment is applied prior to the endotoxemia, it improves hepatosplanchnic perfusion and oxygenation during prolonged endotoxemia, probably through an enhancement in NO synthesis, without causing deleterious systemic side effects [14]. Animal and in vitro models show that vitamin C can act in vascular endothelial cells through the inhibition of Nox and inducible nitric oxide synthase, both of which are induced in sepsis [15, 13]. In addition, in a study involving septic abdominal surgery patients, treatment with 3 intravenous doses of 450 mg/d of vitamin C resulted in the reduction of caspase-3 and poly (ADP-ribose) polymerase levels and the increment of Bcl-2 levels, all of which points to an antiapoptotic effect on peripheral blood neutrophils [16]. This effect could be relevant in the light of evidence showing a possible role of ROS in neutrophil apoptosis and of apoptosis in multiple organ disease syndrome development. In a rat model, it was demonstrated that ascorbic acid administered following a lipopolysaccharide infusion attenuates pro-inflammatory and pro-coagulant states that induce lung vascular injury [17].

When vitamin C is administered by mouth, the relationship between oral dose and plasma concentration is sigmoidal. Its concentration in plasma is tightly controlled and excess of vitamin C is excreted as a function of doses, being completely saturated at doses of 400 mg daily and higher, producing a steady-state plasma concentration by approximately 80 μmol/L [18]. Nevertheless, such plasma ascorbate levels are not enough to scavenge superoxide anion, but only to abrogate its production. Therefore, in clinical situations accompanied by oxidative stress, a marked beneficial effect in the prevention of oxidative damage should not be expected after oral administration of vitamin C. Therefore, intravenous infusion could be considered for this purpose. Indeed, superoxide reacts with NO at a rate 10^5-fold greater than the rate at which superoxide reacts with ascorbic acid [19]. As a consequence, 10 mmol/L ascorbate is needed to support its competition with NO for superoxide. In patients undergoing elective percutaneous coronary intervention, impaired microcirculatory reperfusion is improved by vitamin C infusion suggesting that oxidative stress is implicated in such a phenomenon [20]. Also, in patients subjected to thrombolysis following acute myocardial infarction, superoxide dismutase, in the blood was found to be significantly reduced whereas the activity of the oxidant enzyme, xanthine oxidase, and malondialdehyde levels were found to be significantly increased. However, oral supplementation of vitamin C in post reperfusion patients restored these parameters back to normal or near normal levels [21]. Despite higher ascorbate doses would be needed to reach a better protective effect, it should be taken into account that its biological properties other than that ROS scavenging may have some beneficial effects. On this line, the major enzymatic source of ROS occurs via NADPH oxidase, an enzyme subjected to down-regulation by vitamin C [22]. In addition, vitamin C prevents the oxidation of tetrahydrobiopterin (BH_4), a coupling cofactor of NO synthase that is highly sensitive to oxidation. When BH_4 is oxidized, eNOS activity becomes uncoupled, resulting in the production of superoxide instead of NO, thus enhancing the oxidative damage. Peroxynitrite, the product of superoxide and NO reaction, uncouples eNOS by oxidation of BH_4; ascorbate does not fully protect BH4 from oxidation but recycles BH3. radical back to BH_4 [23]. Finally, it is noteworthy that vitamin C could also abrogate the beneficial effects of ischemic preconditioning; a phenomenon induced by a series of brief sublethal episodes of ischemia and reperfusion prior to a potentially lethal episode of ischemia that renders the heart more resistant to myocardial infarction [24]. A randomized, double-blind, placebo-controlled trial showed that the supplementation of 500 mg/d of vitamin C and 400 IU/d of vitamin E through enteral feeding in critically ill patients, resulted in a significant reduction in mortality [25]. In addition, in an animal model, supplementation with vitamins C and E prevented endotoxin-induced renal oxidative tissue damage [26]. It should be emphasized that a recent metaanalysis reported that high intravenous doses of vitamin C, rendering plasma levels twice higher than those enough to scavenge superoxide, have been administered without causing adverse effects in patients [27]. Recently, it has remarked that herefore; it may be possible to improve microvascular function in sepsis by using intravenous vitamin C as an adjunct therapy [28].

In summary, the beneficial effects of vitamin C to critically ill patients is characterized by increased bioavailability of NO, stabilization of tetrahydrobiopterin and eNOS, decreased production of superoxide anion and even its scavenging at higher ascorbate concentrations, and recycling of α-tocopherol from its free radical form α-tocopheroxyl. All these effects contribute to improve vascular function and systemic organ perfusion, thus diminishing the risk of multiple organ disease syndrome.

3.2 Vitamin E

Vitamin E, mainly α-tocopherol, is the major peroxyl radical scavenger in biological lipid phases such as membranes or low-density lipoproteins [29]. The antioxidant action has been ascribed to its ability to act chemically as a free radical chain-breaking molecule, thereby inhibiting lipid peroxidation through its own conversion into an oxidized product, α-tocopheroxyl. Then, α-tocopherol can be restored by reduction of the α-tocopheroxyl radical with redox-active reagents like vitamin C or ubiquinol [30]. The role of α-tocopherol in sepsis has been very poorly studied. However, the occurrence of oxidative stress points to the prevalence of a pro-oxidant status in this pathological condition. It is known that sepsis induces an imbalance in hepatic vasoregulatory gene expression and that α-tocopherol ameliorates altered expression of vasodilators through its free radical scavenging activity [31]. Furthermore, it was reported that sepsis is associated with a significant decrease in plasma vitamin E levels, but its exogenous administration lessens this phenomenon through NADPH oxidase inactivation, what associates with a reduction of monocyte-macrophage cytokine production in response to endotoxin [32].

In patients with sepsis, vitamin E has been included in an immunonutrition formula for early enteral pharmaconutrition, together with glutamine dipeptides, vitamin C, beta-carotene, selenium, zinc, and butyrate, resulting in significantly faster recovery of organ function compared with control patients [33]. On this line, myocardial damage can also be reduced through antioxidant supplementation, as showed by the attenuation of sepsis-related myocardial contractile dysfunction in rats, following the administration of vitamin C, vitamin E, vitamin A, and zinc [34]. Furthermore, in another prospective randomized trial, supplementation with vitamin E (1000 IU, 3 times a day per naso- or orogastric tube feeding) and vitamin C (1000 mg, 3 times a day, intravenously) was associated to a reduction in the occurrence of pulmonary morbidity and multiple organ failure, also reducing the duration of mechanical ventilation and length of ICU stay [35]. These studies are consistent with the view that a combined antioxidant compound mixture has an enhanced beneficial effect on critically ill patients.

Finally, in a rat model of sepsis, it was recently reported that the newly synthetic vitamin E derivative E-Ant-S-GS inhibited the secretion of cytokine, and thereby reduced organ damage in the experimental model of cecal ligation and puncture-induced sepsis, thus showing anti-inflammatory actions and organ-protective effects consistent with the potential clinical use of this compound as a therapeutic agent against systemic inflammation [36, 37].

3.3 Melatonin

Melatonin, based on its properties as chronobiotic (sleep modulation), antioxidant, and/or analgesic, all of which have been confirmed in numerous experimental studies, offers perspectives of beneficial effects in a variety of pediatric therapies [38]. Endogenous melatonin is primarily recognized for regulation of the sleep-awake cycle, but considerably higher levels have potent antioxidant activity [39], acting specifically in mitochondria [7]. It is a versatile molecule, synthesized not only in the pineal gland, but also in many other organs. Melatonin is a powerful, broad-spectrum, endogenously produced ROS scavenger [40] and its derivatives are also effective as antioxidants [41]. It also synergizes with vitamin C, vitamin E and glutathione in the scavenging of free radicals. In animal models of sepsis, administration of melatonin has been shown to reduce circulatory failure, lung injury, and intestinal apoptotic damage, also improving survival [42]. Melatonin supplementation reduces postoperative oxidative stress in newborns. Furthermore, Gitto et al [43] studied the effect of melatonin administration in septic newborns, showing a reduction in oxidative stress parameters and a possible improvement in survival. Since newborns and particularly those delivered preterm have less protection against oxidation and are highly susceptible to free radical-mediated oxidative damage, melatonin, because of its antioxidant properties, could be useful to reduce oxidative stress in neonates with sepsis, asphyxia, respiratory distress, or surgical stress [44]. In neonatal therapy, the antioxidant properties of melatonin have been the basis for its administration to newborns to reduce oxidative stress [38].

Experimental studies have shown that melatonin ameliorates respiratory syncytial virus-induced disease and lung inflammatory injury in mice via inhibition of oxidative stress and proinflammatory cytokine production and may constitute a novel therapeutic agent in virus-induced pulmonary infection [45]. Melatonin activates a number of antioxidant mechanisms. Thus, its treatment, as well as that with pineal proteins, in a model of adult female Wistar rats significantly up-regulated the antioxidant enzyme activity and gene expression, and the levels of reduced glutathione, whereas lipid peroxidation remained unaffected [46, 47].

In the critically ill patient, abnormalities have been identified in mitochondrial functions, such as defects in the electron transport chain/oxidative phosphorylation system, Krebs's cycle enzymes, and ATP production. These disturbances have all been suggested as the primary causative factors in the pathogenesis of sepsis. I is of major interest that melatonin is selectively taken up by mitochondrial membranes, a function not shared by other antioxidants [48, 49]. In animal models, it was demonstrated that melatonin treatment blunted sepsis-induced inducible mitochondrial nitric oxide synthase isoforms, prevented the impairment of mitochondrial homeostasis under sepsis, and restored ATP production [50]. It was remarked that these properties of melatonin should be considered in clinical sepsis.

Although melatonin treatment has been widely used as an effective and useful adjuvant for several therapies, its adverse time-dependent effects are still obscure and require further study. Side effects of melatonin treatments in children have not been reported [38], but the actual required dose is unclear. Indeed, the tolerability and pharmacokinetics of melatonin remain to be established.

3.4 N-Acetylcysteine

N-acetylcysteine, a glutathione precursor, has marked antioxidant properties. Its direct antioxidant activity has been demonstrated through the thiol group, ability for scavenging even hydroxyl free radicals [51] and to increase GSH reserves. Most studies have been performed in animal models, mainly rats. There is evidence supporting a potentially beneficial effect of early administration of N-acetylcysteine in sepsis-related reduction of regional blood flow. However, the isolated use of NAC could have some limitations due to its pro-oxidant effects, probably by its interaction with iron [52]. This could explain that administration of N-acetylcysteine plus the iron chelator deferoxamine in rats has been associated with a reduction of macrophage cytokine release and mitochondrial dysfunction, thereby improving survival [53]. In an experimental model of sepsis induced using non sterile fecal content and *Escherichia coli*, N-acetylcysteine prevented the mortality of animals. These data confirm the validity of the use of NAC in the treatment of sepsis [54].

High doses of N-acetylcysteine might exert protective effects on systemic hemodynamics and on the reactivity to catecholamines in humans challenged by lipopolysaccharide. This action of the antioxidant N-acetylcysteine is paralleled by humoral anti-inflammatory mechanisms and may be useful in patients with systemic inflammation [55].

Group B streptococcus infections in nonpregnant adults have been increasing, particularly in alcoholics where there is an increased risk of lobular invasion and mortality. In an established rat model it was demonstrated that chronic ethanol ingestion impaired macrophage internalization of inactivated infectious particles in vitro and enhanced bidirectional protein flux across the alveolar epithelial-endothelial barriers, increasing the risk of infection; but dietary N-acetylcysteine improved in vivo clearance of infectious particles, attenuated acute lung injury, and disseminated infection [56]. Treatment of rats with LPS significantly increased spontaneous platelet adhesion, but pretreatment of rats with the antioxidant N-acetylcysteine prevented the increase of non-activated platelet adhesion, and significantly reduced the inhibitory effect of LPS on thrombin-stimulated adhesion [57].

In addition, N-acetylcysteine has been used associated with other protective agents. Considering that the mitochondrial respiratory chain is altered in critically ill patients, in the brain of rats after cecal ligation and perforation, a combination of N-acetylcysteine/deferoxamine, taurine and RC-3095 showed to be an effective treatment of sepsis. The results demonstrated inhibition of mitochondrial complexes I and II, and that the treatments were able to reverse this inhibition in all brain areas. On the other hand, complexes III and IV were not affected by sepsis [58].

The effect of pretreatment with N-acetylcysteine on inflammatory response was studied in a rat model of sepsis induced by cecal ligation and puncture. The results showed an amelioration of sepsis syndrome by reduction of the proinflammatory and increase of the anti-inflammatory cytokine levels and accession of cellular antioxidants [59].

Plasma-induced ROS production by human umbilical vascular epithelial cells is associated with an intracellular decrease in reduced glutathione. Both ROS levels and cell death decreased when N-acetylcysteine or glutathione were added before exposing the cells to plasma. These data suggest a pivotal role of alterations in glutathione in damage caused by sepsis-generated ROS in endothelial cells [60].

3.5 Selenium

The essential trace element selenium (Se), particularly in the form of selenoproteins, plays an important role in host defense by humans in cell redox homeostasis [61]. Named after the Greek moon goddess, Selene, this micronutrient occurs in little amounts in our body. Most of it is in the liver, kidneys, and pancreas and, in men, the testes and seminal vesicles. Se protects cell against membrane lipid peroxidation, proteins and DNA oxidation, and slows the biochemical aging process. Of special interest is its benefit to the cardiovascular system. Epidemiological studies have reported an increased incidence of cardiovascular disease, strokes and other cardiovascular damage in low-Se areas. However, there is currently insufficient available evidence to recommend Se supplements for the prevention of coronary heart disease. Se-containing proteins include antioxidant enzymes necessary for the removal of ROS and free radicals. Thus, it is a structural component of glutathione peroxidase (GSH-Px), a cellular enzyme catalyzing the breakdown of hydroperoxides and the ROS hydrogen peroxide. The growing interest in Se research has led to the discovery of at least 30 selenoproteins; however, the biochemical functional roles of some of these selenoproteins are still unknown. Besides being found in the form of selenoproteins, in biological materials Se can exist in many different chemical forms either as organic Se compounds, such as selenomethionine and dimethylselenide, and inorganic selenites and selenates. In foods, Se is predominantly present as selenomethionine, which is an important source of dietary Se in humans, and also as a chemical form that is commonly used for Se supplements in clinical trials. Concern for potential deficiency diseases associated with low Se status has led to the establishment of the recommended daily requirements for Se in many countries. However, excess Se intakes through supplementation and its potential misuse could also pose a risk of adverse health effects if its use is not properly regulated. Selenium can induce two fundamental types of effects: antioxidant, through its incorporation into selenoenzymes; and pro-oxidant, through the direct effects of selenocompounds. As an antioxidant, it may limit oxidative damage to host cells and as a pro-oxidant, it may provide a transient anti-inflammatory effect by inducing apoptosis of reactive inflammatory cells and potentially damage invading microorganisms.

Serum Se is mainly contained in liver derived selenoprotein P (SePP) which controls the expression of antioxidative selenoproteins. Downregulation of SePP biosynthesis or removal of circulating SePP from blood underlies the negative acute phase response of serum Se in critical illness [62]. Currently, doses below the tolerable upper intake level (400 microg) may be used in supplementation. Higher doses (up to the level of no adverse effect, 800 microg) may be of interest and need to be studied further. The pro-oxidant effects of selenocompounds, especially sodium selenite, which vary depending on the compound, dose, and concentration, also need to be assessed further for their toxicity and potential therapeutic use in patients with septic shock [63].

It should be mentioned that at high doses the direct pro-oxidant effect of selenocompounds could contribute to explain its toxicity. Inorganic selenium compounds have effects on iron-mediated DNA damage, Na_2SeO_3 and SeO_2 exhibit antioxidant and pro-oxidant activities depending on concentrations of both the compound and hydrogen peroxide.

Increasing interest in selenium supplementation to critical patients has been supported on the basis of its antioxidant properties. In critically ill surgical patients, lower plasma selenium concentrations have been found to correlate with tissue damage, the presence of infection, organ dysfunction/failure, and increased ICU mortality. In a prospective, randomized, placebo-controlled, multiple-center trial, Angstwurm et al [64] studied the effect of the supplementation with sodium-selenite at a dose of 1000 μg initially, followed by a continuous infusion of 1000 μg/d for 14 days. An increment of GSH-Px-3 activity and a decrease in mortality rate in supplemented patients were observed. Furthermore, they noted a direct correlation between selenium concentrations and survival rate. However, in another prospective, multicenter, placebo-controlled, randomized, double-blind study, supplementation with sodium selenite at a dose of 4000 μg initially, followed by a continuous infusion of 1000 μg/d for 9 days, showed no improvement in the outcome of septic shock patients [65]. These contradictory results could be a consequence of a different timing in the initiation of supplementation, heterogeneity of patient groups, or the result of a different initial dose, through prooxidant effects or nuclear factor kappaB (NF-κB) modulation.

Selenium (Se), mainly through its incorporation into selenoproteins, plays an important role in inflammation and immunity. The loss of serum proteins resulting from the systemic inflammatory effects of sepsis may contribute to the precipitous loss of serum selenium during septic shock. Its plasma levels should be adequate both for initiating immunity and in regulating excessive immune responses and chronic inflammation. Selenium deficiency has been correlated with an impaired immune response; therefore, supplemental selenium replacement may improve immune function. Se deficiency is related to increased oxidative stress, but protein-folding and calcium flux may also be impaired in immune cells [66].

In terms of the risk of a new infection, it was reported that during critical illness there may be a benefit from supplementing 500 μg of selenium daily for at least five days [67]. High-dose parenteral selenite administered by continuous infusion reduces illness severity and lowers incidence of hospital-acquired pneumonia in critically ill patients with systemic inflammatory response syndrome [68]. This is a novel therapy having no short-term adverse events. However, it was recently found that despite high-dose Se substitution in patients with sepsis increased plasma Se and GSH-Px levels, it was not found a reduction in mortality [69]. Indeed, more studies aimed to elucidate the doses, schemes of administration and precise indications for critically ill patients are still lacking.

3.6 Allopurinol

The significant redox imbalance occurring in critical illness and particularly sepsis is associated with and arises from an increased production of oxidant species and a decrease in endogenous antioxidant defenses. Xanthine oxidase activation as a source of oxidative stress, together with the mitochondrial respiratory electron transport chain, the respiratory burst associated with neutrophil activation, and arachidonic acid metabolism, account for this imbalance. Xanthine oxidase is one of the major endogenous sources of superoxide in the cell and plays a role in superoxide generation in response to LPS [70]. Experimental studies demonstrated that LPS treatment resulted in increased activity of xanthine oxidase [71, 72]. Furthermore, the xanthine oxidase inhibitor allopurinol markedly protects against endotoxemic liver injury and indicates that reactive oxygen species (ROS) mediate synthesis of chemokines and leukocyte adhesion in the liver in vivo [73]. There are few data in the literature regarding the beneficial effect of allopurinol treatment. It is of great importance to keep in mind the possible and potentially harmful side effects of allopurinol therapy [74]. Allopurinol although inhibiting the activity of the enzyme, can actually reduce the enzyme by transfer of an electron to oxygen, thus generating superoxide. It is unclear the relevance of this finding for in vivo situations. Considering the pharmacodynamics of allopurinol and oxypurinol, the maximum inhibitory concentration is reached with doses by 300 mg allopurinol [75]. In general, allopurinol does not have a number of serious side effects, and the cellular and molecular mechanisms of the side effects are incompletely understood. It was reported that renal toxicity is related to impairment of pyrimidine metabolism.

LPS administration to mice gives rise to a systemic inflammation leading to the formation of another source of free radicals from xanthine oxidase-derived oxidizing species in vivo. Thus, tissue carboxypeptidase B, a pancreatic metallocarboxypeptidase, in the septic spleen forms a radical in the presence of xanthine oxidase. The above-mentioned events might result in significant loss of its activity and concomitant accumulation of C5a in the spleen, thus indicating a mechanism by which the inflammatory conditions may be maintained [71]. Due to the major role of xanthine oxidase in this mechanism of oxidative damage, it should be expected that allopurinol alleviate the deleterious organ effect.

3.7 Polyphenols

Polyphenols are a family of chemicals found in food and beverages derived from plants, such as cocoa, green tea, turmeric, and soya, as well as in medicinal herbs. Recently, the ability of wine polyphenols to modulate the activity of endogenous antioxidant system has been documented [76]. These phytochemicals exhibit anti-inflammatory and vascular-protective properties in clinical and preclinical studies and can exert an antioxidant effect through the promotion of the expression of some antioxidant enzymes. Polyphenols are thought to be a possible therapeutic resource against sepsis because of their known protective and anti-inflammatory effects in animal models of sepsis [77]. Wine polyphenols have demonstrated Most of these studies have been performed in rats. The oral or systemic administration of polyphenols protects rodents from endotoxinemia and microbial sepsis. Under these circumstances, polyphenols reproducibly attenuate microvascular hyperpermeability, tissue infiltration by leukocytes, oxidative and nitrosative stress, tissue injury, organ dysfunction, shock and vasoplejia, lactate production, and mortality. Importantly, efficacy is maintained in some cases even when treatment is initiated hours after the onset of sepsis. The most studied polyphenol is resveratrol, a phenolic compound derived from stilbene that reduces sepsis-induced remote organ injury, at least in part, through its ability to balance oxidant-antioxidant status, to inhibit neutrophil infiltration and to regulate the release of inflammatory mediators [78].

As renal microvascular failure during sepsis is correlated with the generation of reactive nitrogen species, the therapeutic potential of resveratrol, a vasodilator also capable of scavenging reactive nitrogen species, was investigated using the cecal ligation and puncture murine model of sepsis-induced acute kidney injury. Resveratrol when given following this procedure reversed the decline in cortical capillary perfusion, assessed by intravital microscopy, in a dose-dependent manner. It produced the greatest improvement in capillary perfusion, renal blood flow and the glomerular filtration rate, without raising systemic pressure. It was argued that resveratrol may have a dual mechanism of action to restore the renal microcirculation and scavenge reactive nitrogen species [79], thus protecting the renal tubular epithelium even when administered after the onset of sepsis [80].

Oral treatment with resveratrol reduced the levels of lipid peroxidation in the small intestine and colon following the administration of LPS, despite LPS caused a decrease in resveratrol absorption. When resveratrol bioavailability after i.p. administration was compared to that observed after oral administration, a different profile of resveratrol metabolites was found in plasma [81]. In addition, LPS-induced iron mobilization from plasma to kidney was abolished by resveratrol treatment. All these results suggest that resveratrol exerted strong antioxidant properties against LPS-induced nephrotoxicity and that its mode of action seemed to involve iron shuttling proteins [82]. Furthermore, the effects of LPS of inducing increased erythrocyte lipid peroxidation and depression of catalase activity were abrogated by resveratrol. This polyphenol can exert different protective effects. In plasma, LPS-induced deleterious effects, such as increased malondialdehyde via NO elevation and decreased iron level, were reversed by a subacute resveratrol pre-treatment via a NO independent way. Resveratrol exhibited potent protective effect on LPS-induced acute phase response in rats [83]. This polyphenol does not inhibit the activation or translocation of NF-κB/Rel proteins but inhibits NF-κB/Rel-dependent transcription by impairing the transactivation potential of p65 [84].

Despite the promising effects of resveratrol and other polyphenols derived from the animal models, their supplementation and clinical use is still limited by the fact that more pharmacokinetic and toxicological data are still lacking.

3.8 Other Antioxidants

Statins appear to be beneficial in sepsis through restoration of the microvascular tone and maintenance of microvascular integrity, an effect mediated by the increment in NO concentrations in vascular endothelium, this way reversing endothelial dysfunction [85]. This effect is consistent with the ability of statins to inhibit the activation of the NADPH pathway.

Vitamin A is obtained from the diet either as all-trans-retinol, retinyl esters, or β-carotene. It has long been known to have antioxidant and immunomodulatory properties. Accordingly, deficiency of this vitamin is associated with inflammation. Vitamin A supplementation reduces the pathophysiological effects of endotoxin in animals [86], an anti-inflammatory effect that could depend, at least in part, on NF-κB inhibition [87]. However, although vitamin A has known antioxidant properties, there is evidence pointing also to effects through binding to nuclear receptors.

L-arginine supplementation in sepsis is controversial. Septic shock has been alternatively viewed as an L-arginine-deficient state or as a syndrome caused by excess nitric oxide, an end-product of L-arginine metabolism. Unexpectedly, L-arginine similarly increased mortality, and worsened shock [88]. Likely, this response is due to increased activity of inducible nitric oxide synthase, consistent with enhanced production of the highly peroxidant peroxynitrite. Therefore, supplemental parenteral L-arginine, at doses above standard dietary practices, should be avoided in critically ill patients with septic shock.

L-Alanyl-L-glutamine supplementation improves clinical outcome in critically ill patients [89], likely including in its mechanisms the antioxidant effect conferred by being a precursor of GSH. Glutamine reduces infectious complications in large-sized trials. Glutamine, GSH, and selenium are linked with the most potent antioxidant enzyme family—glutathione peroxidase—at some stage of their synthesis and metabolism, while lipoic acid might be a generic regenerator [90].

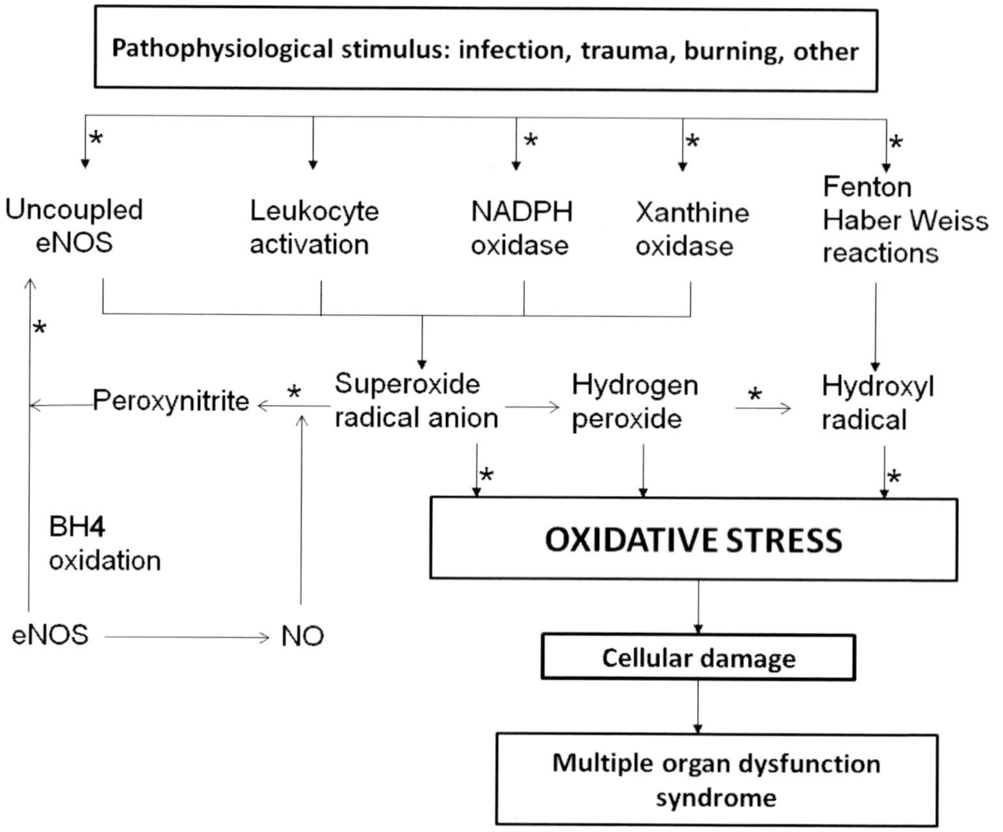

Figure 12-1. Diagram representing a hypothesis to account for the role of oxidative stress in the worsening of critically ill patients and the effects of exogenous antioxidants in abrogating the pathophysiological mechanisms of oxidative damage. NO, nitric oxide; eNOs, endothelial nitric oxide synthase; NADPH, reduced nicotine adenine dinucleotide phosphate; BH4, tetrahydrobiopterin; * site of action of antioxidant molecules.

Treatment with the polymeric iron chelator deferoxamine significantly increases survival of septic subjects and alters the expression of bax, an apoptosis regulating protein in certain organs, such as heart, liver and kidney [91]. The toxic effects of free iron are substantiated by its ability to catalyze via Fenton reaction the generation of damaging hydroxyl free radicals [92]. N-acetylcysteine plus deferoxamine reduces the consequences of septic shock in the rat, by decreasing oxidative stress and limiting neutrophil infiltration and mitochondrial dysfunction, thereby improving survival [53].

In addition, the association of eicosapentaenoic acid and micronutrients has significant anti-inflammatory effects. In critically ill patients, some prospective randomized controlled trials support parenteral supplementation of high doses of vitamin C, E and trace elements [93]. Other antioxidants are still on the clinical benchmark level, awaiting well-designed clinical trials.

Finally, we present a diagram supporting the potential use of antioxidants to improve the clinical outcome of the critically ill patient (see Figure 12-1).

CONCLUSIONS AND PERSPECTIVES

The antioxidant defense system of the body normally counteracts the effects of ROS and RNS, known to cause damage to many cellular components, but in critically ill patients the antioxidant capacity is overwhelmed. Plasma antioxidant micronutrient concentrations are depressed during critical illness and especially during sepsis, as the result of losses, low intakes, dilution by resuscitation fluids, and redistribution to extravascular tissues, creating a circulating antioxidant defense deficit. Hence, provision of antioxidant supplementation to these patients may help in abrogating the effects of the reactive species. This novel therapy should be expected to contribute in limiting tissue and organ damage caused by sepsis mediators, thus improving the clinical outcome of patients. However, no study has yet provided conclusive evidence of such beneficial effect in these clinical settings. Despite the clinical evidence shows that there are several factors which might determine the efficacy of antioxidant supplementation, more studies are still lacking. There is a need for large multicentre prospective randomized control trials to assess the effects of different types and doses of antioxidant supplementation in selected groups of patients with different types of critical illness.

Strategies using combinations of antioxidant micronutrients or drugs constitute a more efficient treatment than the use of either alone. This paradigm is based on the fact that these compounds act in different points of the deleterious pathway, and synergistically. Therefore, the association allows improving the therapeutic effectiveness in severe illness. Optimal effects may be expected with a combination of micronutrients at levels similar to those found in a normal diet for healthy people. In contrast, a single antioxidant given at high doses may have a limited benefit and could even have negative consequences in subjects with high risk of pathologies. In addition, short-term interventions appear to be free of deleterious effects, otherwise occurring in long-term exposure.

Melatonin, acting specifically in mitochondria, is a promising molecule that deserves the attention of future research, due to the relevance of this organelle in the cascade of pathophysiological events leading to multiple organ dysfunction syndrome. In addition, the efficacy of vitamin C in concentrations high enough to abrogate the combination of superoxide and NO has yet to be explored. Further research is required to determine the optimal micronutrient combinations and the doses required according to the timing of intervention and severity of disease. When such problems will be resolved hopefully results about antioxidant therapy in critical illness will be more univocal and promising.

REFERENCES

[1] Brealey D, Brand M, Hargreaves I, Heales S, Land J, Smolenski R, Davies NA, Cooper CE, Singer M. Association between mitochondrial dysfunction and severity and outcome of septic shock. *Lancet* 2002;360:219–223.

[2] Brigelius-Flohé R, Flohé L. Basic principles and emerging concepts in the redox control of transcription factors. *Antioxid Redox Signal* 2011;15:2335–2381.

[3] Víctor VM, Espulgues JV, Hernández-Mijares A, Rocha M. Oxidative stress and mitochondrial dysfunction in sepsis: a potential therapy with mitochondria-targeted antioxidants. *Infect Disord Drug Targets* 2009;9:376-389.

[4] Ogilvie AC, Groeneveld AB, Straub JP, Thijs LG. Plasma lipid peroxides and antioxidants in human septic shock. *Intens Care Med* 1991;17:40–44.

[5] Harrois A, Huet O, Duranteau J. Alterations of mitochondrial function in sepsis and critical illness. *Curr Opin Anaesthesiol* 2009;22:143–149.

[6] Rinaldi S, Landucci F, De Gaudio AR. Antioxidant therapy in critically septic patients. *Curr Drug Targets* 2009;10:872-880.

[7] Galley HF. Bench-to-bedside review: Targeting antioxidants to mitochondria in sepsis. *Crit Care* 2010;14:230.

[8] Schorah CJ, Downing C, Piripitsi A, Gallivan L, Al-Hazaa AH, Sanderson MJ, Bodenham A. Total vitamin C, ascorbic acid, and dehydroascorbic acid concentrations in plasma of critically ill patients. *Am J Clin Nutr* 1996;63:760–765.

[9] Ichim TE, Minev B, Braciak T, Luna B, Hunninghake R, Mikirova NA, Jackson JA, Gonzalez MJ, Miranda-Massari JR, Alexandrescu DT, Dasanu CA, Bogin V, Ancans J, Stevens RB, Markosian B, Koropatnick J, Chen CS, Riordan NH. Intravenous ascorbic acid to prevent and treat cancer-associated sepsis? *J Transl Med* 2011, 9:25.

[10] De Backer D, Donadello K, Taccone FS, Ospina-Tascon G, Salgado D, Vincent JL. Microcirculatory alterations: potential mechanisms and implications for therapy. Ann Intensive Care 2011;1:27.

[11] Secor D, Li F, Ellis CG, Sharpe MD, Gross PL, Wilson JX, Tyml K. Impaired microvascular perfusion in sepsis requires activated coagulation and P-selectin-mediated platelet adhesion in capillaries. *Intensive Care Med* 2010;36:1928-1934.

[12] Tyml K, Li F, Wilson JX. Delayed ascorbate bolus protects against maldistribution of microvascular blood flow in septic rat skeletal muscle. *Crit Care Med* 2005;33:1823-1828.

[13] Tyml K, Li F, Wilson JX. Septic impairment of capillary blood flow requires nicotinamide adenine dinucleotide phosphate oxidase but not nitric oxide synthase and is rapidly reversed by ascorbate through an endothelial nitric oxide synthase-dependent mechanism. *Crit Care Med* 2008;36:2355-2362.

[14] Poeze M, Bruins MJ, Kessels F, Luiking YC, Lamers WH, Deutz NE. Effects of L-arginine pretreatment on nitric oxide metabolism and hepatosplanchnic perfusion during porcine endotoxemia. *Am J Clin Nutr* 2011;93:1237-1247.

[15] Wu F, Wilson JX, Tyml K. Ascorbate protects against impaired arteriolar constriction in sepsis by inhibiting inducible nitric oxide synthase expression. *Free Radic Biol Med* 2004;37:1282-1289.

[16] Ferrón-Celma I, Mansilla A, Hassan L, Garcia-Navarro A, Comino AM, Bueno P, Ferrón JA. Effect of vitamin C administration on neutrophil apoptosis in septic patients after abdominal surgery. *J Surg Res* 2009;153:224-230.

[17] Fisher BJ, Seropian IM, Kraskauskas D, Thakkar JN, Voelkel NF, Fowler AA 3rd, Natarajan R. Ascorbic acid attenuates lipopolysaccharide-induced acute lung injury. *Crit Care Med* 2011;39:1454-1460.

[18] Graumlich JF, Ludden TM, Conry-Cantilena C, Cantilena LR Jr, Wang Y, Levine M. Pharmacokinetic model of ascorbic acid in healthy male volunteers during depletion and repletion. *Pharm Res* 1997;14:1133-1139.

[19] Jackson TS, Xu A, Vita JA, Keaney JF Jr. Ascorbate prevents the interaction of superoxide and nitric oxide only at very high physiological concentrations. *Circ Res* 1998;83:916-922.

[20] Basili S, Tanzilli G, Mangieri E, Raparelli V, Di Santo S, Pignatelli P, Violi F. Intravenous ascorbic acid infusion improves myocardial perfusion grade during elective percutaneous coronary intervention: relationship with oxidative stress markers. *JACC Cardiovasc Interv* 2010;3:221-229.

[21] Bhakuni P, Chandra M, Misra MK. Effect of ascorbic acid supplementation on certain oxidative stress parameters in the post reperfusion patients of myocardial infarction. *Mol Cell Biochem* 2006;290:153-158.

[22] Ulker S, McKeown PP, Bayraktutan U. Vitamins reverse endothelial dysfunction through regulation of eNOS and NAD(P)H oxidase activities. *Hypertension* 2003;41:534-539.

[23] Kuzkaya N, Weissmann N, Harrison DG, Dikalov S. Interactions of peroxynitrite, tetrahydrobiopterin, ascorbic acid, and thiols: implications for uncoupling endothelial nitric-oxide synthase. *J Biol Chem* 2003;278:22546-22554.

[24] Tsovolas K, Iliodromitis EK, Andreadou I, Zoga A, Demopoulou M, Iliodromitis KE, Manolaki T, Markantonis SL, Kremastinos DT. Acute administration of vitamin C abrogates protection from ischemic preconditioning in rabbits. *Pharmacol Res* 2008;57:283-289.

[25] Crimi E, Liguori A, Condorelli M, Cioffi M, Astuto M, Bontempo P, Pignalosa O, Vietri MT, Molinari AM, Sica V, Della Corte F, Napoli C. The beneficial effects of antioxidant supplementation in enteral feeding in critically ill patients: a prospective, randomized, double-blind, placebo-controlled trial. *Anesth Analg* 2004;99:857–863.

[26] Kanter M, Coskun O, Armutcu F, Uz YH, Kizilay G. Protective effects of vitamin C, alone or in combination with vitamin A, on endotoxin-induced oxidative renal tissue damage in rats. *Tohoku J Exp Med* 2005;206:155-162.

[27] Padayatty SJ, Sun AY, Chen Q, Espey MG, Drisko J, Levine M. Vitamin C: intravenous use by complementary and alternative medicine practitioners and adverse effects. *PLoS One* 2010;5:e11414.

[28] Wilson JX, Wu F. Vitamin C in sepsis. *Subcell Biochem* 2012;56:67-83.

[29] Terentis AC, Thomas SR, Burr JA, Liebler DC, Stocker R. Vitamin E oxidation in human atherosclerotic lesions. *Circ Res* 2002;90:333–339.

[30] Shi H, Noguchi N, Niki E. Comparative study on dynamics of antioxidative action of alpha-tocopheryl hydroquinone, ubiquinol, and alpha-tocopherol against lipid peroxidation. *Free Radic Biol Med* 1999;27:334–336.

[31] Kim JY, Lee SM. Effect of alpha-tocopherol on the expression of hepatic vascular stress genes in response to sepsis. *J Toxicol Environ Health A* 2005;68:2051–2062.

[32] Durant R, Klouche K, Delbosc S, Morena M, Amigues L, Beraud JJ, Canaud B, Cristol JP. Superoxide anion overproduction in sepsis: effects of vitamin e and simvastatin. *Shock* 2004;22:34-39.

[33] Beale RJ, Sherry T, Lei K, Campbell-Stephen L, McCook J, Smith J, Venetz W, Alteheld B, Stehle P, Schneider H. Early enteral supplementation with key pharmaconutrients improves Sequential Organ Failure Assessment score in critically ill patients with sepsis: outcome of a randomized, controlled, double-blind trial. *Crit Care Med* 2008;36:131-144.

[34] Carlson D, Maass DL, White DJ, Tan J, Horton JW. Antioxidant vitamin therapy alters sepsis-related apoptotic myocardial activity and inflammatory responses. *Am J Physiol Heart Circ Physiol* 2006;291:H2779–2789.

[35] Nathens AB, Neff MJ, Jurkovich GJ, Klotz P, Farver K, Ruzinski JT, Radella F, Garcia I, Maier RV. Randomized, prospective trial of antioxidant supplementation in critically ill surgical patients. *Ann Surg* 2002;236:814–822.

[36] Koga H, Hagiwara S, Inomata M, Kono Y, Oyama Y, Kai S, Nishida T, Noguchi T. The New Vitamin E Derivative, ETS-GS, Protects Against Cecal Ligation and Puncture-Induced Systemic Inflammation in Rats. *Inflammation* 2012;35:545-555.

[37] Kono Y, Inomata M, Hagiwara S, Shiraishi N, Noguchi T, Kitano S. A newly synthetic vitamin E derivative, E-Ant-S-GS, attenuates lung injury caused by cecal ligation and puncture-induced sepsis in rats. *Surgery* 2012;151:420-426.

[38] Sánchez-Barceló EJ, Mediavilla MD, Reiter RJ. Clinical uses of melatonin in pediatrics. *Int J Pediatr* 2011;2011:892624.

[39] Galano A, Tan DX, Reiter RJ. Melatonin as a natural ally against oxidative stress: a physicochemical examination. *J Pineal Res* 2011;51:1-16.

[40] Tan DX, Manchester LC, Reiter RJ, Qi WB, Karbownik M, Calvo JR. Significance of melatonin in antioxidative defense system: reactions and products. *Biol Signals Recept* 2000;9:137-59.

[41] Lowes DA, Almawash AM, Webster NR, Reid VL, Galley HF. Melatonin and structurally similar compounds have differing effects on inflammation and mitochondrial function in endothelial cells under conditions mimicking sepsis. *Br J Anaesth* 2011;107:193-201.

[42] Reynolds FD, Dauchy R, Blask D, Dietz PA, Lynch D, Zuckerman R. The pineal gland hormone melatonin improves survival in a rat model of sepsis/shock induced by zymosan A. *Surgery* 2003;134:474-479.

[43] Gitto E, Karbownik M, Reiter RJ, Tan DX, Cuzzocrea S, Chiurazzi P, Cordaro S, Corona G, Trimarchi G, Barberi I. Effects of melatonin treatment in septic newborns. *Pediatr Res* 2001;50:756-760.

[44] Gitto E, Pellegrino S, Gitto P, Barberi I, Reiter RJ. Oxidative stress of the newborn in the pre- and postnatal period and the clinical utility of melatonin. *J Pineal Res* 2009;46:128-139.

[45] Huang Z, Rose AH, Hoffmann PR. The Role of Selenium in Inflammation and Immunity: From Molecular Mechanisms to Therapeutic Opportunities. *Antioxid Redox Signal* 2012;16:705-743.

[46] Rodriguez C, Mayo JC, Sainz RM, Antolín I, Herrera F, Martín V, Reiter RJ. Regulation of antioxidant enzymes: a significant role for melatonin. *J Pineal Res* 2004;36:1-9.

[47] Bharti VK, Srivastava RS. Effect of pineal proteins at different dose level on fluoride-induced changes in plasma biochemicals and blood antioxidants enzymes in rats. *Trace Elem Res* 2011;141:275-282.

[48] Srinivasan V, Pandi-Perumal SR, Spence DW, Kato H, Cardinali DP. Melatonin in septic shock: some recent concepts. *J Crit Care* 2010;25:656.e1-6.

[49] Srinivasan V, Spence DW, Pandi-Perumal SR, Brown GM, Cardinali DP. Melatonin in mitochondrial dysfunction and related disorders. *Int J Alzheimers Dis* 2011;2011:326320.

[50] Escames G, López LC, Ortiz F, López A, García JA, Ros E, Acuña-Castroviejo D. Attenuation of cardiac mitochondrial dysfunction by melatonin in septic mice. *FEBS J* 2007;274:2135-2147.

[51] Agnihotri N, Mishra PC. Mechanism of scavenging action of N-acetylcysteine for the OH radical: a quantum computational study. *J Phys Chem B* 2009;113:12096-12104.

[52] Sprong RC, Winkelhuyzen-Janssen AM, Aarsman CJ, van Oirschot JF, van der Bruggen T, van Asbeck BS. Low-dose N-acetylcysteine protects rats against endotoxin-mediated oxidative stress, but high-dose increases mortality. *Am J Respir Crit Care Med* 1998;157(4 Pt 1):1283-1293.

[53] Ritter C, Andrades ME, Reinke A, Menna-Barreto S, Moreira JC, Dal-Pizzol F. Treatment with N-acetylcysteine plus deferoxamine protects rats against oxidative stress and improves survival in sepsis. *Crit Care Med* 2004;32:342-349.

[54] de Mello RO, Lunardelli A, Caberlon E, de Moraes CM, Christ Vianna Santos R, da Costa VL, da Silva GV, da Silva Scherer P, Buaes LE, da Silva Melo DA, Donadio MV, Nunes FB, de Oliveira JR. Effect of N-Acetylcysteine and Fructose-1,6-Bisphosphate in the Treatment of Experimental Sepsis. *Inflammation* 2011;34:539-550.

[55] Schaller G, Pleiner J, Mittermayer F, Posch M, Kapiotis S, Wolzt M. Effects of N-acetylcysteine against systemic and renal hemodynamic effects of endotoxin in healthy humans. *Int J Pediatr* 2011;2011:892624.

[56] Tang SM, Gabelaia L, Gauthier TW, Brown LA. N-acetylcysteine improves group B streptococcus clearance in a rat model of chronic ethanol ingestion. *Alcohol Clin Exp Res* 2009;33:1197-1201.

[57] Casarin AL, Lopes-Pires ME, Morganti RP, Antunes E, Marcondes S. Reactive oxygen and nitrogen species modulate the ex-vivo effects of LPS on platelet adhesion to fibrinogen. *Life Sci* 2011;89:773-778.

[58] Cassol OJ Jr, Rezin GT, Petronilho FC, Scaini G, Gonçalves CL, Ferreira GK, Roesler R, Schwartsmann G, Dal-Pizzol F, Streck EL. Effects of N-acetylcysteine/deferoxamine, taurine and RC-3095 on respiratory chain complexes and creatine kinase activities in rat brain after sepsis. *Neurochem Res* 2010;35:515-521.

[59] Senoglu N, Yuzbasioglu MF, Aral M, Ezberci M, Kurutas EB, Bulbuloglu E, Ezberci F, Oksuz H, Ciragil P. Protective effects of N-acetylcysteine and beta-glucan pretreatment on oxidative stress in cecal ligation and puncture model of sepsis. *J Invest Surg* 2008;21:237-243.

[60] Huet O, Cherreau C, Nicco C, Dupic L, Conti M, Borderie D, Pene F, Vicaut E, Benhamou D, Mira JP, Duranteau J, Batteux F. Pivotal role of glutathione depletion in

plasma-induced endothelial oxidative stress during sepsis. *Crit Care Med* 2008;36:2328-2334.

[61] Sakr Y, Reinhart K, Bloos F, Marx G, Russwurm S, Bauer M, Brunkhorst F. Time course and relationship between plasma selenium concentrations, systemic inflammatory response, sepsis, and multiorgan failure. *Br J Anaesth* 2007;98:775–784.

[62] Hollenbach B, Morgenthaler NG, Struck J, Alonso C, Bergmann A, Köhrle J, Schomburg L. New assay for the measurement of selenoprotein P as a sepsis biomarker from serum. *J Trace Elem Med Biol* 2008;22:24–32.

[63] Vincent JL, Forceville X. Critically elucidating the role of selenium. *Curr Opin Anaesthesiol* 2008;21:148-154.

[64] Angstwurm MW, Engelmann L, Zimmermann T, Lehmann C, Spes CH, Abel P, Strauss R, Meier-Hellmann A, Insel R, Radke J, Schüttler J, Gärtner R. Selenium in Intensive Care (SIC): results of a prospective randomized, placebo-controlled, multiple-center study in patients with severe systemic inflammatory response syndrome, sepsis, and septic shock. *Crit Care Med* 2007;35:118-126.

[65] Forceville X. Effects of high doses of selenium, as sodium selenite, in septic shock patients a placebo-controlled, randomized, double-blind, multi-center phase II study--selenium and sepsis. *J Trace Elem Med Biol* 2007;21(Suppl 1):62-65.

[66] Huang SH, Cao XJ, Liu W, Shi XY, Wei W. Inhibitory effect of melatonin on lung oxidative stress induced by respiratory syncytial virus infection in mice. *J Pineal Res* 2010;48:109-116.

[67] Andrews PJ, Avenell A, Noble DW, Campbell MK, Croal BL, Simpson WG, Vale LD, Battison CG, Jenkinson DJ, Cook JA; Scottish Intensive care Glutamine or seleNium Evaluative Trial Trials Group. Randomised trial of glutamine, selenium, or both, to supplement parenteral nutrition for critically ill patients. *BMJ.* 2011;342:d1542.

[68] Manzanares W, Biestro A, Torre MH, Galusso F, Facchin G, Hardy G. High-dose selenium reduces ventilator-associated pneumonia and illness severity in critically ill patients with systemic inflammation. *Intensive Care Med* 2011;37:1120–1127.

[69] Valenta J, Brodska H, Drabek T, Hendl J, Kazda A. High-dose selenium substitution in sepsis: a prospective randomized clinical trial. *Intensive Care Med* 2011;37:808–815.

[70] Nakai K, Kadiiska MB, Jiang JJ, Stadler K, Mason RP. Free radical production requires both inducible nitric oxide synthase and xanthine oxidase in LPS-treated skin. *Proc Natl Acad Sci U S A* 2006;103:4616-4621.

[71] Chatterjee S, Lardinois O, Bonini MG, Bhattacharjee S, Stadler K, Corbett J, Deterding LJ, Tomer KB, Kadiiska M, Mason RP. Site-specific carboxypeptidase B1 tyrosine nitration and pathophysiological implications following its physical association with nitric oxide synthase-3 in experimental sepsis. *J Immunol* 2009;183:4055-4066.

[72] Chinnaiyan AM, Huber-Lang M, Kumar-Sinha C, Barrette TR, Shankar-Sinha S, Sarma VJ, Padgaonkar VA, Ward PA. Molecular signatures of sepsis: multiorgan gene expression profiles of systemic inflammation. *Am J Pathol* 2001;159:1199-1209.

[73] Xiang L, Klintman D, Thorlacius H. Allopurinol inhibits CXC chemokine expression and leukocyte adhesion in endotoxemic liver injury. *Inflamm Res* 2003;52:353-358.

[74] Hung CC, Liu WC, Kuo MC, Lee CH, Hwang SJ, Chen HC. Acute renal failure and its risk factors in Stevens-Johnson Syndrome and Toxic Epidermal Necrolysis. *Am J Nephrol* 2009;29:633–638.

[75] Graham S, Day RO, Wong H, McLachlan AJ, Bergendal L, Miners JO, Birkett DJ.Pharmacodynamics of oxypurinol after administration of allopurinol to healthy subjects. *Br J Clin Pharmacol* 1996;41:299–304.

[76] Rodrigo R, Miranda A, Vergara L. Modulation of endogenous antioxidant system by wine polyphenols in human disease. *Clin Chim Acta* 2011;412:410-424.

[77] Shapiro H, Lev S, Cohen J, Singer P. Polyphenols in the prevention and treatment of sepsis syndromes: rationale and pre-clinical evidence. *Nutrition* 2009;25:981-297.

[78] Kolgazi M, Sener G, Cetinel S, Gedik N, Alican I. Resveratrol reduces renal and lung injury caused by sepsis in rats. *J Surg Res* 2006;134:315-321.

[79] Holthoff JH, Woodling KA, Doerge DR, Burns ST, Hinson JA, Mayeux PR. Resveratrol, a dietary polyphenolic phytoalexin, is a functional scavenger of peroxynitrite. *Biochem Pharmacol* 2010;80:1260-1265.

[80] Holthoff JH, Wang Z, Seely KA, Gokden N, Mayeux PR. Resveratrol improves renal microcirculation, protects the tubular epithelium, and prolongs survival in a mouse model of sepsis-induced acute kidney injury. *Kidney Int* 2012;81:370-378.

[81] Larrosa M, Azorín-Ortuño M, Yañez-Gascón MJ, García-Conesa MT, Tomás-Barberán F, Espín JC. Lack of effect of oral administration of resveratrol in LPS-induced systemic inflammation. *Eur J Nutr* 2011;50:673-680.

[82] Sebai H, Ben-Attia M, Sani M, Aouani E, Ghanem-Boughanmi N. Protective effect of resveratrol on acute endotoxemia-induced nephrotoxicity in rat through nitric oxide independent mechanism. *Free Radic Res* 2008;42:913-920.

[83] Sebai H, Ben-Attia M, Sani M, Aouani E, Ghanem-Boughanmi N. Protective effect of resveratrol in endotoxemia-induced acute phase response in rats. *Arch Toxicol* 2009;83:335-340.

[84] Pendurthi UR, Meng F, Mackman N, Rao LV. Mechanism of resveratrol-mediated suppression of tissue factor gene expression. *Thromb Haemost* 2002;87:155-162.

[85] McGown CC, Brookes ZL. Beneficial effects of statins on the microcirculation during sepsis: the role of nitric oxide. *Br J Anaesth* 2007;98:163-175.

[86] Iversen MH, Hahn RG. Acute effects of vitamin A on the kinetics of endotoxin in conscious rabbits. *Intensive Care Med* 1999;25:1160-1164.

[87] Austenaa LM, Carlsen H, Hollung K, Blomhoff HK, Blomhoff R. Retinoic acid dampens LPS-induced NF-kappaB activity: results from human monoblasts and in vivo imaging of NF-kappaB reporter mice. *J Nutr Biochem* 2009;20:726-734.

[88] Kalil AC, Sevransky JE, Myers DE, Esposito C, Vandivier RW, Eichacker P, Susla GM, Solomon SB, Csako G, Costello R, Sittler KJ, Banks S, Natanson C, Danner RL. Preclinical trial of L-arginine monotherapy alone or with N-acetylcysteine in septic shock. *Crit Care Med* 2006;34:2719-2728.

[89] Déchelotte P, Hasselmann M, Cynober L, Allaouchiche B, Coëffier M, Hecketsweiler B, Merle V, Mazerolles M, Samba D, Guillou YM, Petit J, Mansoor O, Colas G, Cohendy R, Barnoud D, Czernichow P, Bleichner G. L-alanyl-L-glutamine dipeptide-supplemented total parenteral nutrition reduces infectious complications and glucose intolerance in critically ill patients: the French controlled, randomized, double-blind, multicenter study. *Crit Care Med* 2006;34:598-604.

[90] Berger MM, Chioléro RL. Antioxidant supplementation in sepsis and systemic inflammatory response syndrome. *Crit Care Med* 2007;35(9 Suppl):S584-590.

[91] Messaris E, Antonakis PT, Memos N, Chatzigianni E, Leandros E, Konstadoulakis MM. Deferoxamine administration in septic animals: improved survival and altered apoptotic gene expression. *Int Immunopharmacol* 2004;4:455-459.

[92] Ganz, T. Hepcidin, a key regulator of iron metabolism and mediator of anemia of inflammation. *Blood* 2003;102:783–788.

[93] Fukushima R, Yamazaki E. Vitamin C requirement in surgical patients. *Curr Opin Clin Nutr Metab Care* 2010;13:669-676.

In: Oxidative Stress and the Critically Ill Patient
Editors: Ramón Rodrigo and Bettina von Dessauer
ISBN: 978-1-62081-576-2

Chapter XIII

MYOCARDIAL DYSFUNCTION

Pedro Alvarez*[*], *Ana María Bañales, and Agustín Gatica
Intensive care, Hospital metropolitano, Santiago, Chile

1. ABSTRACT

Cardiac function depends on multiple factors. Preload, afterload, heart rate and contractility are the most recognizable. Myocardial dysfunction is a clinical syndrome characterized by heart abnormalities. It accompanied by renal, neural and hormonal alterations. Commonly, occurs in a heart that has been previously damaged by multiple factors. The increases of arterial blood pressure and coronary heart disease are the most important risk factors.

In addition of the description of hemodynamic characteristics, in this chapter we show that heart failure is not only the consequence of a hemodynamic process which involves the retention of water and salt, but a complex syndrome with significant neurohumoral alterations that contribute towards the symptoms and progression of the disease.

Exist various methods for evaluate the myocardial dysfunction. Nevertheless, hemodynamic monitoring which is performed with a transthoracic echocardiogram, is the most frequently used in the present, due to the amount of morphofunctional information which this test provides, high accessibility and lower cost.

Reactive oxygen species (ROS) and reactive nitrogen species (RNS) have several potentially important effects on endothelial function and are implicated in physiological regulation and contractility alterations. Free radicals contribute to mitochondrial dysfunction by a range of mechanisms and induce both necrotic and apoptotic cell death. This is consistent with the negative relationship between higher values of lipid peroxidation biomarkers and low values of ventricular function in critically ill patients.

Reversibility of myocardial dysfunction during a period from 7 to 10 days in survivors is other typical manifestation of septic myocardial dysfunction. Hence, one can speculate that development of such a type of myocardial dysfunction as a temporary protective compensatory mechanism could be advantageous for of an individual patient. A large body of evidence about mechanisms of myocardial dysfunction was described;

[*]Master student, Faculty of Medicine, University of Chile

endothelial dysfunction with consequent microcirculatory and mitochondrial dysfunction and role of circulating factors are considered to be the most important.

ABBREVIATIONS

ROS	reactive oxygen species
RNS	reactive nitrogen species
AMP	adenosine monophosphate
ATP	adenosine triphosphate
ANP	atrial natriuretic peptide
BNP	brain natriuretic peptide
CI	cardiac index
CO	cardiac output
CPR	c protein reaction
EF	ejection fraction
ET	endothelin
HF	heart failure
MDA	malondialdehyde
NP	natriuretic peptide
NPC	natriuretic peptide type C
LV	left ventricular
RAAS	renin-angiotensin-aldosterone system
ROS	reactive oxygen species
SVR	systemic vascular resistence
TNF-α	tumor necrosis factor α
XO	xantino oxidase

2. INTRODUCTION

Sepsis is a serious medical condition and a direct cause of death in critical patients [1]. The incidence and frequency of sepsis is increasing due to the higher prevalence of elderly population, larger number of immuno-compromised patients and the fact that more patients are admitted to intensive care units every day. Despite the higher investments on intensive care units and the aggressive treatments available, mortality from severe sepsis or septic shock has only had a small reduction and still ranges from 30 to 50% [1, 2].

Sepsis is a complex disease and is a manifestation of the host immune, inflammatory and coagulation response to infection. Severe sepsis is defined as sepsis with organ dysfunction, while septic shock is sepsis with persistent hypotension despite of resuscitation with fluids [1, 2]

Recent definitions recognize the importance of myocardial depression and include a low cardiac index (CI) or echocardiographic evidence of cardiac dysfunction as criteria for diagnosing severe sepsis [3].

Before the introduction of invasive cardiovascular monitoring, it was widely thought that there were two different phases in septic shock. Patients with septic shock initially went through a hyper dynamic phase (warm shock) characterized by warm skin, tachycardia with concomitant hypotension followed by cold shock, with poor peripheral perfusion, a thready pulse, cool extremities, which lead ultimately to death.

Current studies demonstrating an association between a high CI and higher survival rate support this theory. Other studies showed that patients with septic shock who were not hypovolemic had hyperdynamic circulation with a normal or elevated cardiac output (CO) and a low systemic vascular resistance (SVR). However, it was not until the introduction of the pulmonary artery catheter with its ability to accurately measure CO and estimate left ventricular (LV) filling pressures that it was demonstrated that patients with septic shock who were resuscitated adequately with fluids consistently had hyperdinamic circulation with warm peripheries, high CO and low SVR. However, despite the increase in CO and maintenance of a normal stroke volume, many also suffer from intrinsic myocardial dysfunction. This manifests as a reduction in ejection fraction (EF), which is a clinically useful quantitative measurement of ventricular performance. Although EF depends on afterload and preload, the assessment of the myocardium in patients with sepsis using independent techniques also reveals significant myocardial dysfunction.

Endothelial dysfunction is responsible for resistance to vasopressor agents. Contractile response of arteries and arterioles to norepinephrine or phenylephrine is decreased in sepsis; this effect is mediated by circulating factors. A variety of factors have been demonstrated to be useful.

|Venous return is also decreased in sepsis. This reduction in venous tone appears to be grater than the arterial one. Venous congestion is not equally distributed, with the splanchnic more prone to develop venous pooling. Portal hypertension is also seen with venous pooling in sepsis. The combination of venous pooling and increased permeability traduced in peripheral edema results in severe hypovolemia. Venous compliance is decreased in septic patients so that central venous pressure may underestimate the severity of hypovolemia. Consequences of hypovolemia include lower, inadequate cardiac output and redistribution of regional blood flow, particularly at expenses of splanchnic and renal beds [4]

3. Management of Sepsis-Induced Myocardial Dysfunction

Nowadays, the best treatment available for myocardial dysfunction in sepsis is the correct treatment of sepsis and the adequate multi-disciplinary to assure an adequate perfusion pressure and blood flow to cover global and regional metabolic demands [4].

The use of inotropes may be necessary if the cardiac output persists insufficient, despite even when the volemia filling pressures have been restored.

3.1 Fluid Resuscitation

Fluid resuscitation is one of the cornerstones in treatment of patients in intensive care units. Fluid replacement is used with the purpose of optimizing cardiac output without increasing the risk of pulmonary edema. Bolus doses of 250 – 500 ml of a crystalloid solution are usually given, with careful monitoring to ensure that there is no increase in pulmonary capillary pressure leading to hypoxemia.

A central issue in the pathophysiology and therapy of sepsis and septic shock that is still controversial is the double-edged effect of fluid loading on the cardiovascular system as a whole and the heart chambers in particular. The study of Kumar et al showed that large volumes of saline infused to normal, no septic volunteers significantly decreased SVR en 17% and increased CI with a reduction in end-systolic volume and increase in stroke volume index but with no change in end-diastolic volume, the explanation for this could be the decrease in SVR occurred most likely because of the effects of hemodilution in blood viscosity, SVR also could decrease through neuroendocrine pathways stimulated by the increase in stroke volume and CO was induced by the Frank-Starling effects of preload on the heart [4].

In any case, although fluid resuscitation is the suggested first line of treatment to restore blood pressure, CO, and tissue perfusion in septic shock, it may also further decrease SVR. A low SVR and the need for large fluid resuscitation are associated with increased mortality in septic shock patients as well as in experimental sepsis irrespective of whether CI is high, normal or low [3, 5]

Sepsis is associated with major changes in the microcirculation and capillary permeability, leading to interstitial edema, which is more significant in the lungs but affects all tissues [6]. However, is typical to develop subcutaneous edema and body cavity, indicating the presence of increased vascular permeability. Tissue edema is not benign: the accumulation of parenchymal and interstitial fluid could affect the function of organs due to an increased distance required for oxygen diffusion and the compromise of microvascular perfusion secondary to increased interstitial pressure. Is no coincidence that a sign of septic shock recovery is spontaneous diuresis during edema reduction, while the vascular integrity is restored. Since endothelial cells line all blood vessels, vascular fluid leakage and tissue edema that occur in sepsis are signs of endothelial dysfunction. It is easy to imagine how the damage of microvascular endothelium may predispose not only to the leakage of vascular fluids and edema but also to shock, microvascular thrombosis and organ failure, common tables that precede death in patients with severe sepsis. So far, it is unknown whether endothelial damage or dysfunction and edema in sepsis are simply an epiphenomenon or an important component of its pathophysiology. It is important to answer this question. If the loss of endothelial integrity contributes to disease and death in sepsis, it is very important to understand the mechanisms involved and would allow to develope new treatments [6]

3.2 Vasopressor Therapy

Vasopressors should be titrated to maintain an adequate perfusion pressure over 65 mmHg. Delayed capillary refill, oliguria, and impaired consciousness all suggest tissue hypoperfusion as does lactic acidosis and an elevated lactate/pyruvate ratio, traducing a decrease in cytoplasmic and mitochondrial redox state.

For those patients with persistently low CO despite adequate LV filling pressures, dobutamine remains the first- choice agent, in an attempt to achieve a central venous oxygen saturation greater than 70% . This catecholamine with selective β_1 effects increases stroke volume, heart rate and CI in septic patients. However, sepsis induced impaired β-adrenergic receptor stimulation of cAMP may cause the myocardium to be less responsive to catecholamines. Inotropic agents that act independently of β-adrenoreceptors may therefore have an important role in treating sepsis-related myocardial dysfunction [5, 6]

As sepsis-induced myocardial dysfunction may reflect cardiac hibernation and be an adaptive response, the judicious use of catecholamines is recommended. Adrenergic stimulation leads to an increase in cardiac work and may damage cardiomyocytes. In addition; the use of norepinephrine has been associated with myocardial depression [5, 6]

Levosimendan, a calcium sensitizer and a K+-ATP channel opener, plays a significant role in the treatment of myocardial depression although its use in sepsis has not yet been established. Compared to other inotropic agents, it has been shown to improve myocardial contractility without increasing oxygen requirements, together with anti-apoptotic and anti-inflammatory properties.

However, experience with levosimendan in patients with septic shock is limited. Levosimendan compared with dobutamine improves the hemodynamic parameters in septic patients with myocardial dysfunction; and while there is evidence that it reduces mortality, further studies are needed to verify this [5, 6]

4. Evaluation of Myocardial Dysfunction

The evaluation of left ventricular dysfunction during sepsis is particularly complex, due to the multiple factors involved and the temporality with which they appear [7]. In the initial stage, non-ischemic myocardial damage is produced, which can evolve in a sub-clinical manner and manifest itself with the appearance of compromised hemodynamic functions (low blood pressure), also including the intervention of vasodilation and hypovolemia. It is difficult to evaluate systolic function, because the ejection fraction may not reflect the real inotropic state of the heart due to how much it depends on preload (usually low) and afterload, highly diminished during sepsis.

Currently, hemodynamic monitoring is performed through a transthoracic echocardiogram given the enormous amount of morphofunctional information this exam provides, its non-invasive nature and its decisive role in therapeutic management and survival rate [7, 8]. The echocardiogram evaluates both systolic and diastolic function. There are many indexes and scores for each function. It can be performed in an isolated fashion, associated with other exams or even in conjunction with the information obtained through monitoring with a Swan-Ganz catheter in order to comprehend and enable rational management of each particular patient's hemodynamics.

The structural information provided by the transthoracic echocardiogram allows us to evaluate the size of the cavities and the presence of valve failure and its severity, as well as the severity of stenosis, which could otherwise go undetected in a critical patient as they are out of the reach of the Swan-Ganz catheter. It also evaluates the presence of lumps, tumors, burst blood vessels, etc., which can be decisive towards the appearance of a particular hemodynamic scenario and decisive when it comes time to choose the correct therapeutic solution.

Ideally, hemodynamic information should reflect contractility, yet this information can only be obtained in an invasive procedure, through pressure-volume loop analysis, a method that is unfeasible in common clinical practice [7]. In its stead, alternative, albeit less reliable indexes are used, which depend on preload, afterload and heart rate, such as ejection fraction, systolic index and cardiac output. The calculation of ventricular DP/DT based on the mitral insufficiency jet has been incorporated for patients that present such conditions and it has shown a good correlation with the invasive measurement [7].

Echocardiogram cardiac output consists of measuring the flow through an orifice. It is calculated by measuring the integral of flow velocity at any of the ventricular outlets, multiplied by heart rate and the area of the outlet. Systolic volume can also be calculated as the flow at a ventricular outlet level by measuring with a pulsed Doppler. It is the time-based integral of velocity multiplied by the area of the ventricular outlet. Cardiac output measurement has a good correlation with the invasive measurement, even in critical patients [7].

Ejection fraction is the index used the most in clinical practice; however, it has many constraints that are not sufficiently considered and which can lead to errors in diagnosis and prescribed therapy. The first thing that must be said is that measuring ejection fraction requires an experienced examiner as it is highly influenced by preload and afterload, as well as by the presence of mitral insufficiency, not to mention its severity and chronicity. It has a poor correlation with functional capacity, maximum consumption of oxigen or ventricular filling pressures. Despite these constraints, ejection fraction is used frequently due to its ease of retrieval and prognostic value.

DP/DT calculation corresponds to a time-based ventricular pressure elevation velocity and it is the most accurate measurement for ventricular inotropism. Its limitation lies in the fact that it is an invasive measurement not available in everyday clinical practice. Nevertheless, DP/DT can be obtained when there is mitral insufficiency by using the spectral curve to calculate the time it takes the curve to reach from 1mts/sec to 3mts/sec. [7, 8, 9]

The TEI index is a global cardiac function index that evaluates both systolic and diastolic function [7, 8]. It is calculated by adding the time it takes for isovolumetric relaxation and isovolumetric contraction, divided by ejection time.

Ventricular dysfunction causes a prolongation of isovolumetric contraction time and of isovolumetric relaxation time, with a shortening of ejection time; therefore, this index is prolonged the greater the ventricular dysfunction is. There are not many papers that study the prognostic value of the TEI index in critical patients. In the clinical trials involving patients with dilated myocardiopathy and severe systolic dysfunction, TEI index greater than 0.75, has been proven to be a predictor of survival [9, 10].

Diastole is the period of time within the cardiac cycle that takes place between the closing of the aortic valve to the closing of the mitral valve. During the isovolumetric relaxation phase, the heart loses its rigidity. The speed with which it loses rigidity or relaxes corresponds to the dp/dt (-) or tau constant. The speed with which the ventricle fills up after mitral opening will depend on the instantaneous pressure gradient present between the auricle and the ventricle and the compliance (dV/Dp) of the ventricular chamber. Alterations in relaxation or ventricular compliance cause alterations in diastolic filling and can be investigated through an echocardiogram. There are many other factors that intervene in ventricular filling, such as auricular contraction, the pericardium, ventricular interaction, heart rate, etc. The severity of the diastolic dysfunction is directly related to the prognosis of patients with heart failure [10, 11]

An experimental model for sepsis using lab animals managed to document that the presence of ventricular dilation was associated to greater survival and said dilation was related to the indemnity of the diastolic function [10, 11].

Diastolic filling is divided into rapid or early filling and slow or late filling. Spectral curves reflect the instantaneous pressure gradients between the auricular and the ventricular cavity. Using a pulsed Doppler at the edge of the mitral valve records the rapid flow (E wave) and the slow filling (A wave), which are obtained thanks to auricular contraction. Under normal conditions, approximately 80% of ventricular filling is performed during the early or rapid filling phase (E wave); therefore, E wave shall be greater than A wave. The time it takes the E wave to decelerate and reach 0 is the deceleration time (DT), which reflects ventricular compliance.

When diastolic dysfunction is mild, an alteration is produced in relaxation, resulting in a decrease in velocity of the E wave. Filling will now depend more on auricular contraction (A wave). When diastolic function is greatly deteriorated due to a drop in ventricular compliance, there is an elevation in auricular pressure that consequently leads to an increase in the E wave. This leads to a pseudo-normalization of the E/A ratio. When there are high levels of diastolic dysfunction, very fast ventricular filling takes place with a high E wave and a short DT as a result of the high pressure gradient between AI and VI and the quick balance of the pressures, respectively.

The velocity of the E wave for mitral filling is directly related to the pressure gradient between the left auricle and ventricle and inversely related to the alteration in relaxation. When high pressure in AI and an alteration in ventricular relaxation coexist, the isolated E wave does not allow us to obtain any type of information; therefore, it is corrected with a parameter that specifically measures relaxation, obtained through the use of a tissue Doppler at the mitral ring level. This parameter shall be referred to as the E' or Em wave.[11, 12, 13].

5. Biomarkers in Heart Failure

Today is understood that heart failure (HF) occurs not only as a result of an hemodynamic process of salt and water retention, but as a complex syndrome with significant neurohumoral alterations that contribute to worsen symptoms and to a progression of the disease.

Biomarkers are biological variables that provide information about specific diseases. In heart failure, can be demographic characteristics (age and sex), cardiac imaging (echocardiography, x-ray, scan or magnetic resonance imaging) or even the determination of a specific genetic polymorphism.

The term biomarker often refers to circulating substances which can be determined through analysis that are not considered as standard blood tests used in usual clinical management. Biomarkers of interest in the HF can be grouped broadly according to the current knowledge of their role in the pathophysiology of the disorder: the best-known subgroup is the neurohormones, which includes the natriuretic peptide (PN) heart, the components of the Renin-angiotensin-aldosterone system (RAAS), catecholamines, arginine-vasopressin and the derivatives of endothelial Vasoactive Peptides, endothelin and adrenomedullin and urocortinas; markers of inflammation and oxidative stress markers of remodelling of matrix interticial and finally lesion miocitaria markers like the troponin.

5.1 Natriuretic Peptide

Bold et al were the first to publish a description of diuretic effects and natriuretic of an infusion of extract of atrial tissue in rats [14]. Since then, have published a large number of trials in which have suggested the heart as endocrine organ. A clinical trial of Bold et al led to the isolation and cloning of the atrial natriuretic peptide, first member identified in a family of peptides with a potent diuretic action, natriuretic and vasodilatador [14, 15]

The natriuretic peptides are a group of similar peptide structure but genetically different substances. 4 Types of natriuretic peptides have been identified so far. Of these, the most important are the atrial natriuretic peptide (ANP) and brain (BNP), of cardiac origin and the peptide type C (NPC) of endothelial origin [16].

In patients with heart failure, circulating plasma concentrations of ANP, BNP and terminal fragments of their pro-hormones (NT-pro - ANP and NT-proBNP) are high due to the cardiac hormone system that is activated by the increase of the stretch of the wall [15, 16].

As well as in the Atrial, the main stimulus that controls the synthesis and release of ANP in the ventricles is the stress of wall. The cardiac ventricles contribute significantly to the movement of the ANP in experimental animals, patients with heart failure and left ventricular hypertrophy [15, 16]

In humans, the ventricular release of ANP is increased in dilated cardiomyopathy and elevated plasma concentrations are both the Atria and the ventricles. However, while the ANP concentration is higher in the Atrium, given the increased ventricular mass, the ventricular myocardium reaches being the main circulating synthesis of ANP and NT-proANP in HF [17]

While in the normal human heart the ANP is secreted mainly by the headphones myocytes, the BNP is produced by both the Atrial and the ventricles. In normal subjects, the plasma concentrations of BNP are lower than the ANP. However, compared to the ANP and the NTproANP, the BNP and NT-proBNP reach much greater in the case of this disease [17, 18].

In humans, the acute intravenous saline overload and postural changes that modify the atrial pressure increase values of ANP, but not of BNP, while chronic overload-based diets rich in salt for days result in increased plasma concentrations of BNP [18]. These findings suggest that PNA is a hormone of rapid response, while concentrations of BNP would better reflect the chronic cardiac overload. Therefore, the BNP and NT-proBNP appear to be more likely markers of chronic ventricular dysfunction than the ANP [17, 18]

5.2 Catecholamines

The increase of norepinephrine in the peripheral blood was one of the first neurohormonal alterations detected in heart failure. The origin of its activation is multifactorial; on one hand, the decrease in cardiac output, through the activation of vascular baroreceptors, increases their release in the central nervous system; on the other hand, the RAAS activation also activates the release of norepinephrine. This increase in release, along with the reduction of its reabsorption in the nerve terminals, gives rise to an increase in plasma concentrations of norepinephrine [18, 19, 20]. With the sympathetic activation increases heart rate and contractility, increasing cardiac output; In addition, causes an important peripheral vasoconstriction that helps maintain blood pressure. However, this implies an increase in the consumption of oxygen and heart work that contributes in long term to progressive deterioration of LVfunction.

In addition, noradrenaline can cause myocardial and cell death by apoptosis, necrosis aggravating ventricular dysfunction. For this reason, it is believed to contribute actively to the prognosis of these patients [18, 19, 20].

The high values of norepinephrine are associated, classically, a worse prognosis in heart failure and increased mortality in these patients [18, 19, 20]

5.3 Angiotensin II

Angiotensin II is part of the RAAS. Nowadays known that has a vasoconstrictor effect, stimulates myocardial fibrosis and hypertrophy, reabsorption of fluid, proinflamatory activity and stimulate the secretion of other hormones with similar action as aldosterone and vasopressin. Therefore, has been given a very important role in the progression of heart failure, associating their high levels in blood with increased morbidity and cardiovascular mortality. It also suggests a better prognosis in these patients by modifying the blood concentration of angiotensin II.

5.4 Endothelin

Endothelin (ET) is a peptide with potent vasoconstrictor effect released by the endothelium. There are 3 types of ET. The ET-1 is detected in the endothelial cells, the ET-2 is prevalent in the gastrointestinal tract, kidney, and in small amounts in myocardium, placenta and uterus. ET-3 possesses low levels in blood and would not have the importance of the 2 first. High concentrations of this peptide are described primarily in brain, kidney, adrenal, lung and bowel. The ET-1 is highly specific for ET-A receptor and is widely distributed in vascular smooth muscle cells.

The union of ET-1 to the ETA receptor produces most of the hypertensive effects of this peptide. Unlike the ETA receptor, the ETB responds equally to all isoforms of endothelins.

In heart failure where ET values are high, this elevation is correlated with the severity of IC and associated pulmonary hypertension [20]

5.5 Inflammatory Markers

Numerous experimental observations indicate that the inflammatory mediators are important in the pathogenesis of heart failure, contributing to cardiac remodeling and vascular disorders. Various studies have shown increases in the levels of plasma inflammatory cytokines such as interleukins 1 and 6, tumor necrosis factor α (TNF-α) and C protein reaction (PCR), taking also a factor associated prognosis [21, 22, 23]

In experimental models of Endothelial dysfunction, the increase of reactive oxygen species (ROS) and myocardial remodeling is associated with higher levels of inflammatory mediators, which support their participation in the pathophysiology of the IC [21, 22, 23]. Particularly, the concentrations of TNF-α appears to provide prognosis information in patients with IC. Levine et al. (1990) was the first to demonstrate that the concentrations of TNF- α were significantly higher in patients with IC, compared with control patients. They also noted that concentrations increased TNF-α are associated with a greater severity of the disease. Thus, in experimental studies administration of TNF-α has induced left ventricular dysfunction and cardiomyopathy, has stimulated the left ventricular remodeling and has enhanced the apoptosis. Also have been recipients of TNF - α (TNFR-1 and TNFR-2) and will have been able to detect soluble in circulation forms. In addition, these soluble receptors appear to be regulators of the activity of TNF-α in patients with HF, so that the rise in their circulating concentrations is associated with an adverse evolution [22, 23]

6. Relationship between Oxidative Stress Occurrence and HF

Oxidative stress in HF contributes to endothelial dysfunction, apoptosis, necrosis and ventricular dysfunction. It have been described some markers of damage by ROS in the HF, mainly the products of lipid peroxidation. Indeed, the MDA levels were negatively correlated with functional parameters, shows an inverse relationship between malondialdehyde (MDA), EF and exercise capacity. Similarly, another study showed correlation between high levels of MDA with sympathetic activation and decrease of the response to exercise [24, 25].

The precise role of ROS in the HF is still a controversial issue. Potential sources of ROS include inflammatory cells and mitochondria of cardiomyocytes and fibroblasts. The predominant enzyme systems in the synthesis seem NADPH oxidase and xantino oxidase (XO) even though; there may be other ways of ROS generation in some particular etiologies. At lmyocardial level, the generation of ROS can be triggered by a large number of stimuli: ischemia and reperfusion, exposure to inflammatory cytokines, Angiotensin II, ET-1, α-adrenergic agonists and mechanical stretch. All these stimuli converge in the activation of the NF kappaB pathway, resulting in amplification of the inflammatory response and increase in the synthesis of ROS mediated by NADPH oxidase and XO [24, 25].

Septic plasma can be viewed as a pool of cytokines, chemokines, and other inflammatory mediators that have the potential to activate several intracellular signaling pathways in cardiac myocytes, some of which may lead to conversion of the cardiac myocytes to a proinflammatory phenotype [26]. Previous studies [27, 28] indicate that septic plasma can convert adult human and rat cardiomyocytes, as well as mouse neonatal myocytes, to a proinflammatory phenotype. The three MAP kinases (ERK1/2, JNKs, and p38 MAP kinase) can be both activated by inflammatory mediators and, in turn, generate inflammatory mediators. This molecules also been regulated by intracellular ROS levels.

6.1 Uric Acid

Uric acid is the final product of the catabolism of purines in humans produced by the enzymatic action of XO. The main enzyme action of the XO is the consecutive catalytic conversion of hypoxanthine to Xanthine and then from Xanthine to uric acid. At the same time, products of these reactions produce ROS as a superoxide anion and hydrogen peroxyde.

Till now, there is no consensus about the role of uric acid in heart failure. On one hand, various basic and clinical studies suggest that it is actively involved in its genesis and progression while other research postulate a beneficial action of the uric acid through an antioxidant activity [29]

Various clinical and epidemiological studies have shown the relationship between the levels of uric acid and several cardiovascular diseases, as arterial hypertension, metabolic syndrome, coronary disease, pre-eclampsia, kidney disease and acute and chronic heart failure. It has also been reported that elevated plasma levels of uric acid in patients with chronic heart failure was associated with increased mortality or need to heart transplant, independent of renal function, plasma sodium, use of diuretics and age of the patient [29].

Conclusions and Perspectives

Despite the identification of various mechanisms contributing to cardiac dysfunction (such as cardiodepressant mediators, mitochondrial dysfunction, or apoptosis), we are far from understanding their exact impact. Each theory has a major flaw that challenges its principles. Cardiodepressant, such as TNF-α, IL-1β, IL-6, etc., are known to be elevated early during sepsis, but return to normal levels within 2 to 3 days. Thus, cytokine/chemokine involvement in early cardiodepression seems possible. However, because cardiodepression is usually reversed only 7 to 10 days after sepsis onset in humans, myocardial suppression by cytokines/chemokines during the late stages of sepsis seems highly unlikely, unless these mediators are predominantly stored inside cardiomyocytes and exert their functions mainly without being secreted. However, this would infer functions of mediators without their interactions with surface receptors.

The link between inflammatory response and development of the critically ill state is the oxidative stress occurrence. The imbalance between the production of ROS and their effective removal by non-enzymatic and enzymatic antioxidants systems could induce endothelial dysfunction with alterations of vascular tone, increases in cell adhesion properties (leukocytes and platelet adhesion), increase in vascular wall permeability and a pro-coagulant state. Increasing evidence supports the idea that the principal cause of myocardial dysfunction during sepsis is cell injury and mitochondrial dysfunction. ROS and RNS contribute to mitochondrial dysfunction by a range of mechanisms and induce both necrotic and apoptotic cell death. This is consistent with the negative relationship between higher values of lipid peroxidation biomarkers and low values of ventricular function in critically ill patients

Further research into reducing cardiomyocyte damage via oxidative stress, reducing pro-inflammatory responses induced by TLR-4/NF-κB signaling, decreasing mitochondrial dysfunction, and improving cellular respiration thereby decreasing apoptosis are examples of areas that may be future therapeutic targets.

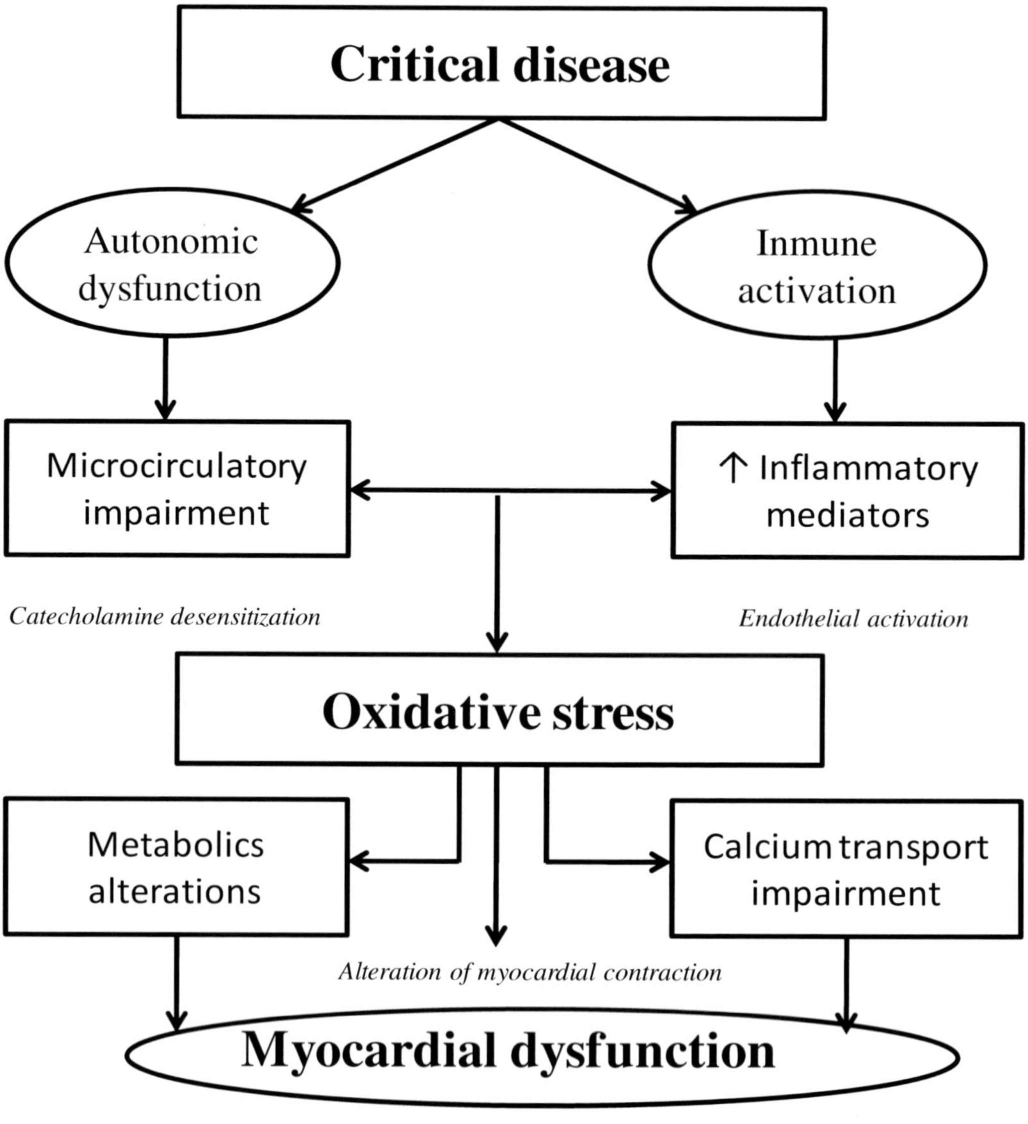

Figure 1. schematic representation of the mechanisms that link the occurrence of oxidative stress in the development of myocardial dysfunction in critically ill patients.

REFERENCES

[1] Hunter H, Doddi M. Sepsis and the heart. *Br J Anaesth 2010; 104: 3 -11.*

[2] Annane D, Bellissant E, Cavaillon JM. Septic shock. *Lancet 2005; 365: 63-78*

[3] Dellinger, RP, at al. Surviving Sepsis Campaign: International Guidelines for Management of Severe Sepsis and Septic Shock: 2008. *Crit Care Med 2008; 36:296-327.*

[4] Andresen M, Regueira T. Disfuncion miocardica en la sepsis. *Rev Med Chile 2010; 138: 888-896*

[5] Vaitsis J, H Michalopoulou H, Thomopoulos C. Use of levosimendan in myocardial dysfunction due to sepsis. *Critical Care 2009, 13(Suppl 1):P165*

[6] Rincón JA, Martínez J, Monteon I, Córdova VH. Tratamiento de la depresión miocárdica por sepsis con levosimendan. Serie de casos y revisión de bibliografía. *Med Int Mex 2010; 26(4): 324-336*

[7] Rabuel C, Mebazaa A. Septic shock: a heart story since the 1960s. *Intensive Care Med 2006; 32: 799-807.*

[8] Harvey S, Young D, Brampton W, Cooper Ab, Doig G, Sibbald W, Rowan K. Pulmonary artery catheters for adult patients in intensive care (Review). *Cochrane Database Syst Rev. 2006 jul 19; Issue 3.*

[9] Poelaert J, Declerck C, Vogelaers D, Colardyn F, Visser CA. Left ventricular systolic and diastolic function in septic shock. *Intensive Care Med 1997, 23: 553-60.*

[10] Parker MM, Shelhamer JH, Bacharach SL, Green MV, Natanson C,Frederick Tm, et al. Profound but reversible myocardial depressionin patients with septic shock. *Ann Intern Med. 100(4): 483-90.*

[11] Parker MM, Suffredini AF, Natanso NC, Ognibene FP, Shelhamer JH,Parrillo JE. Responses of left ventricular function in survivors and nonsurvivors of septic shock. *J Crit Care 1989; 4(1): 19-25.*

[12] A Vieillard-Baron, S Prin, K Chergui, O Dubourg, F Jardin.Hemodynamic Instability in Sepsis. Bedside Assessment by Doppler Echocardiography. *Am J Respir Crit Care Med 2003; 168:1270-6*

[13] Vieillard-Baron A, Chergui K, Rabiller A, Peyrouset O, Page B, JardinF et al. Superior vena caval collapsibility as a gauge of volume status in ventilated septic patients. *Intensive Care Med. 2004; 30(9): 1734-9.*

[14] De Bold AJ, Borenstein HB, Veress AT, Sonnenberg H. A rapid and potent natriuretic response to intravenous injection of atrial myocardial extract in rats. *Life Sci.* 1981;28:89-94.

[15] Lang RE, Thölken H, Ganten D, Luft FC, Ruskoaho H, Unger T. Atrial natriuretic factor-a circulating hormone stimulated by volume loading. *Nature.* 1985;314:264-6.

[16] Ruskoaho H. Tholken H, Lang R. Increase in atrial pressure releases atrial natriuretic peptide from isolated perfused rat hearts. *Pfluegers Arch.* 1986;407:170-4.

[17] Lemus J, McGuire D. Natriuretic peptide in cardiovascular disease. *Lancet* 2003;362:316-22.

[18] Lang CC, Coutie WJ, Khong TK, Choy AM, Struthers AD. Dietary sodium loading increases plasma brain natriuretic peptide levels in man. *J Hypertens. 1991;9:779-82.*

[19] Buckley MG, Markandu ND, Sagnella GA, McGregor GA. Brain and atrial natriuretic peptides: a dual peptide system of potential importance in sodium balance and blood pressure regulation in patients with essential hypertension. *J Hypertens*. 1994;12:809-13.

[20] Roing Mingell E. Utilidad clínica de los marcadores neurohumorales en insuficiencia cardiaca. *Rev Esp Cardiol* 2004; 54:347-56.

[21] Satoh S, Oyama J, Suematsu N. Increased productivity of tumor necrosis factor-alpha in helper T cells in patients with systolic heart failure. *Inter J Cardiol 2005; 26: 1298-304.*

[22] Deswall A, Petersen NJ, Feldman A. Cytokines and cytokine receptors in advanced heart failure: an analysis of the cytokine database from the Vesnarinone trial (VEST). *Circulation 2001; 103: 2055-9.*

[23] Rauchhaus M, Doehner W, Francis DP, Davos C, Kemp M, Liebenthal C, et al. Plasma cytokine parameters and mortality in patients with chronic heart failure. *Circulation. 2000;102:3060-7.*

[24] Griendilg KK, Sorescu D, Ushio M. NAD(P)H oxidase: role in cardiovascular biology and disease. *Circ Res* 2000; 86: 494-501.

[25] Landmesser U, Spiekermann S, Dikalov S. Vascular oxidative stress and endothelial dysfunction in patients with chronic heart failure: role of xanthine-oxidase and extracellular superoxide dismutase. *Circulation. 2002 Dec 10;106(24):3073-8*

[26] Kumar A, Kumar A, Michael P, Brabant D, Parissenti A M, Ramana C V, Xu X, Parrillo J E. Human serum from patients with septic shock activates transcription factors STAT1, IRF1, and NF-kappaB and induces apoptosis in human cardiac myocytes. *J Biol Chem* 2005;280:42619–42626.

[27] Madorin W S, Rui T, Sugimoto N, Handa O, Cepinskas G, Kvietys P R. Cardiac myocytes activated by septic plasma promote neutrophil transendothelial migration: role of platelet-activating factor and the chemokines LIX and KC. *Circ Res* 2004;94:944–951.

[28] Yang M, Wu J, Martin CM, Kvietys PR, Rui T. Important role of p38 MAP kinase/NF-kappaB signaling pathway in the sepsis-induced conversion of cardiac myocytes to a proinflammatory phenotype. *Am J Physiol Heart Circ Physiol* 2008;294:H994-1001.

[29] Alcaíno H, Greig D, Castro P. Acido úrico: una molécula con acciones paradójicas en la insuficiencia cardiaca. *Red Med Chile 2011; 139:505-515.*

INDEX

A

B

C

D

E

F

I

J

K

L

M

N

O

P

Q

R

S

T